MEDICAL ART

PRINCIPLES AND TECHNIQUES FOR THE CREATIVE MEDICAL ARTIST

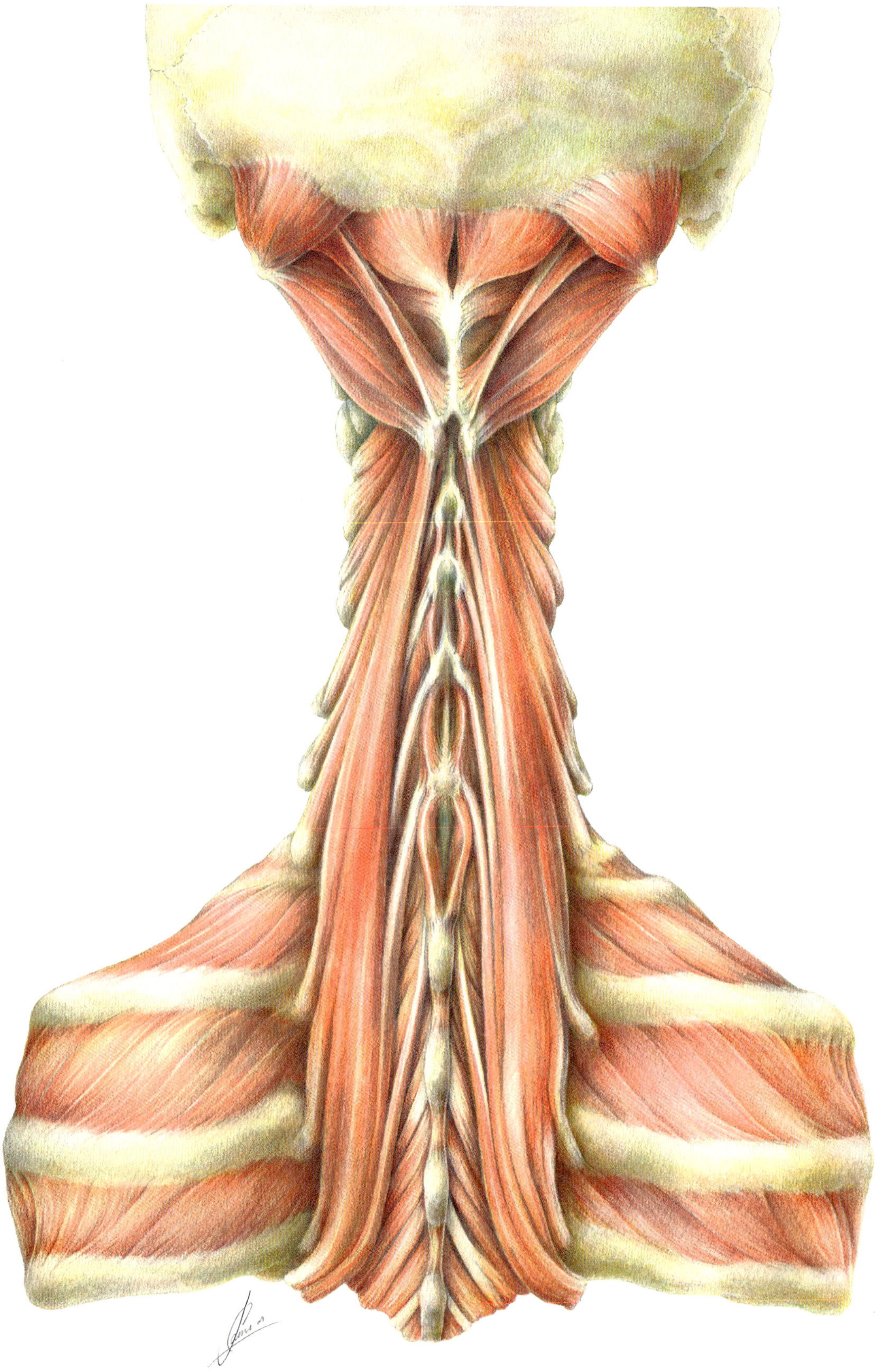

JOANNA
CAMERON

MEDICAL ART

PRINCIPLES AND TECHNIQUES FOR THE CREATIVE MEDICAL ARTIST

THE CROWOOD PRESS

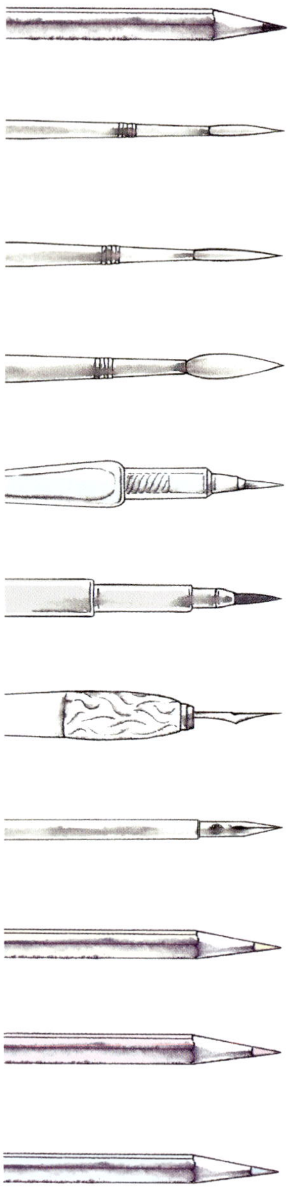

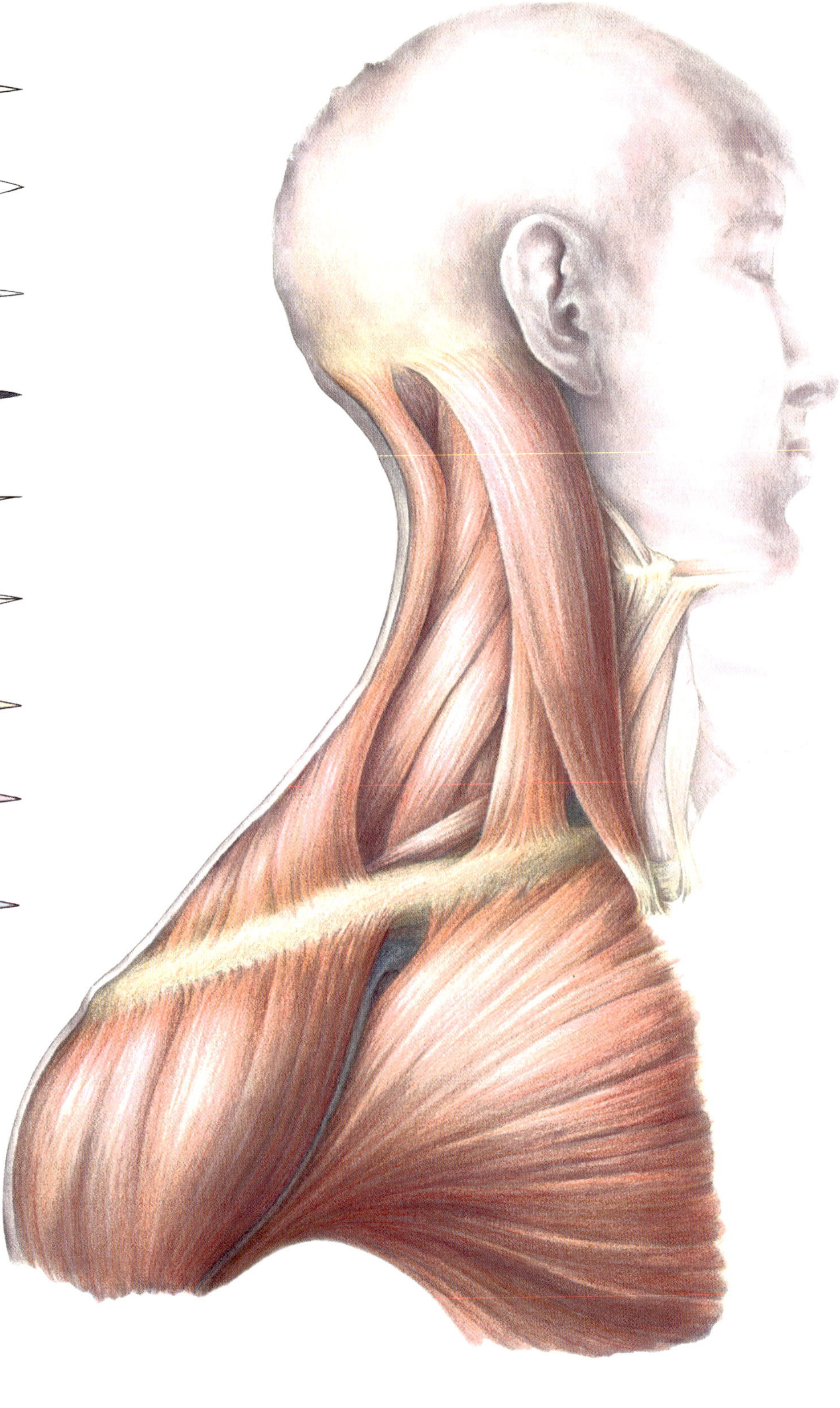

CONTENTS

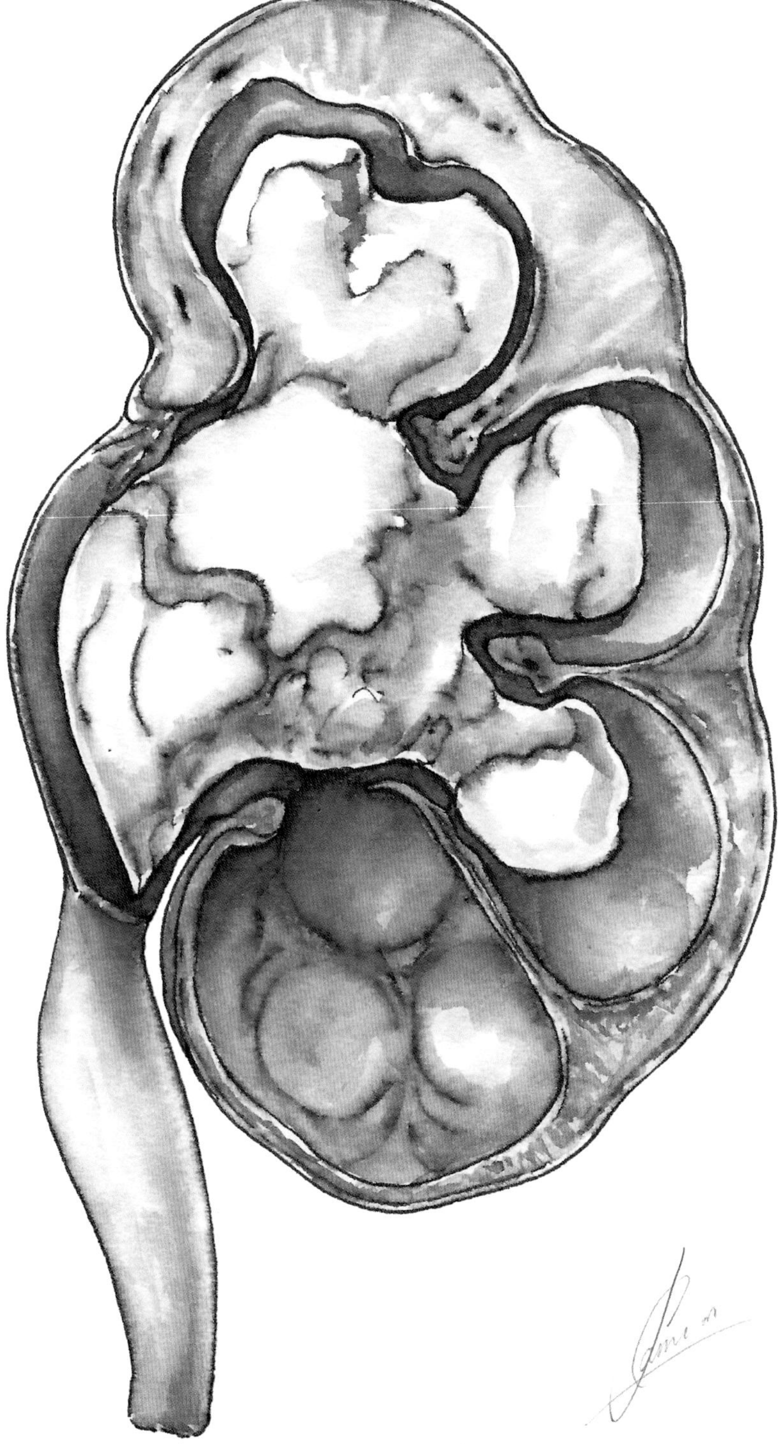

INTRODUCTION

Dispel from your mind the thought that an understanding of the human body in every aspect of its structure can be given in words; the more thoroughly you describe – the more thoroughly you will confuse – it is necessary to draw as well as describe. I advise you not to trouble with words unless you are speaking to blind men.
Leonardo da Vinci, 1452–1519

This practical handbook is aimed at all those wishing to enter the fascinating world of medical art. It introduces those techniques and principles that a student or individual can develop to embark on a path of study when training towards becoming a professional medical artist.

A variety of illustration techniques will be covered, concentrating on those frequently used in medical and scientific illustration. Beginning with direct observational projects, guidance is given on where and how to begin and how to improve your observation and drawing skills, from studying the skeleton and internal bodily structures to the external bony landmarks and skin.

Professional medical artists will encounter every conceivable human anatomical scenario: this is not necessarily a profession for the faint-hearted! Two step-by-step examples include working from fresh mammal specimens, in this instance a lamb's kidney and heart obtained from a local butcher. An introduction to working with specimens will help you to become familiar with observing, holding and drawing real organs, structures and tissues.

We will begin by examining those art essentials and the importance of direct observational drawing, studying light and shadow, and tonal and colour work. Medical artists need to become masters in many different media and techniques, including pencils, inks and watercolours, but first and foremost, they must be excellent at observing and interpreting what they see in their drawings. Nothing can replace time spent through hands-on practical observational experience when it comes drawing, so begin by simply taking your time to look, study and draw. Artists are always looking, often without realising how this is being interpreted, as they tend to have a naturally keen eye combined with an inquiring mind.

A frequent question medical artists encounter is: 'Why draw it? Why not a photograph?' Illustrations often translate very complex and technical information into visually relatable and understandable formats whether for patient information or to accompany a complex anatomical text. Medical artists are called upon to create a wide variety of illustrations, each designed for a particular audience in mind. For example, illustrations created for a patient leaflet on a skin condition will have a very different design and content to those created to accompany a complex medical procedure for surgeons. The medical artist must switch with fluidity and ease through the wide variety of work received as commissions and this becomes a distinct skill. Medical art really has become an 'art in itself'.

Kidney cross-section showing a large staghorn calculi stone. Pen and wash watercolour.

This book will encourage you to practise a range of techniques for creating a variety of artworks in different media, build a portfolio when applying or embarking on a specilaist course in medical art. Medical artists come from a diverse range of backgrounds and include fine artists, illustrators, designers, clinicians, surgeons, midwives, vets and archaeologists, to name a few. Each brings their own personal and unique skills, alongside years of studying and application.

Delving into medical and anatomical subjects opens a never-ending wonderful world of research, discovery, knowledge and enquiry and, of course honing the art of medical illustration techniques. A list of medical art courses can be found in Appendix I. With the constant advances in medical practice and knowledge, often at incredible speed, the specific skills and expertise of a trained and professional medical artist will always be required.

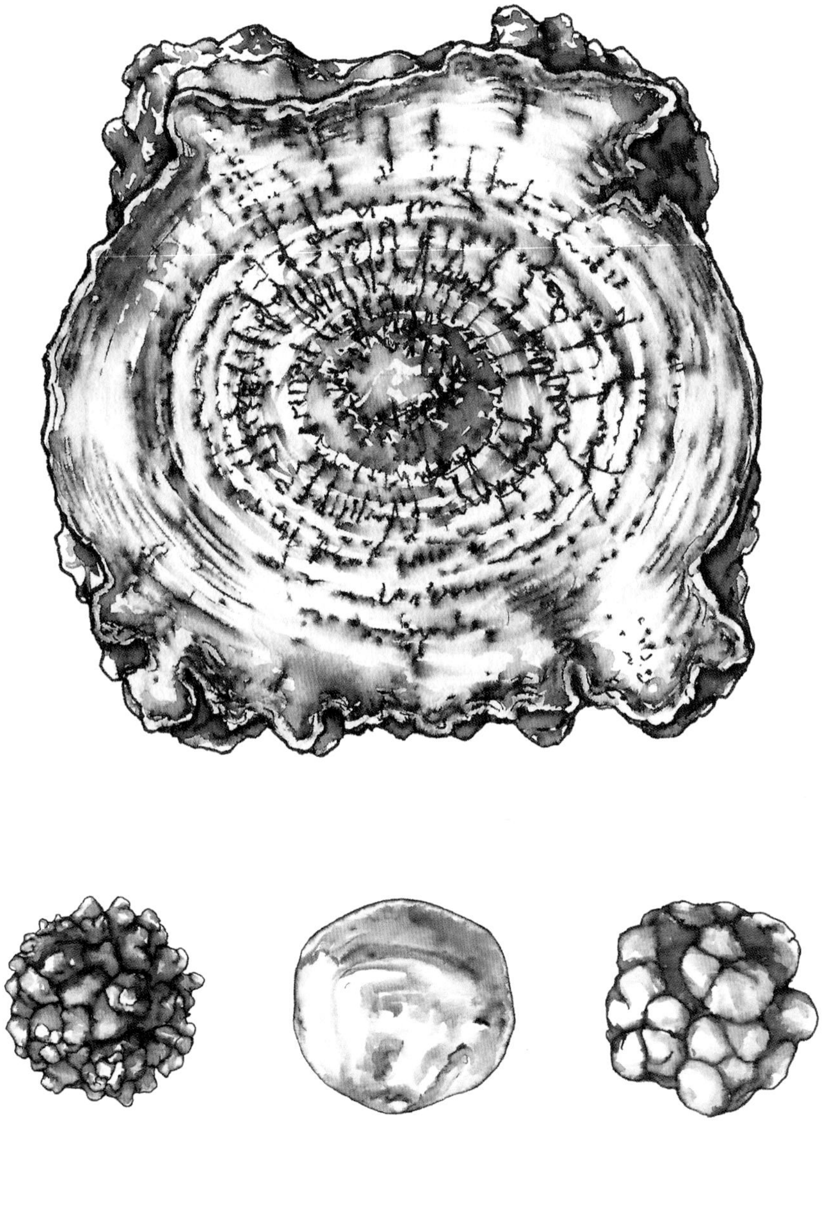

Kidney stones. Pen and wash.

THE ART OF DISCOVERY

Medical art relies on the combination of observation, learning and discussion, drawing together the views of all observers, including the artist, the medical clinician, the patient or the client. All collaborate to visualise and create informative, educational and anatomically accurate medical artworks.

The human figure has been recorded for centuries. Many well-know examples of early historical cave and wall drawings which include human figures, seen in many diverse locations from coastal to underground limestone caves and often found alongside animal depictions.

One of the oldest known records of the human figure in a medical context was found in an ancient Egyptian papyrus, where specific human physical features and symptoms of diseases have been documented. Civilisations will undoubtedly have passed their knowledge down through the generations, but little or no written evidence has survived. From early beliefs concerning our souls through mythology and religions, gradually, more specific questions arose relating to our own human anatomy, leading the early Greek anatomists to dissect and study human bodies to find out how the body worked. Many Greek words are still used today, often in conjunction with Latin, creating the combination of prefixes and suffixes for our modern medical and anatomical terminology (*see* Glossary). Becoming familiar with medical terminology will help immeasurably in studying medical art and anatomy.

Considerable advances in the study of human anatomy have been made since the first century. These were often undertaken hidden from public view for fear the church would not approve. Only when the anatomist and physician Andreas Vesalius created his influential anatomical text, frequently and now simply referred to as the *Fabrica,* did the study of human anatomy become more acceptable. Importantly, within this now famous text were over 200 detailed anatomical woodcut prints created by many skilled artists of the time.

Anatomists and surgeons continued their study and research, for example, investigating how the blood was pumped around the body by the heart and circulatory system. Consequently, texts began to be regularly accompanied by many detailed anatomical drawings to explain their findings.

A well known and more recent example included 300 original detailed woodcuts created by the anatomist, surgeon and artist Henry Vandyke Carter, who illustrated the text for *Gray's Anatomy*, which was written by the anatomist and surgeon Henry Gray. The illustrations can now only be found in earlier editions. Alongside these illustrations, this has undoubtedly become the most famous anatomy text worldwide.

Today, significant discoveries and developments within the fields of medicine and surgery are still being made. Expanding modern technologies including 3D printing, virtual reality (VR) and artificial intelligence (AI) among others are improving patient outcomes. Medical artists are in continual demand for their skills in bringing these new innovative ideas and concepts to life.

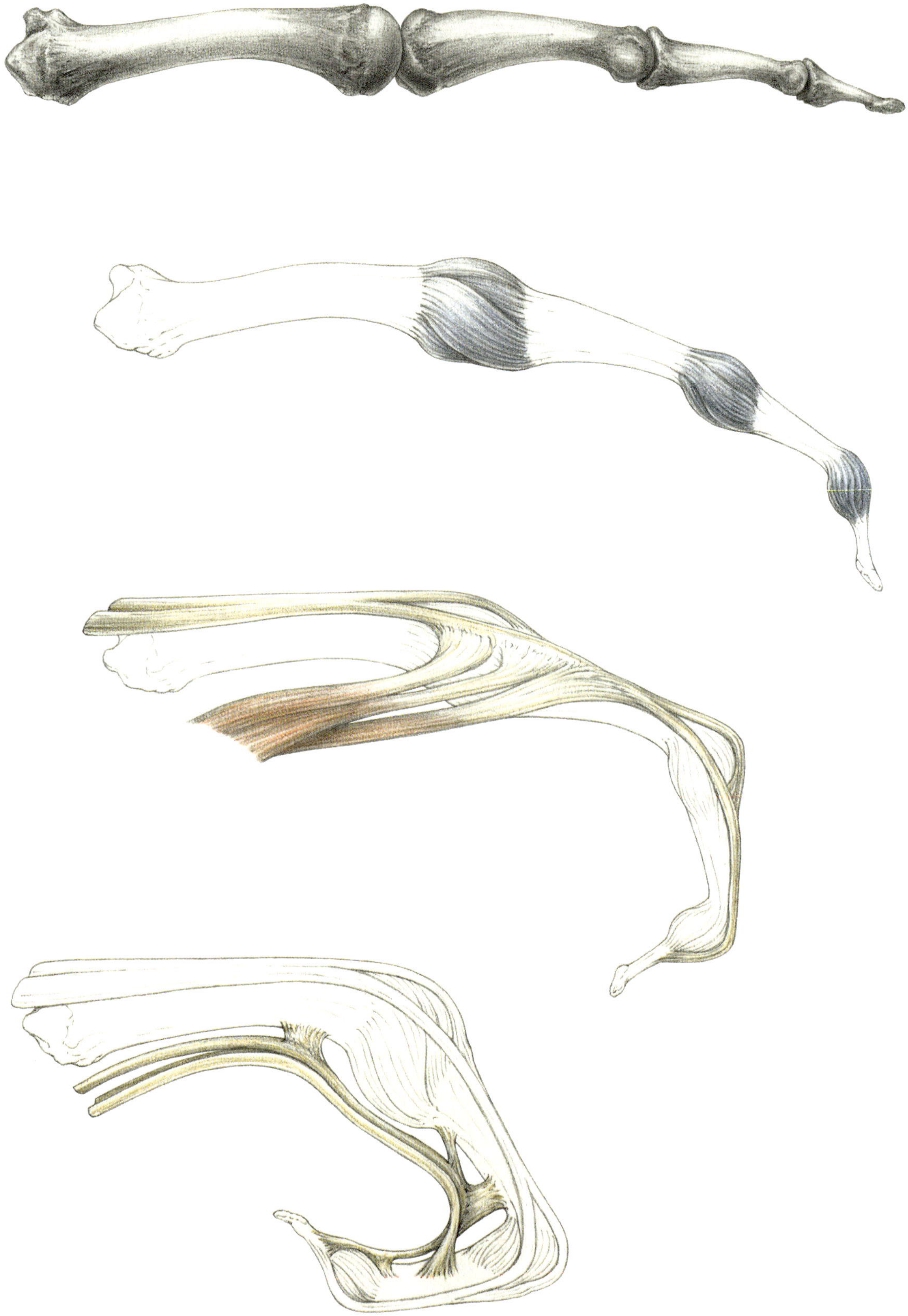

CHAPTER 1

ANATOMICAL TERMINOLOGY

A medical artist needs to become familiar with anatomical form and structures and how they are identified and classified, and this includes the skeletal structures, anatomical systems and internal organs that lie beneath the skin. Key to this is a working knowledge of anatomical terminology – the names given to each muscle, organ, structure and the relationships of structures to each other.

Anatomical and clinical terminology is often derived from a combination of Greek and Latin prefixes and suffixes. There are many freely available resources to familiarise yourself with these. A prefix is attached to the front of a word, the stem is the root or the word itself, while the suffix is added to the end.

A medical artist will be required to converse competently with clinicians and medical editors. Familiarity with the relevant anatomical and medical terminology will also help you to study related texts and discuss the artwork with whoever has commissioned it through its various stages, from initial verbal communications, to written instructions, reading and research, effective planning and completion.

The following terminology and explanations are aimed at artists and include essential terminology and abbreviations you will likely encounter through your medical art training and studies.

ANATOMICAL POSITION

Medical artists need to be aware that anatomical nomenclature is reviewed and occasionally updated for scientific or related clinical requirements. Nomenclature also may vary between countries and languages, so at any one time, more than one version of a particular anatomical term may be used. Consequently, it has been agreed internationally to introduce a standardised approach to names and references for anatomical terms. These terms relate to the 'anatomical position' for the human body (*see* page 12), which has since become the international standard for both human and veterinary anatomy. However, artists should be aware when referring to historical texts, terms and names may have changed over time. If you are preparing labelled anatomical artworks, your supervisor, author and the medical publishing editor can advise and edit any annotation that requires updating.

All anatomical directions, terminology and nomenclature now derive from this now standard 'anatomical position'; where the body is taken as being viewed from the front, standing in the upright position, with both feet on the ground facing forward and the arms down to the sides, with the palms of the hand open, flat and facing forward. Anatomical structures are referenced from this position.

Bones, tendons and ligaments of the finger.
Graphite and coloured pencils with watercolour.

THE THREE BODY PLANES

Anatomical planes are hypothetical planes used to transect the body, they are used to help describe the location of structures or the direction of movements

Sagittal (medial plane) A central line vertically or longitudinally through the body from front to back, dividing the body into left and right areas or any section parallel to this

Coronal (frontal plane) A central line through the body viewed from the side, dividing the body into anterior (front) and posterior (back) areas or any section parallel to this

Transverse, axial, or horizontal plane Any horizontal section where the level needs to be defined

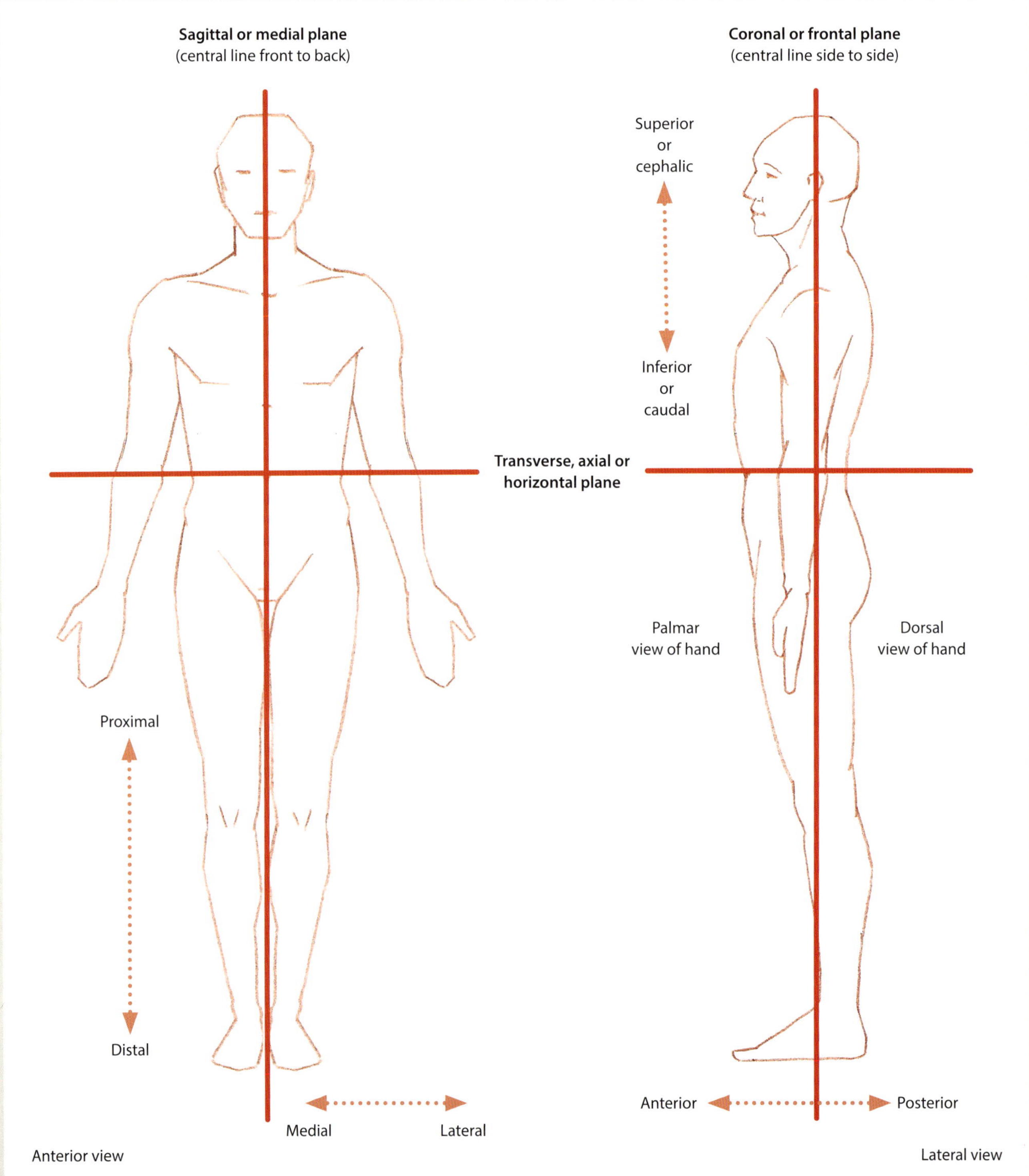

Common terms used to describe relative positions within the body include the following:

Superior Towards the head (also sometimes termed 'cranial')
Inferior Towards the feet (also 'plantar')
Anterior (A) Towards the front (also 'frontal' or 'ventral')
Posterior (P) Towards the back (also 'dorsal')
Anterior to posterior (AP) Direction front to back
Posterior to anterior (PA) Direction back to front
Medial (M) Towards the middle or midline (also 'internal')
Lateral (L) Away from the middle or midline (also 'external')
Distal (D) Away from the body
Proximal Towards or nearer the trunk of the body or point of origin of a part, usually used to describe limbs
Central Close to the centre of the body or the organ
Peripheral (or superficial) Towards the surface of the body or organ
Superficial Nearer the surface of the body or the organ
Deep Away from the surface of the body or the organ
Rostral Towards the front of the brain, nose or mouth
Cranial Closer to the head
Caudal (or deep) Close to the centre of the body or organ

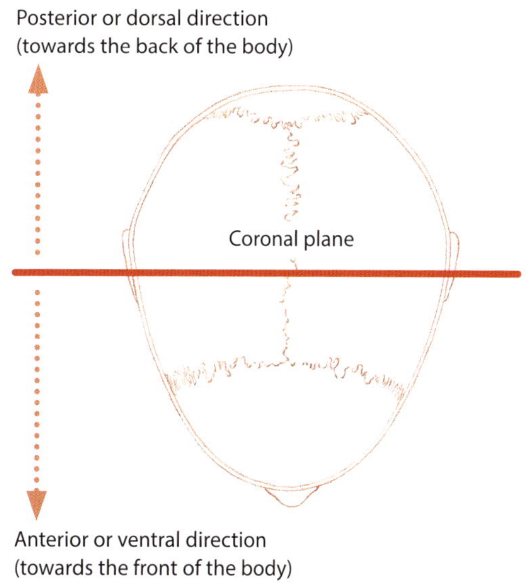

Planes and directional terms for an adult skull viewed from above.

BODY POSITIONS OTHER THAN THE ANATOMICAL POSITION

Supine Lying horizontal, face up
Prone Lying horizontal, face down
Right lateral recumbent Lying horizontal with the left side of the body on the floor
Left lateral recumbent Lying horizontal with the right side of the body on the floor

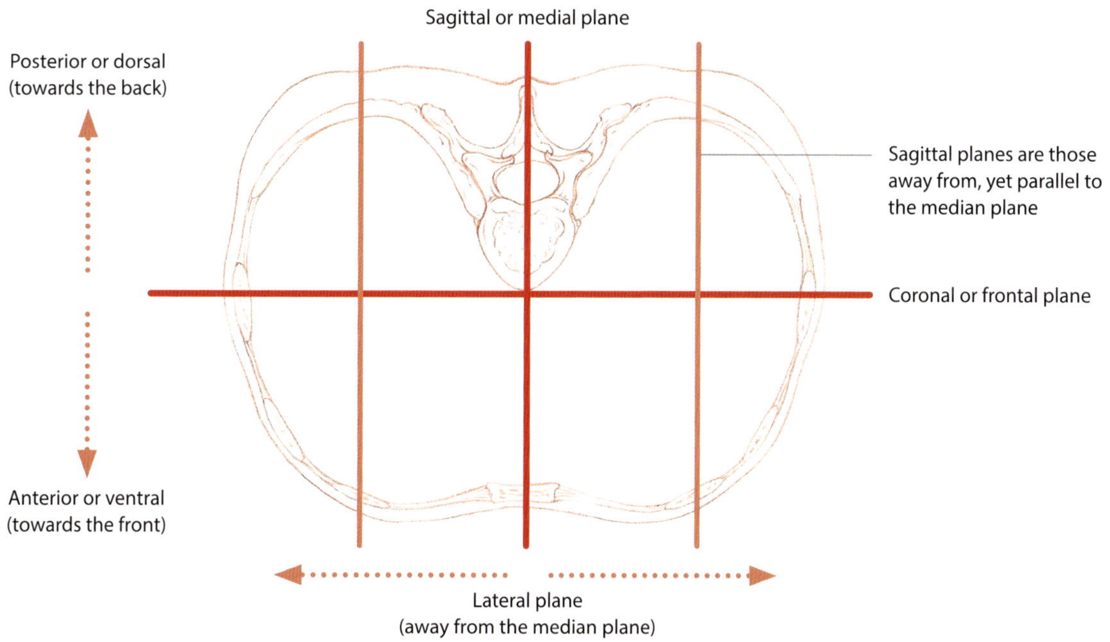

Cross-section through the thorax showing the spine and portions of the ribcage, with planes and anatomical terms indicated.

Movement

The human body is naturally mobile, and there is a whole separate terminology relating to the movement of the bones at the joints. Motions can also be classified according to their planes of movement, such as gliding, angular and linear. Not all muscles or joints have the same extent of movement, however, and some have nomenclature pertaining to a particular body part only, such as eversion and inversion movements of the foot.

Movements can also go beyond what we would expect as the normal range, and these terms begin with the prefix 'hyper', for example, hyperflexion.

For an artist, direct observation by drawing from life (not from photos or digital interpretations), in conjunction with anatomical study is essential; as we see with our eyes, we can begin to interpret our understanding of all that is happening on and below the skin through our artworks.

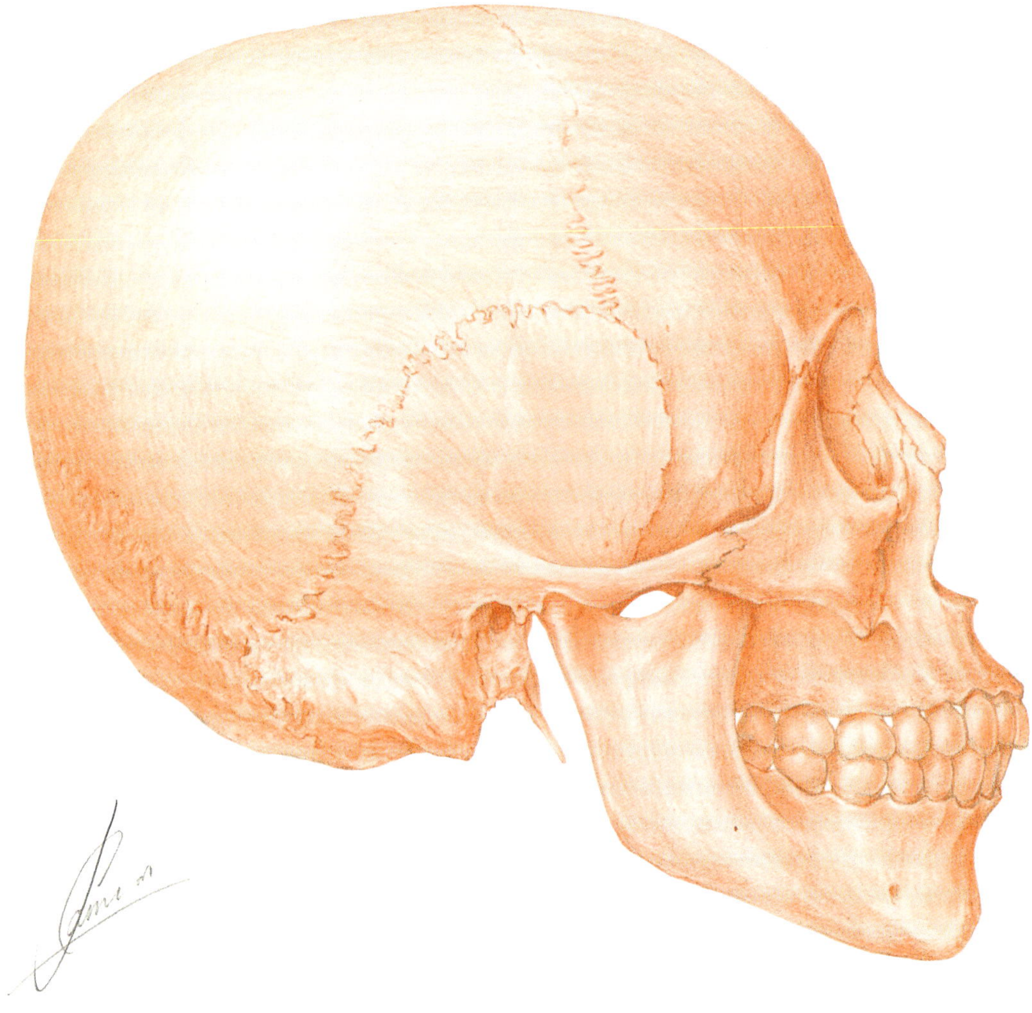

Lateral view of the human skull. Sanguine-coloured pencil.

Abduction Direction of movement away from the median line of the body
Adduction Direction of movement towards the median line of the body
Flexion Bending movement by reducing an angle; for example, bending the legs when moving from a standing to a sitting position
Extension Stretching or extending movement; for example, straightening the legs when changing from a sitting to a standing position
Circumduction Movement of the limb, hand or fingers in a circular motion, using the combination of flexion, adduction, extension and abductions motions
Rotation Pivoting or rotational movement
Eversion Movement of the foot away from the central median plane (*see* Chapter 2)
Inversion Movement of the foot towards the central median plane (*see* Chapter 2)

There are many more anatomical terms relating to specific limbs, organs, movement or positions, as well as to medical specialty. For example in MRI (magnetic resonance imaging) and CT (computerised tomography), reference to the left and right sides are as if you are looking at a photograph, for example the left side is seen on the right in the image.

For medical artists, when receiving instructions for an artwork, it is necessary to be familiar with any medical terms and their meanings for the related discipline. If in doubt, always ask for clarification.

Body Systems

The human body can be divided into named systems, each with its own specialism and function.

Integumentary system The skin is the largest system of the body (*see* Chapter 12)
Skeletal system The structural support inside the body, consisting of the bones and joints that enable movement (*see* Chapter 2)
Muscular system The muscles and tendons, which affect movement and stability at joints (*see* Chapter 11)
Cardiovascular system The circulation of blood around the body, transporting oxygen, nutrients and remaining dioxide
Nervous system The nerves that transmit signals between the brain and the body, and from the body back to the brain
Respiratory system Circulates oxygen from the lungs around the body and clears carbon dioxide.
Lymphatic system A drainage network supporting your immunity
Endocrine system The glands and organs that produce hormones
Digestive system The organs related to the process by which we break down food into nutrients for the body and expel waste
Urinary system Filters the blood and removes any waste products via urine
Reproductive system For the creation of the next generation

Other areas related to terminology and bodily systems are covered in the chapters on bony landmarks for the artist (Chapter 3), the important role skin plays in observation and clinical interpretation (Chapter 12), and the artistic depiction of internal systems and organs (Chapter 13).

Additional Terminology

Afferent or innovates Refers to a structure's approach towards the organ it supplies, for example, a nerve or blood vessel leading to an organ
Efferent Refers to a structure going away from its related organ, for example the venous drainage of an organ
Origin (of muscle) The point of attachment of a muscle to bone; the origin of a muscle does not move during contraction
Insertion (of muscle) The point where the muscle and tendon attach, whether this is to bone or other tissues, and moves when the muscle is contracted; the insertion is usually distal to the origin
Kinesiology The study of the movement of the human body, deriving from the ancient Greek words *kinesis,* meaning 'movement', and *logia*, meaning the 'study of'

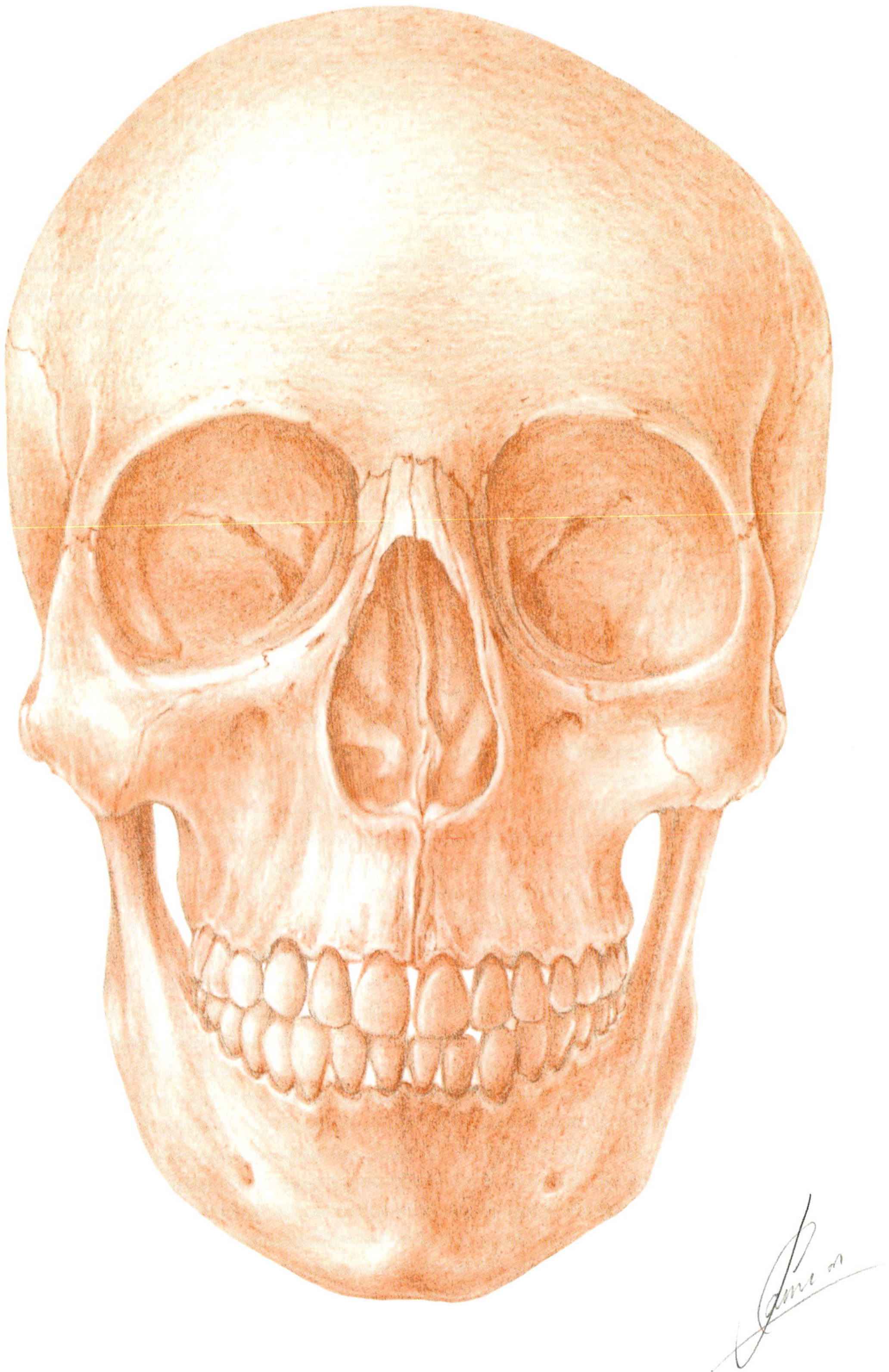

CHAPTER 2

THE SKELETON

The human body is made up of a myriad of cells, each having its own specialised function and form. When cells come together, they form many different types of tissue within the body, for example, bone, cartilage or muscle tissues. Bone is called osseous tissue, strengthened by the accumulation of calcium and other minerals laid down within the tissues as we grow.

Our bony skeleton is the key structural foundation within our bodies, to which muscles and tendons attach for movement and forms protection for many organs such as the heart and the lungs.

Medical artists need to become knowledgeable in many subjects, including skeletal structure, identifiable bony landmarks and body proportions, alongside how each bone may function and relate to their attachments, encompassing their neighbouring structures and organs.

In this book we will examine the skeleton and musculature relevant to the artist, covering many structural anatomical elements and their visual artistic representation; however, this is not a detailed text on anatomy. A few suggested anatomical texts are listed in the appendix for reference. Anatomical terminology is covered in Chapter 1.

In this section and the following chapter, covering body proportions and bony landmarks for the artist, the artworks have been drawn using coloured pencils, which historically have been used for many scientific and medical illustrations. The softness of the colour suits the nature of the human form, creating detailed yet expressive anatomical works.

THE BONY SKELETON

The bony skeleton begins to develop long before we are born, however the growth process continues over many years into adulthood by a process called ossification, whereby cartilage gradually converts into bone. This developmental process creates our individual bodies, giving us our shape and overall proportions. Here and throughout this book, we will concentrate on the adult human skeleton, with a few age variations for comparison.

The principal function of the skeleton is to create a strong support frame for the body. Bones provide protection for our internal organs and are the structures to which our muscles and tendons attach. Bone marrow is also important for creating stem cells (a process called haemopoiesis), a developmental stage for the blood.

We will look at observing and drawing bones in Chapter 9. Combining observation and the study of real skeletal specimens is essential for medical artists.

The adult human skeleton is made up of 206 bones. This number may vary slightly between individuals and does not include additional bones such as the sesamoids. We are born with around 300 bones, initially separated by areas of cartilage that gradually decrease as the bone develops. These 300 bones eventually fuse to form 206 bones that form the human skeleton, making up about 15 per cent of an average person's body weight. A person's bones stop growing when they are between sixteen and twenty.

Anterior view of the human skull. Sanguine-coloured pencil.

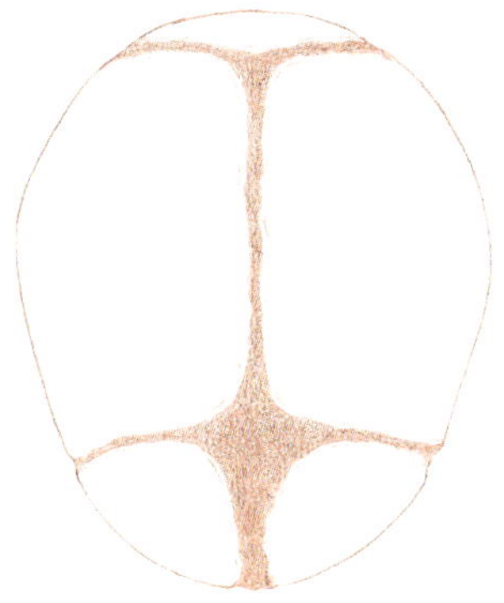

An infant's skull viewed from above. The skull is wider at the back and narrower towards the forehead, giving a slight egg-shaped appearance. The shaded areas indicate cartilage, which will gradually fuse together during childhood.

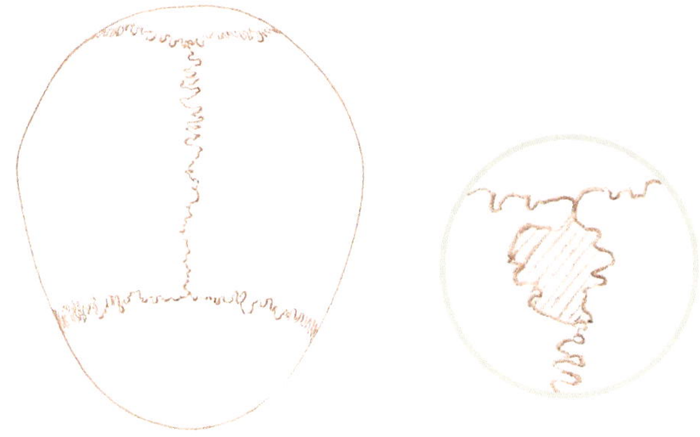

An adult skull viewed from above. When the separate bones fuse together, occasionally an 'island' of bone may be formed between the fused sutures. This is called a 'womain' bone.

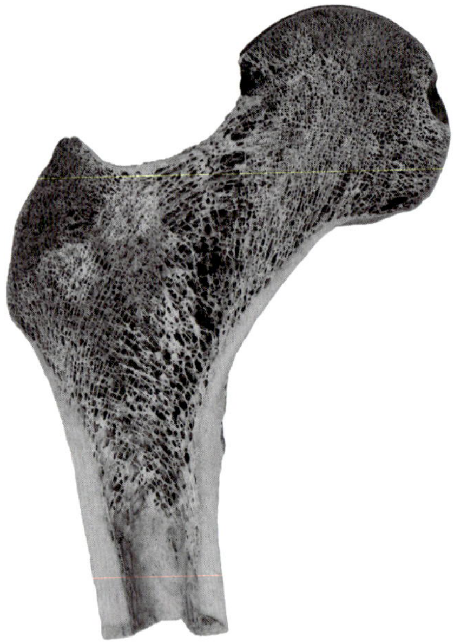

Head of the left adult femur (thigh bone), revealing the strong network of calcified bone.

The skeleton can be divided into two main sections:

Axial skeleton The skull (cranium, facial bones and mandible), the spine (vertebrae, sacrum and coccyx) and the ribcage (ribs and sternum).
Appendicular skeleton The arms and legs, plus the points that connect them to the axial skeleton – the shoulders and pelvic girdle. (*Page 29*).

The axial skeleton provides key structural support for both movement and position. Humans are bipedal; they move on just two legs, which has evolved over millions of years. The skeleton also provides strong protection for all our main organs – the brain within the skull (cranium), the spinal cord within the vertebrae, and the heart and lungs within the ribcage.

The axial skeleton is made up of 80 bones:

Skull The head has 22 bones (fourteen facial bones and eight cranial bones), of which only the mandible, or lower jawbone, is mobile.
Ear Each ear has three ossicles (totalling six). The stapes bone is the smallest bone in the body.
Neck The neck has a single, centrally placed U-shaped bone called the hyoid bone, situated below the tongue and under the mandible.
Spine The spine has 24 vertebrae, with 26 bones in total. Humans fall into the classification of vertebrates – which have a backbone or spine comprising individual vertebrae. The spine has seven cervical vertebrae, twelve thoracic vertebrae and five lumbar vertebrae, concluding with the sacrum and the coccyx (or tailbone), which is made up of four fused bones, a residual feature illustrating humans have evolved and no longer need tails. Each of the vertebrae is separated by a disc made of cartilage. The 23 intervertebral discs provide an essential cushioning effect during movement and flexion of the spine, as well as protecting the spinal cord.
Ribcage There are twelve pairs of ribs, making 24 in total. The upper seven ribs are called 'true' ribs, as they attach directly to the sternum, while the remaining ones are called 'false' or 'floating' ribs, as they don't attach directly to the sternum. The area created between each rib is known as the intercostal space.

THE AXIAL SKELETON

The Skull

The skull is mainly comprised of bones fixed together with sutures, apart from the mandible (the lower jawbone).

The bones that protect the brain are the parietal, temporal, occipital, sphenoid, ethmoid and frontal bones. Other bones comprise the face and include the maxilla (the upper jaw), zygomatic and the nasal bones forming the piriform aperture.

The hyoid bone is rarely if at all, seen on articulated skeletons, as this does not articulate directly with any other bone. It lies below the mandible and anterior to the larynx. If you raise your chin, and place your fingers gently against your throat area and swallow, you may be able to feel it move. The 'Adam's apple' is a separate structure made of cartilage lying below the hyoid bone, called the thyroid cartilage, which is part of the larynx.

Teeth

Humans have teeth in both the upper jaw (maxilla) and lower jaw (mandible), with each person having two sets of teeth throughout their lifetime, the twenty deciduous (baby) teeth appear (erupt) from birth onwards. These include incisors, canines and molars. Over time, these are gradually replaced with a set of 32 permanent teeth which then include premolars, incisors, canines and molars. Teeth are made of calcium, with adult teeth unable to repair or regenerate themselves.

If you lose an adult tooth, you will either have a gap or a replacement fitted by a dentist. Each tooth has its own specific identifying features; details for an excellent guide to their distinguishing features are given in Appendix III.

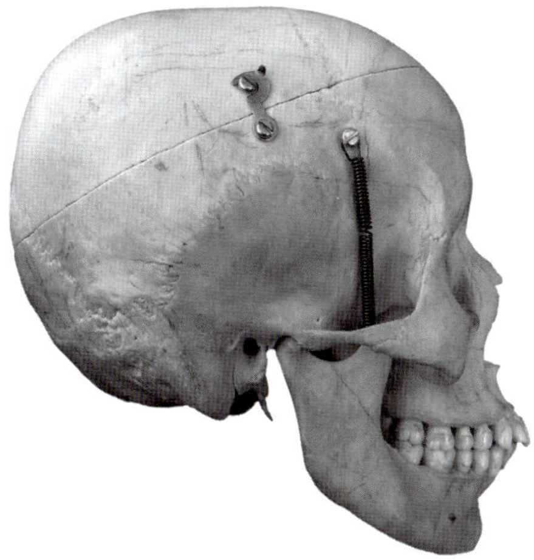

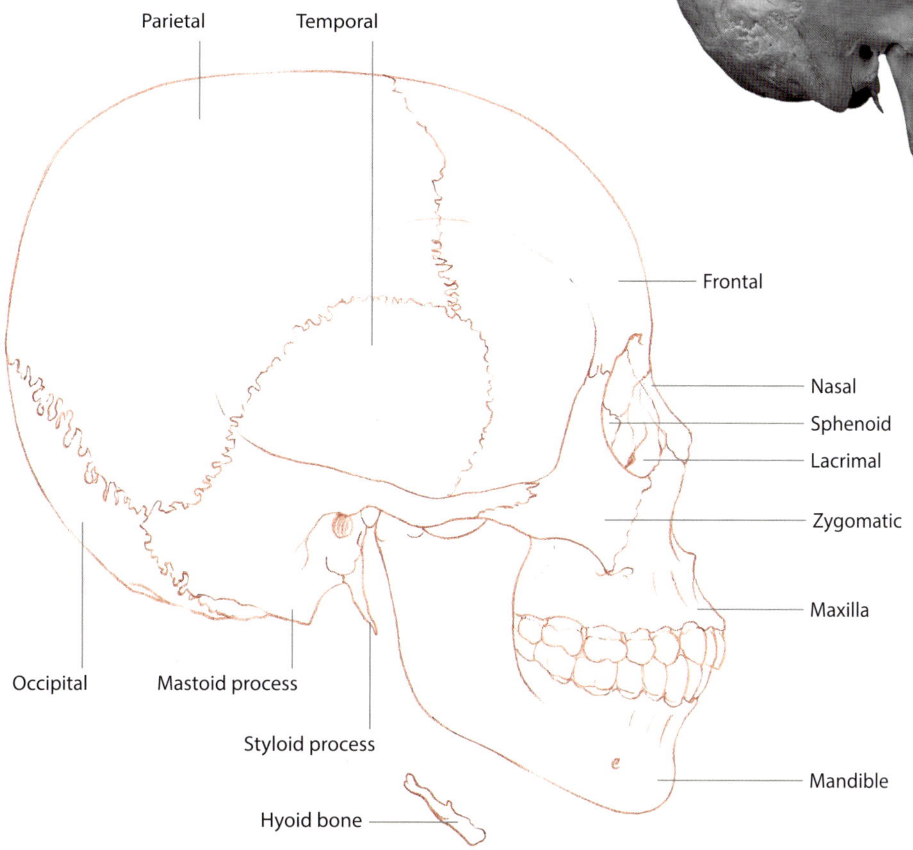

Lateral view of the skull with a real skull for comparison.

The Spine

The vertebral column or spine of the body is made up of 24 separate vertebrae, with a further eight or nine fused vertebrae making up the sacrum and coccyx. The vertebrae gradually increase in size from the cervical vertebrae down to the lumbar vertebrae of the lower back.

The spine can be divided into four distinct curvatures, which for an artist are useful to note. The cervical vertebrae are posteriorly concave (anteriorly convex) and give the greatest range of movement, primarily at C1 and C2. The thoracic vertebrae move the least as they are fixed by the ribs and posteriorly are convex (anteriorly concave). The lumbar vertebrae are the largest and posteriorly are concave (anteriorly convex, with a good range of movement). Finally, the sacrum has a posterior convex curve (anteriorly concave).

The positions of the vertebrae within the body are also useful to note. While the cervical vertebrae sit quite centrally in the neck, the thoracic vertebrae are placed more posteriorly to accommodate the internal organs in the chest; then the lumbar vertebrae are positioned almost centrally again, providing structural support for the body above. The spinal column is surrounded by a strong network of ligaments and muscles, allowing for controlled movement and support.

There are seven cervical vertebrae of the neck, labelled C1 to C7. The first two cervical vertebrae, C1 (the atlas) and C2 (the axis), are called 'atypical', because they are unique in their shape and function. They allow significant rotation of the atlas, up to 70 degrees around the dens of the axis. This allows you to turn your head from side to side.

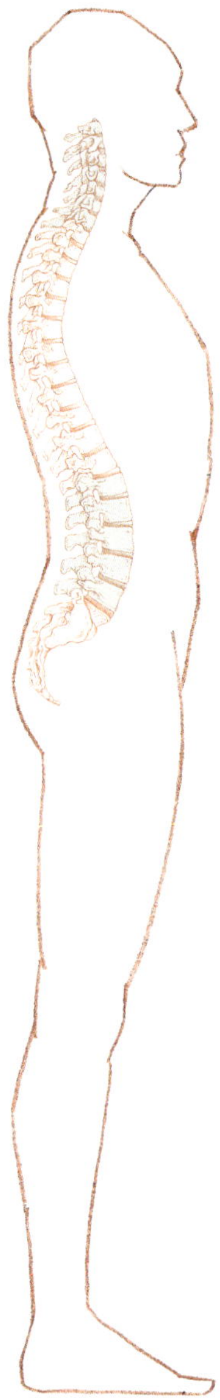

Position of the spine within the body.

Vertebral Discs

Each vertebra is separated from the next by a disc made of cartilage, designed to support the body's weight and give a certain amount of movement. Overall, the spine has 23 flexible intervertebral discs that provide an essential cushioning effect, protecting the spine and the spinal cord during movement. The lumbar region has the largest discs, which compensate for weight bearing and pressure. The transverse processes of the spine prevent the spine from moving too far sideways. Artists need to be aware of the changes in the discs in relation to spinal movements and compression.

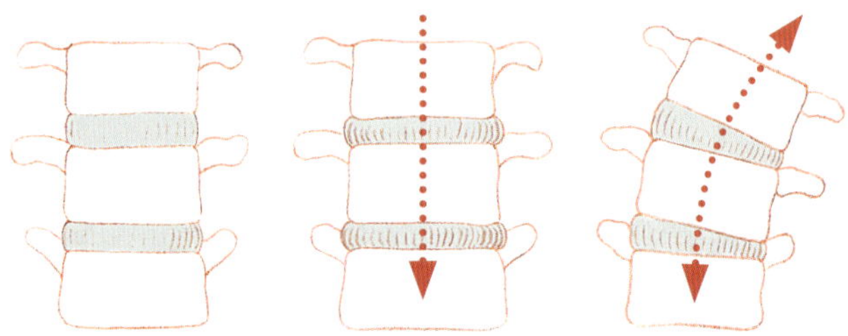

Vertebrae and intervertebral discs in a relaxed position.

The intervertebral discs become wider and flatter under compression.

The flexibility of the intervertebral discs allows movement of the spine.

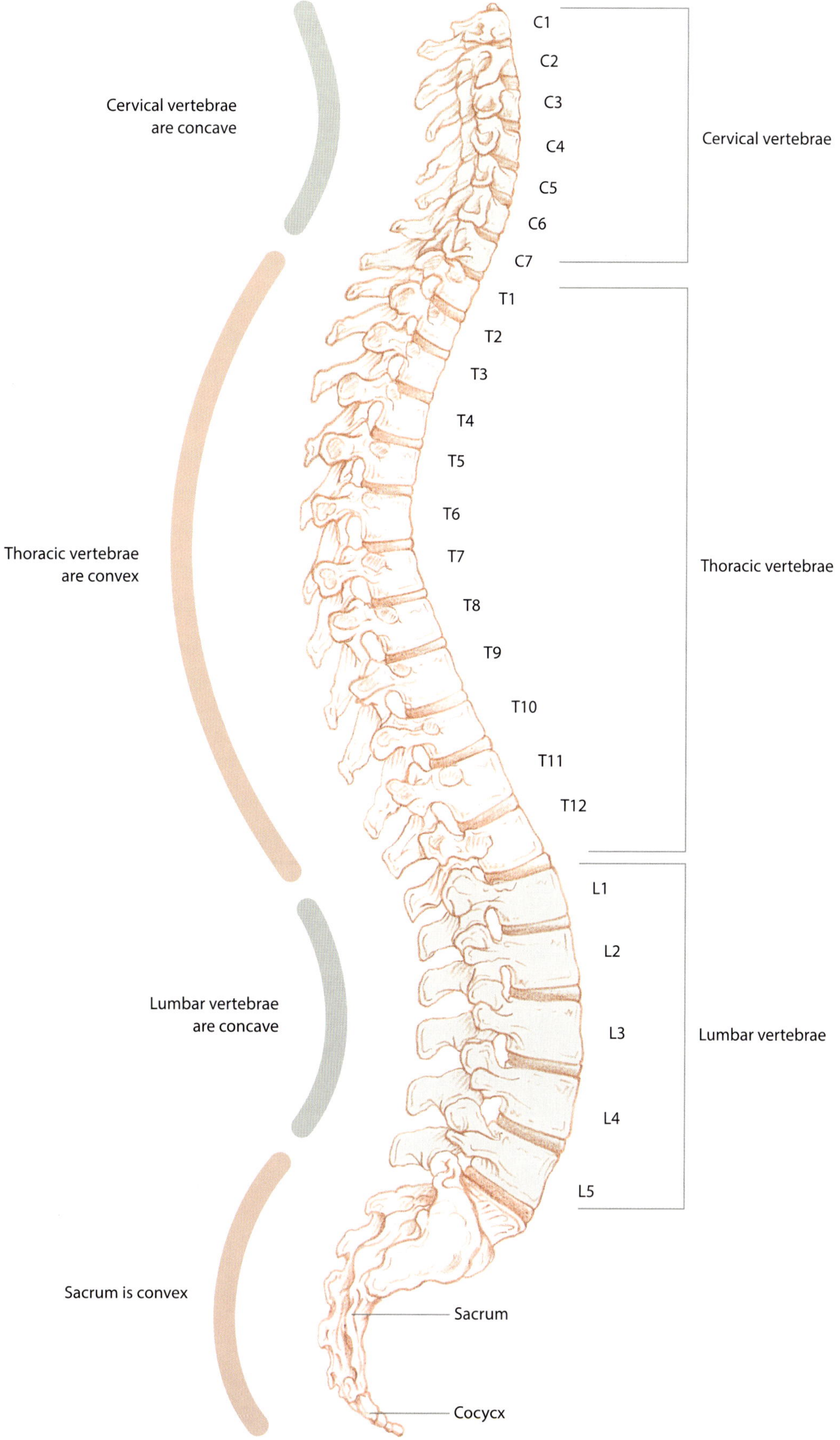

Posterior curvatures of the spinal column.

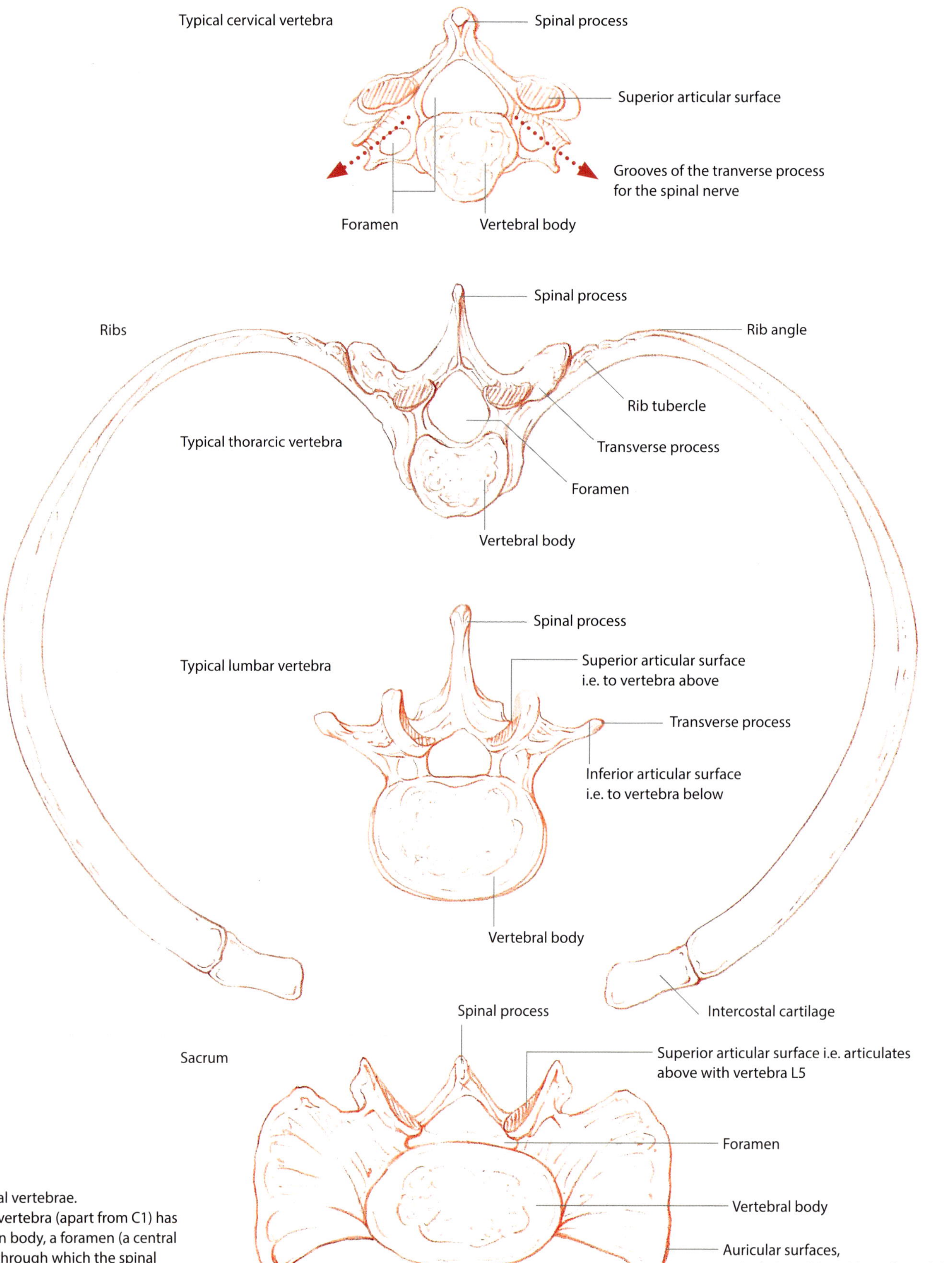

Typical vertebrae.
Each vertebra (apart from C1) has a main body, a foramen (a central hole through which the spinal cord passes), spinal and transverse processes and articular processes which interlock with those vertebrae above and below.

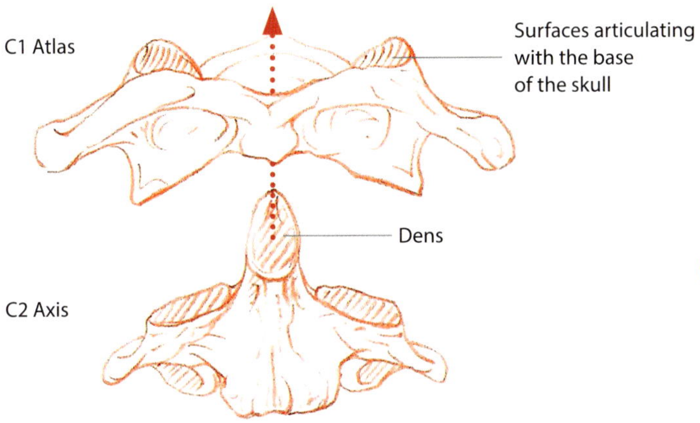

Anterior view of cervical vertebra C1(atlas) and C2 (axis). The dens interlocks inside the foramen of C1.

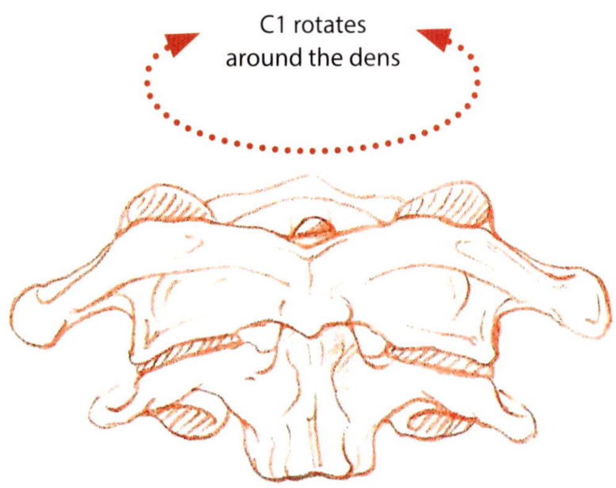

Cervical vertebra C1 can rotate around the dens of the C2 axis, thereby allowing the head to rotate.

The Thorax

The thorax is the upper part of the body, framed by the spine, clavicles, sternum, ribcage and diaphragm that protect the heart and lungs.

For the artist, understanding the structural relationship of the bones of the thorax, and how they are placed below the skin, is key to identifying these and other bony landmarks on the skin surface.

The clavicles (collarbones) are S-shaped bones (viewed from above), medially articulating with the sternum by the sternoclavicular joint. The clavicles are positioned almost horizontally. Laterally they articulate with the acromion of the scapula at the acromioclavicular joint (*see* Chapter 3). The clavicle and the scapula combine to form the shoulder girdle.

Due to its location, the clavicle is one of the weakest and therefore most often fractured or broken bone in the body. It frequently receives the full force of a fall from an outstretched hand or onto the shoulder.

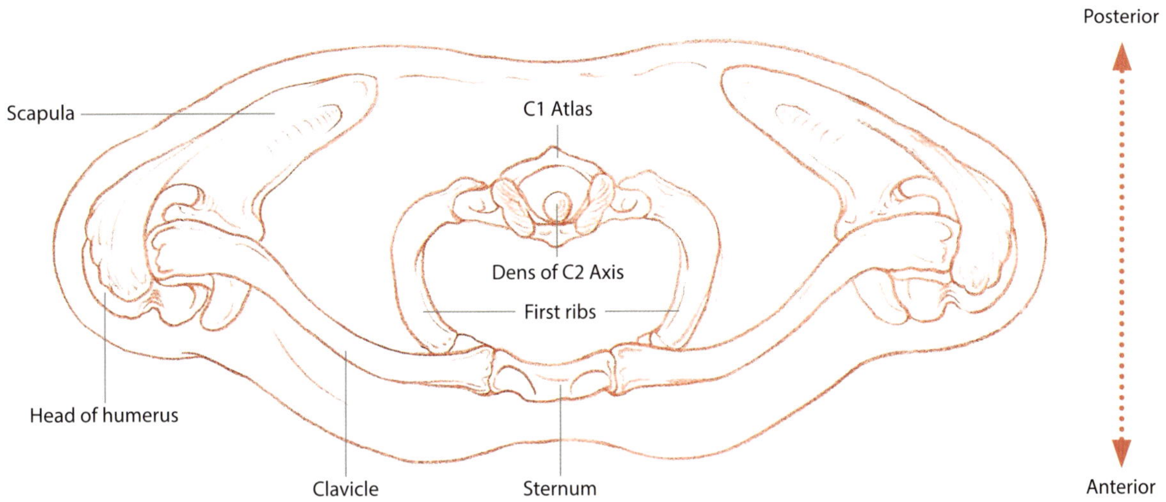

Superior view of the shoulders, showing the structural relationships between the sternum, clavicles, scapulae and first ribs, to the central position of the cervical portion of the spine.

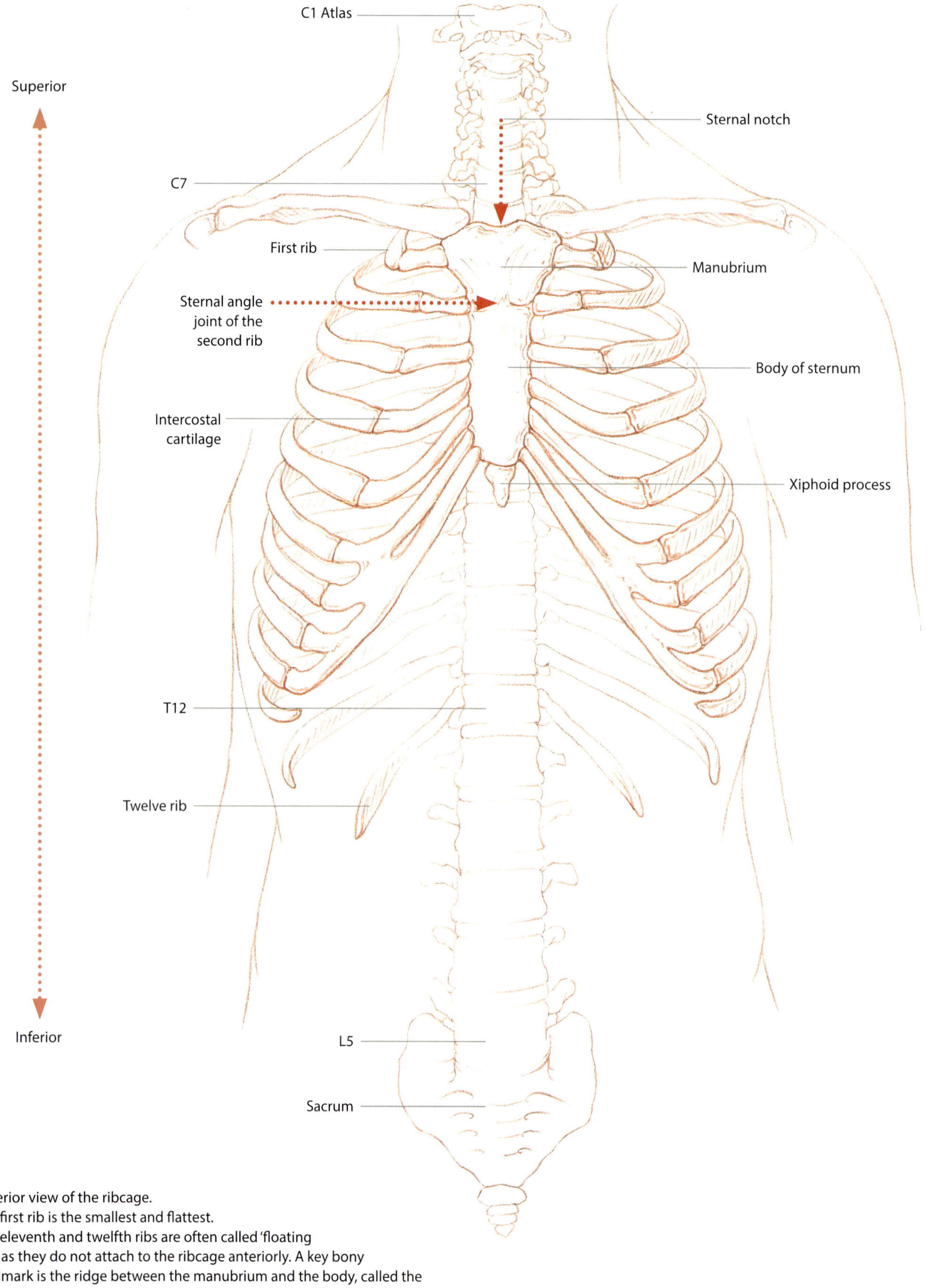

Anterior view of the ribcage.
The first rib is the smallest and flattest.
The eleventh and twelfth ribs are often called 'floating ribs' as they do not attach to the ribcage anteriorly. A key bony landmark is the ridge between the manubrium and the body, called the sternal angle, which can be felt just below the surface of your skin. This bony landmark indicates the level of the second rib.

THE APPENDICULAR SKELETON

This comprises the limbs – arms and legs – and their connecting girdles, such as shoulder and hip bones.

The Arm or Upper Limb

The upper arm bone (humerus) attaches to the scapula (shoulder blade) and runs down to the elbow.

The ulna and radius form the bones of the forearm, between the wrist and the elbow. The radius bone can rotate over the ulna (see below). You will see how this works by rotating your forearm. Place your forearm on a table with your hand palm side up and your thumb pointing away from you. Keep your elbow on the table, then rotate your hand 180 degrees so the palm of the hand becomes flat on the table. This rotation explains how the bone received its name: the radius is half the diameter of a circle, which is the rotational distance of the radius.

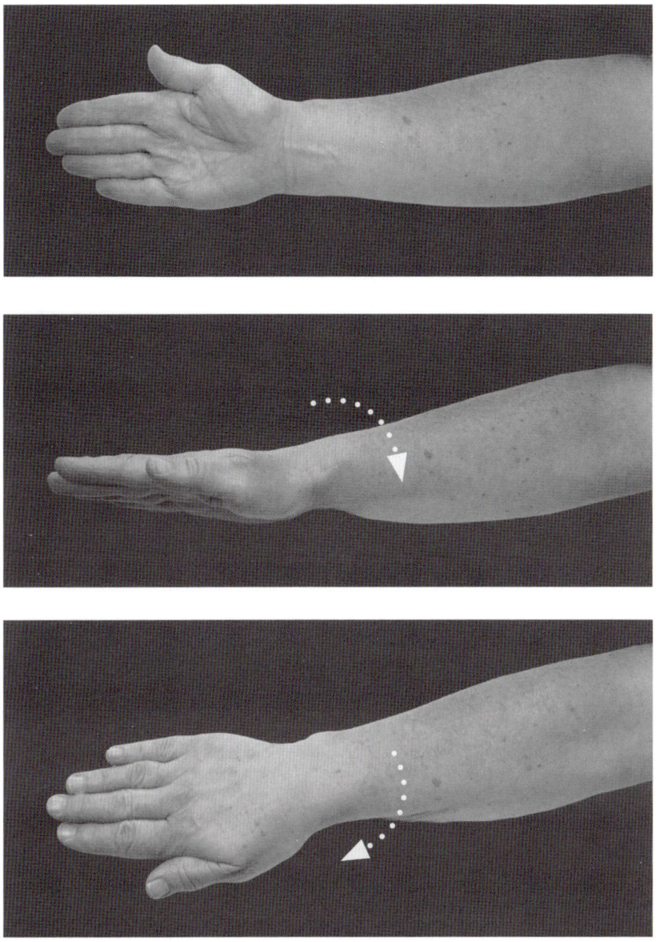

Top: Start with your arm placed on a flat surface, with the palm facing upwards (supination).
Middle: Gradually rotate your arm medially.
Bottom: When the arm has completed the rotation, the palm will face downwards (pronation).

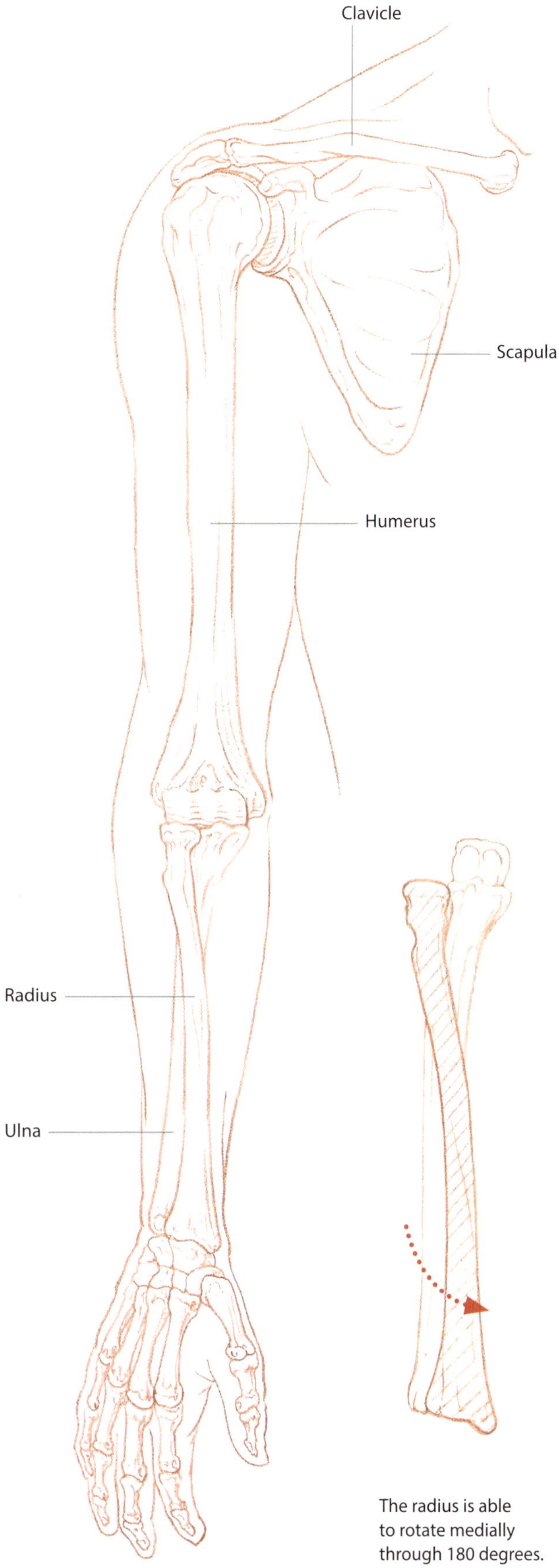

The radius is able to rotate medially through 180 degrees.

Bones of the forearm.

The Wrist and Hand

The wrist and hand contain 27 bones each (making 54 in total). The wrist comprises eight bones in approximately two parallel rows. Those bones closest to the radius and ulna are the scaphoid, lunate, triquetral and pisiform bones. Those positioned towards the fingers or digits of the hand (distal) are the trapezium, trapezoid, capitate and hamate bones.

The bones forming the palm of the hand comprise five metacarpals. These are numbered from 1 to 5, with 5 being the smallest or little finger and the thumb 1. The thumb comprises only two carpal bones, whereas the four fingers each have three.

For artists, the hand is an important anatomical area to study. First, consider the hand without the thumb, so the wrist and fingers create a flat paddle. Then add the thumb, which is unique in having a saddle joint (the only one in the body), which allows the circumduction movement of the thumb, moving forward, back and sideways and, specifically, to oppose the fingers to form a grip.

Saddle joint. Trapezium and first metacarpal bones of the thumb.

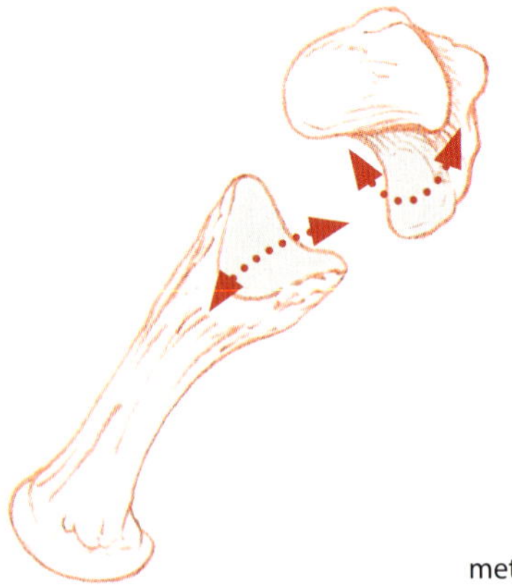

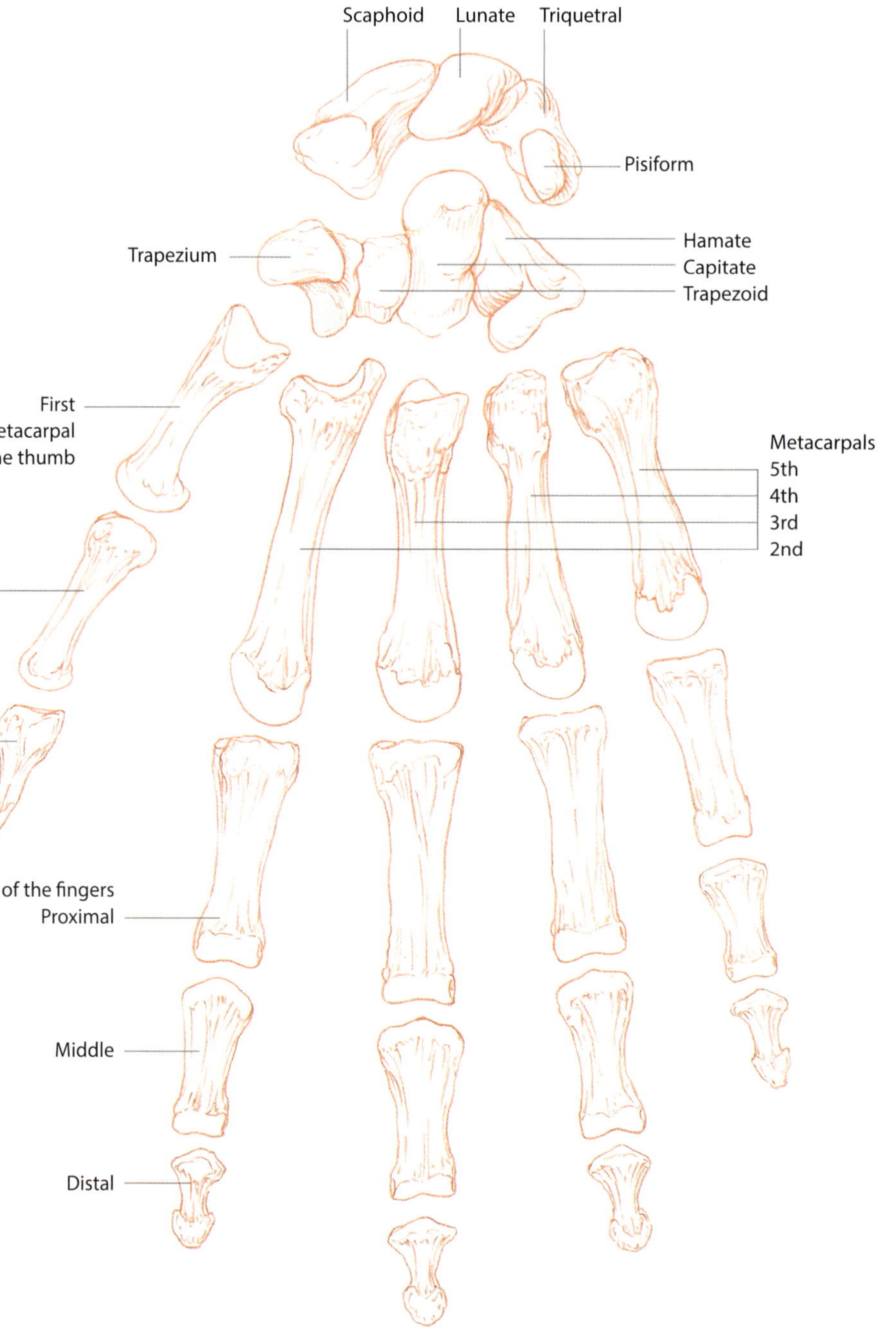

Palmar view of the right hand, showing the bones of the wrist and hand.

Movements of the Thumb

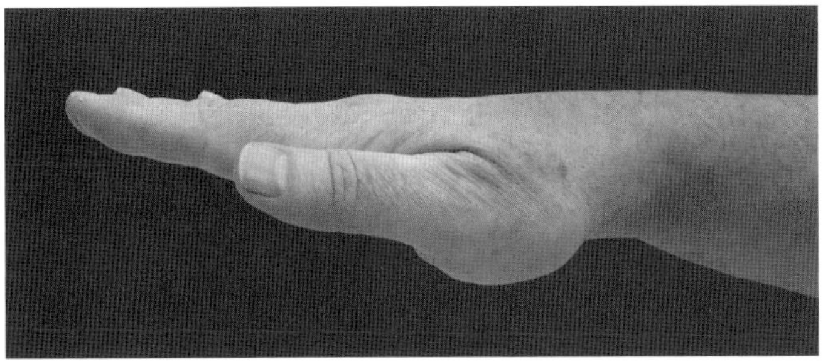

Adduction of the thumb (above) – positioned close beside the hand.
Abduction of the thumb (right) – positioned away from the hand.

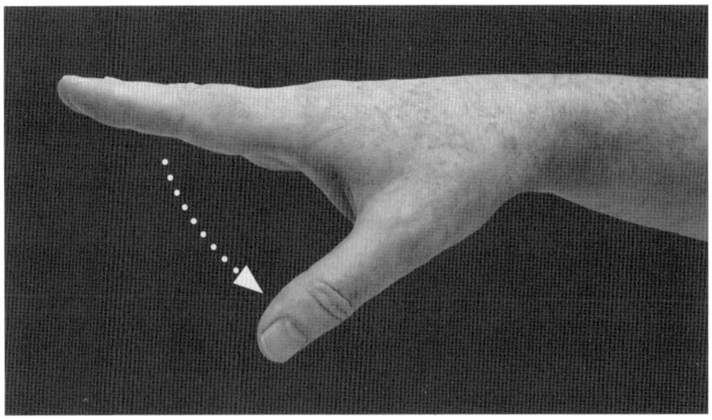

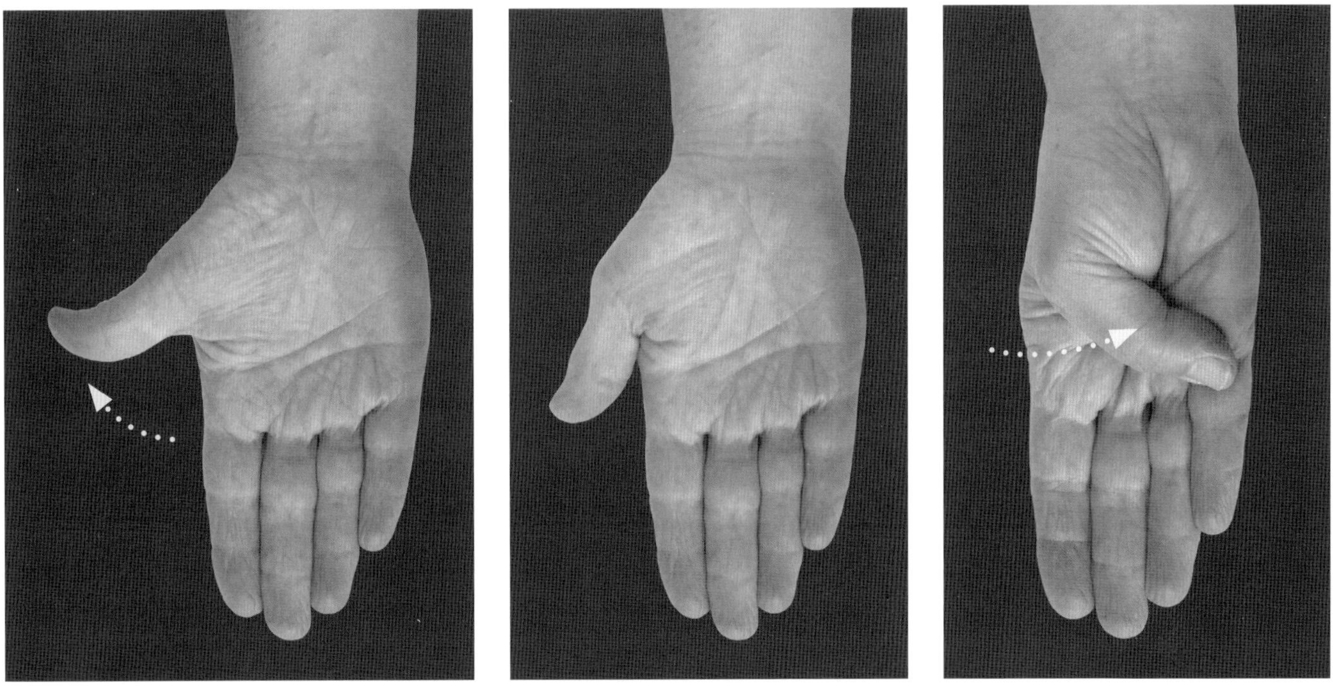

Extension of the thumb (left) – positioned away from the hand. The thumb in a relaxed position (central). The thumb flexed across the palm (right).

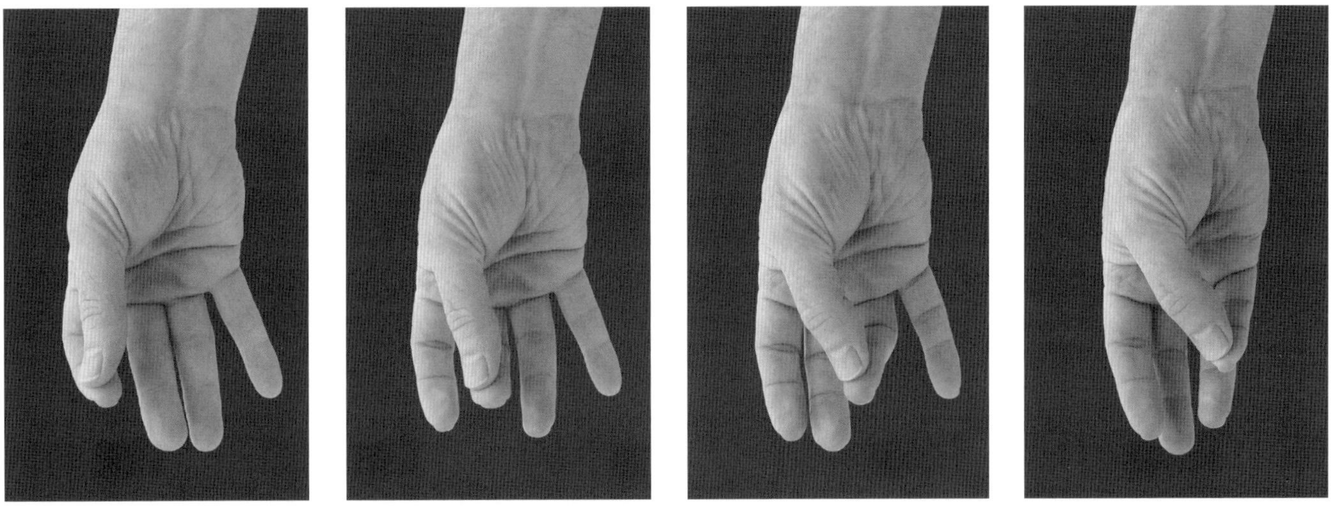

Opposition movements of the thumb, towards the first, second, third and fourth fingers.

The Leg or Lower Limb

The leg is the longest limb of the body, comprising four main bones, excluding the foot. The femur or thigh bone is the longest and strongest bone in the body, while the lower leg comprises the patella or kneecap and the tibia and fibula.

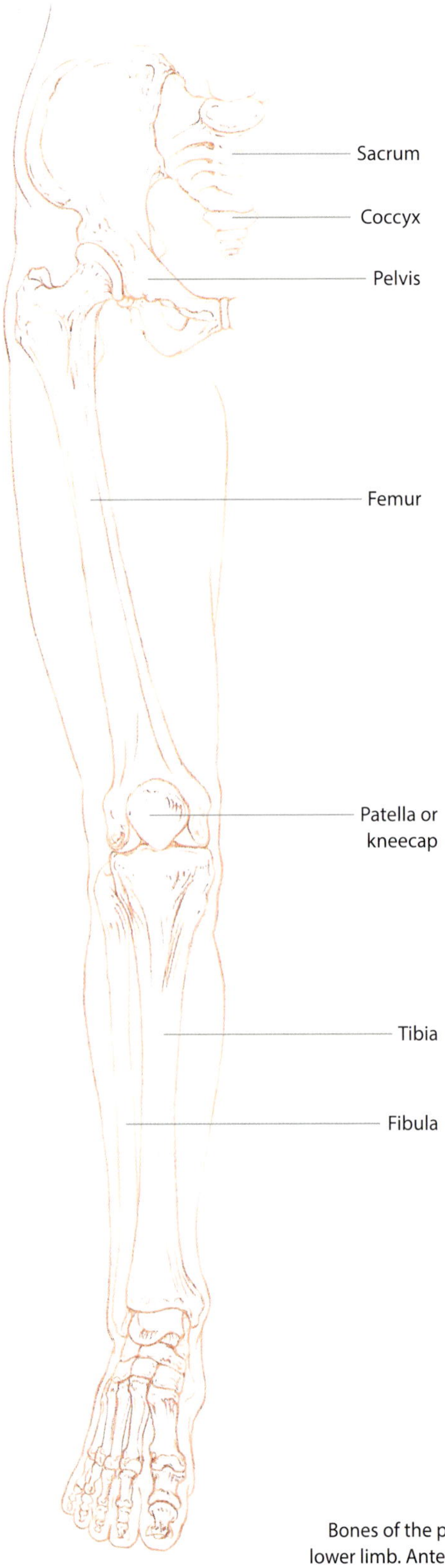

Bones of the pelvis and lower limb. Anterior view.

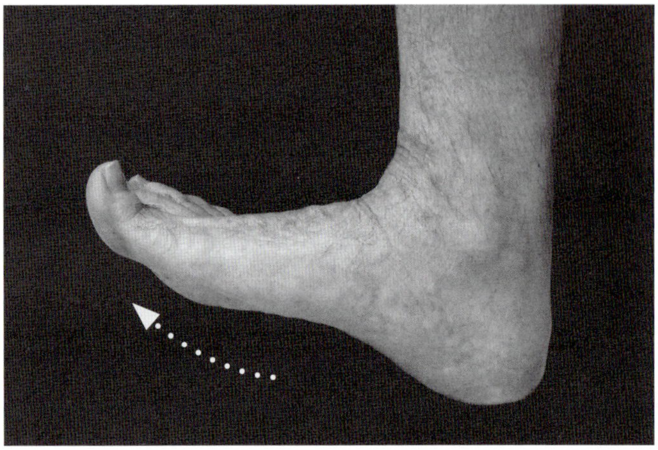

The foot in dorsiflexion. Medial view (above) and lateral view (below).

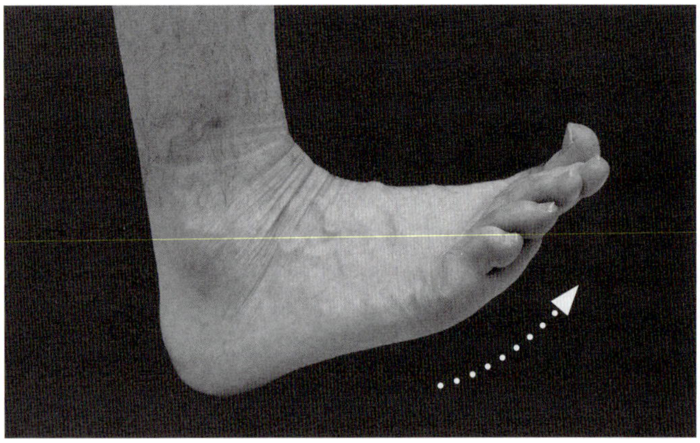

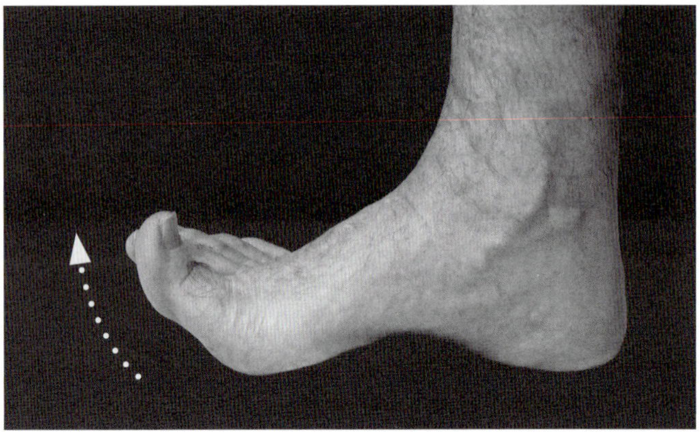

The big toe in extension. Medial view (above) and lateral view (below).

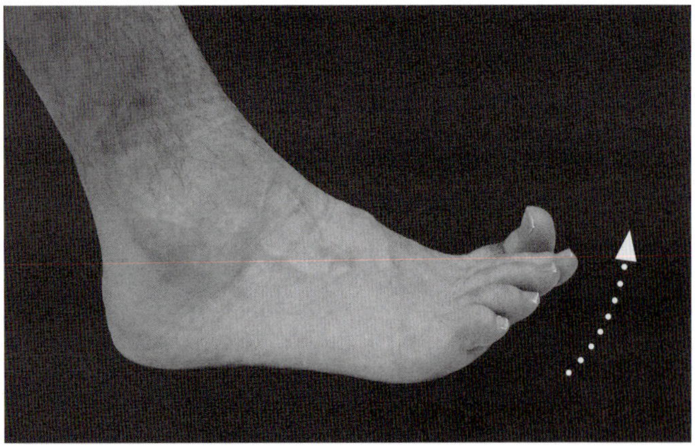

The Foot

Each foot has 26 bones, which can be divided into three main sections: the seven irregular tarsus bones, the five metatarsal bones and the fourteen phalanges (two phalanx bones for the big toe and the twelve phalanges forming the bones of the remaining four toes). The calcaneus bone of the heel is the largest bone in the foot.

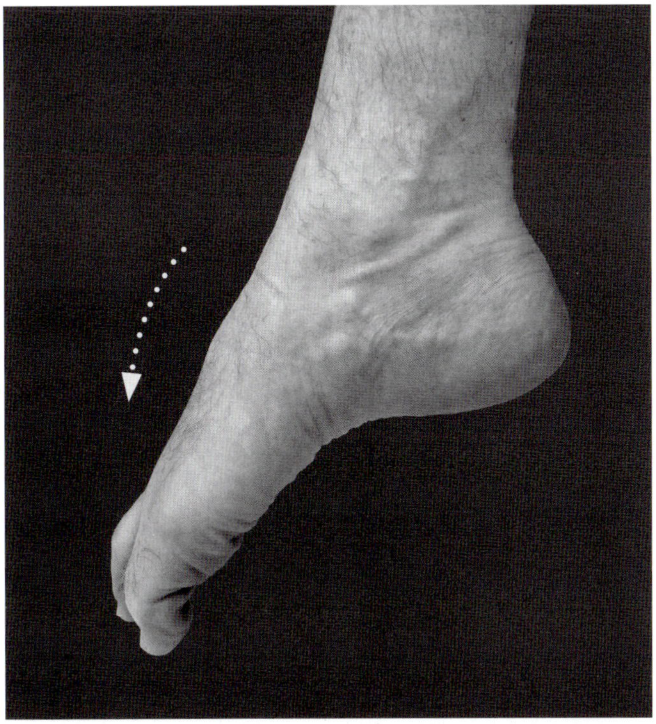

The foot in plantar flexion. Medial view (above) and lateral view (below).

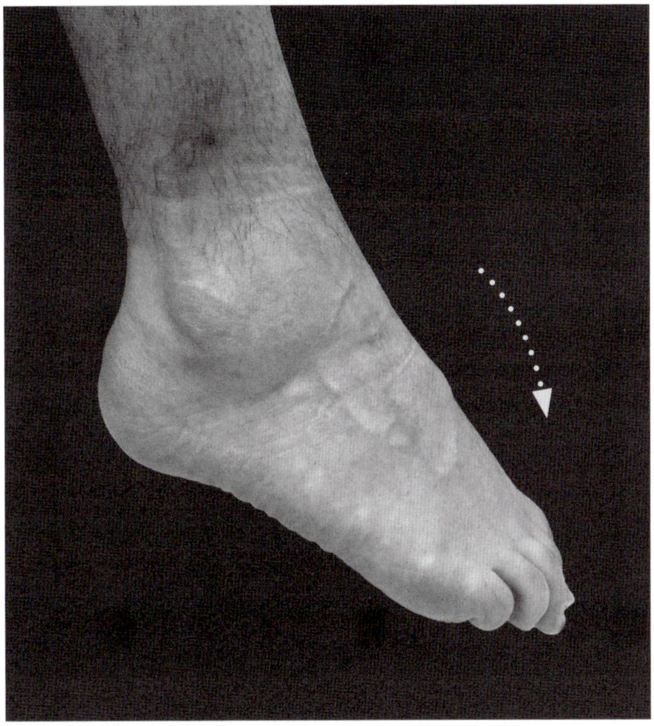

Bones of the right foot. Superior view.

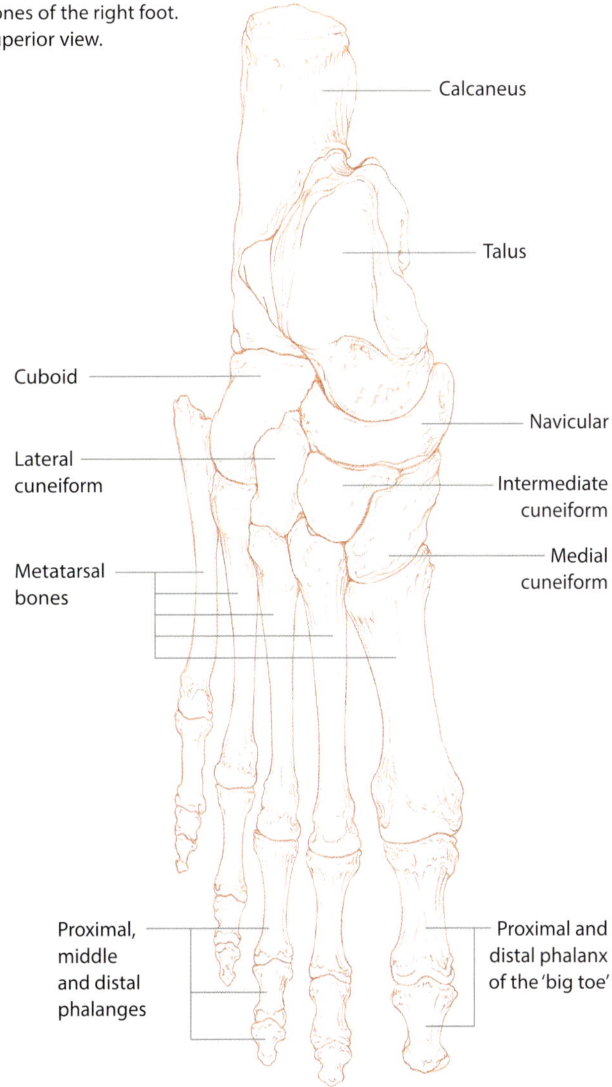

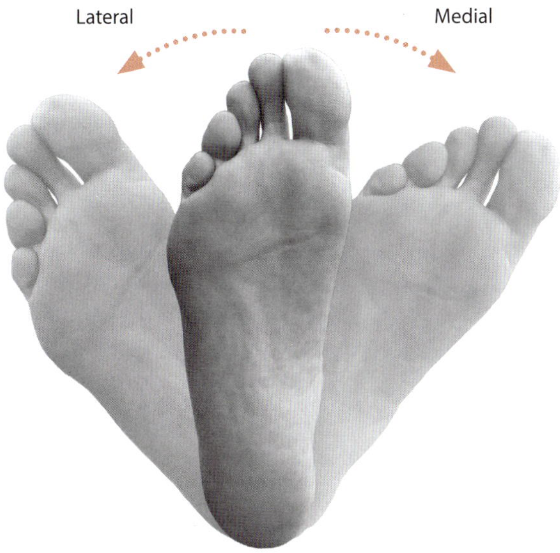

Lateral and medial rotation of the foot.

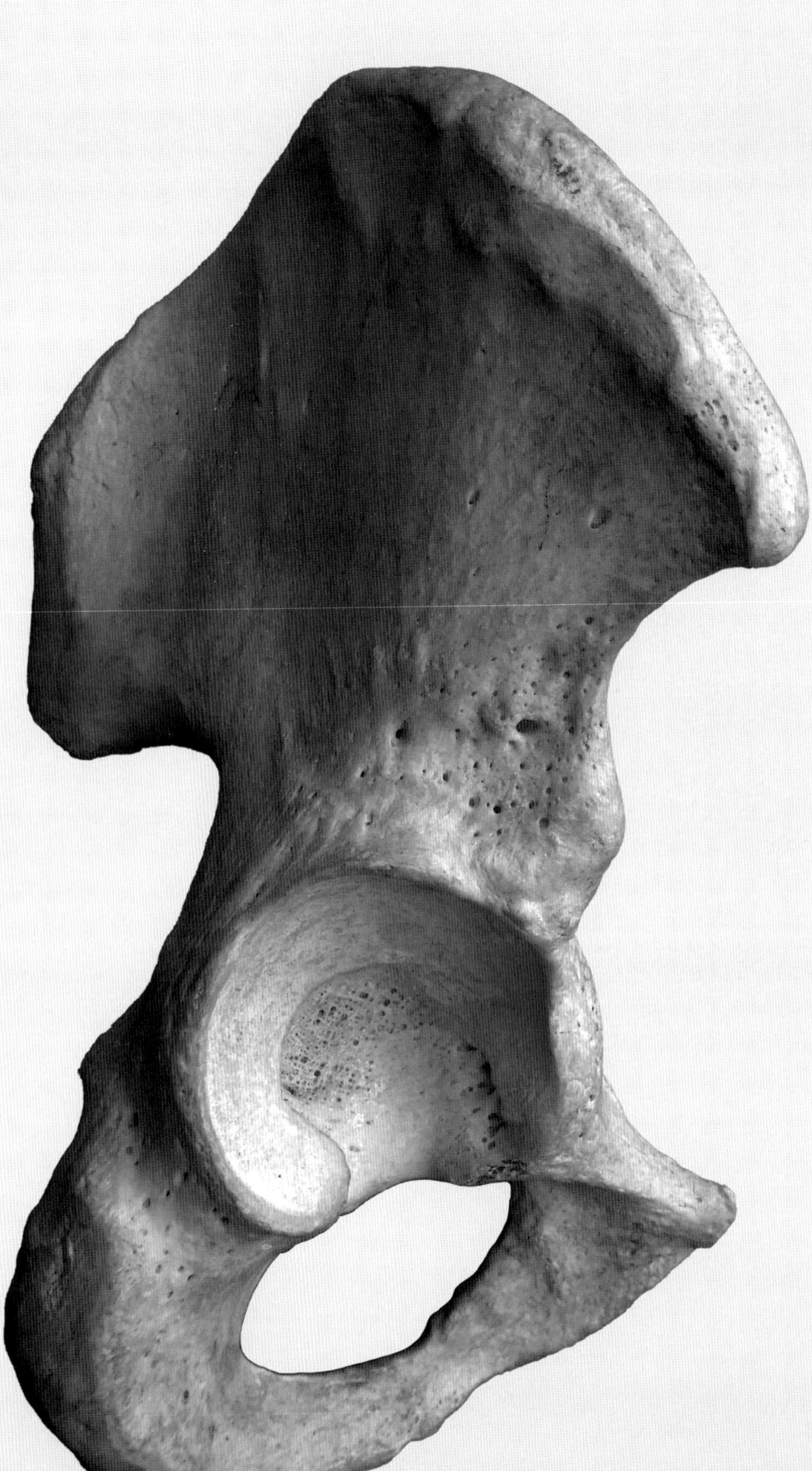

CHAPTER 3

PROPORTIONS AND BONY LANDMARKS

For the purposes of this text, our starting point is a 'normal' human body standing in the 'anatomical position' (*see* Chapter 1). We can then expand this to include body proportions, physical bony landmarks, underlying features and other anatomical points that will be useful for a medical artist. Each reference will accumulatively aid you in creating anatomically correct drawings and illustrations. The terms of orientation, planes and movement for the human body have been covered in Chapter 2.

ABOVE AND BELOW THE SKIN

Many bones and muscles can be felt just below the skin, or visually explored with the aid of a mirror. By this practical method, you can start to identify distinct features and bony structures. For example, move your hand and, stretch your fingers, and observe how the bones move and which tendons you can see. Each feature contributes to our overall shape and form. From the horizontal clavicles (collarbones) to our protruding kneecaps (the patella), down to the sharp angular ridge down the shin bone (the fibula), you can begin to identify many bony elements of the skeleton and how they connect to each other.

Firstly, we will look further at the body and its relative proportions. These have been studied for centuries, with many notable historical advances, for example during the Renaissance period. Leonardo da Vinci's famous illustration of the *Vitruvian Man* illustrates the ideal proportions of a man's body, drawn with arms outstretched, with his legs spaced apart to fit perfectly within a circle.

All the ratios and schematic guides illustrated here should be taken purely as a starting point. Every human body you observe and draw will have its own distinct features in terms of height, form, shape, size and colour, each with its own relative proportions. We all come in an infinite number of variations, with every human body having its own unique characteristics.

For the artist, dividing the human body into eight divisions with the head representing one eighth, forms a simple yet convenient guide for creating identifiable proportions of the body *(see page 32)*. There are many other anatomical ratios and proportional relationships throughout the body, which can collectively assist with drawing. A selection of proportional guides relating to the body are covered in this chapter.

Medical artists are frequently required to draw whole or parts of the body, for example, illustrating surgical procedures. A patient may be partially or completely covered by sheets or clothing. Understanding the proportions of the human body and its integral proportions will help you create accurate drawings whether you can see specific features or not.

Lateral view of the right hip bone.

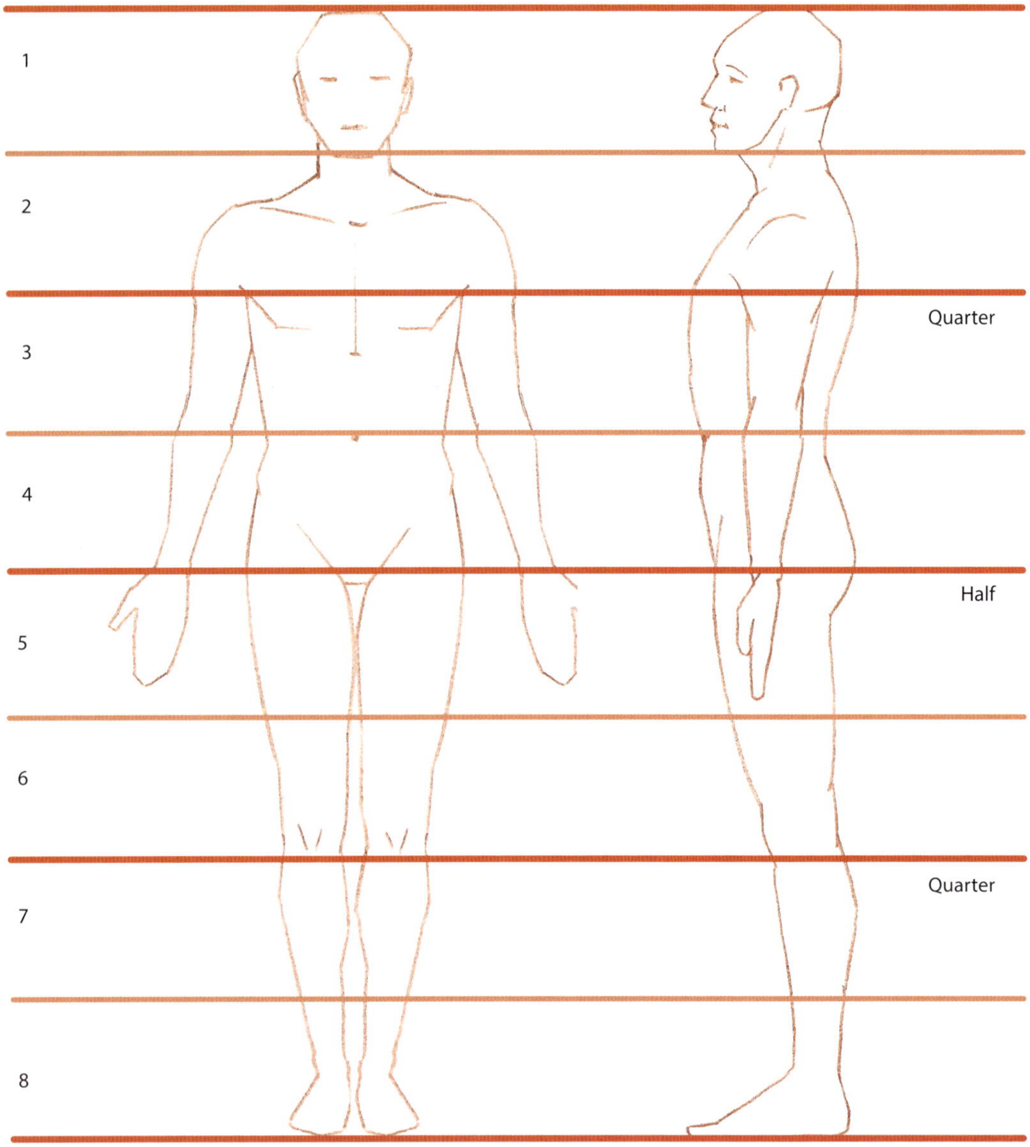

Schematic drawing showing a proportional guide where the body in this example has been divided into eight portions, working from the head as the first single portion. The body then can be divided into two halves at the pubic bone and quarters just below the line of the armpits and then again just below the kneecaps. The top eighth runs to below the chin and three-eighths to the umbilicus (tummy button).

A schematic guide showing a useful guide for artists whereby the head can be divided into two halves, with the eye placed centrally between the top of head and the bottom of the chin. Always be aware individual head proportions may vary, however, this guide can form a good starting point for illustrations and drawing portraits.
When the mouth is in a relaxed position, take a vertical line (indicated by the dotted lines) from the centre of the iris of each eye down to the outer width of the mouth, being a proportional guide for drawing the mouth.

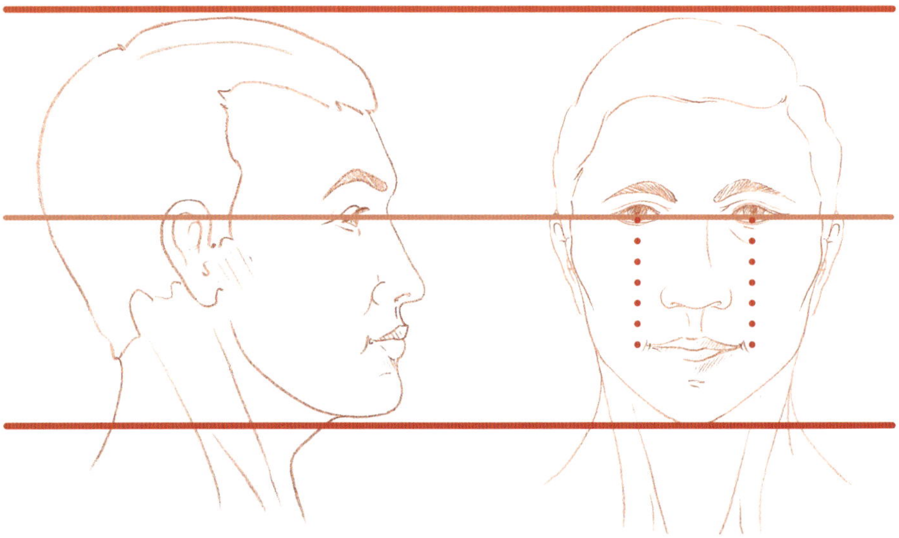

Head and Skull

The key bony landmarks of the head are:

1. Frontal brow ridge Ridges of the forehead and the upper or supra-orbital ridge above the eye, form the frontal bone
2. Nasal ridge The front portion is cartilage *(see page 37)*
3. Orbital edge of the eye socket Either side of the nose, these form the frontal maxilla (upper jawbone)
4. Zygomatic arch A prominent feature also known as the cheekbone (comprised partly of the zygomatic bone and partly of the temporal bone)
5. Frontal mandible protuberance The chin, in the middle of the lower jawbone
6. Jaw line of the mandible
7. The mastoid process Base of the temporal bones on each side of the skull, behind the earlobes
8. The occipital protuberance The rear lower part of the skull

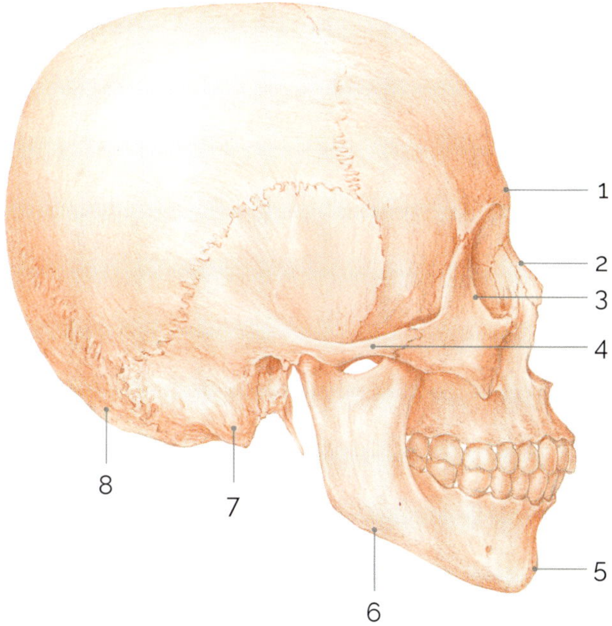

Proportions of the Face

These schematic drawings and the following series of photographs will cover various proportions of the face, for example the face in relation to the hand and foot (below right) and where the head fits within a square (see page 34). Further illustrated examples relate to the eyes, ears, nose and mouth. Each comparison will provide you with additional proportions and points of reference to help build proportionally accurate anatomical drawings.

Our faces are rarely symmetrical, with variations, however slight, from one side to the other, alongside differences in shape and individual character.

Try the example below: with your hand open and flat, place the centre of your wrist against your chin. Your middle finger will reach the centre of your forehead, giving you an instant guide for a hand-to-head ratio.

The foot is proportionately slightly longer than the head, with the hand length reaching only the fifth, or little toe.

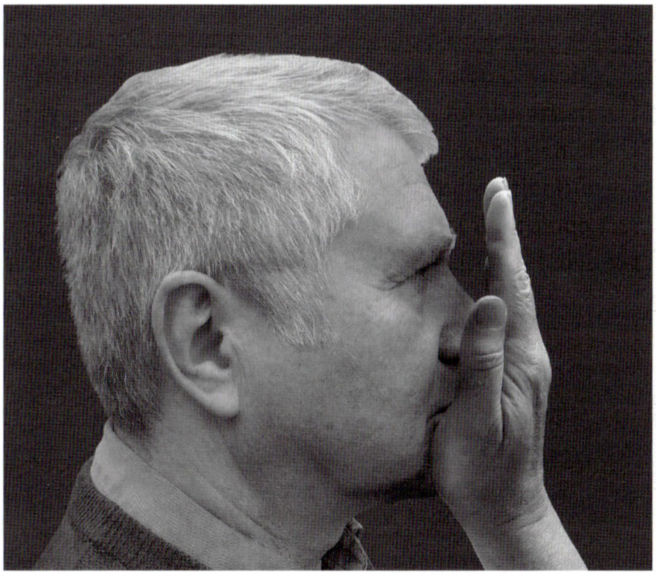

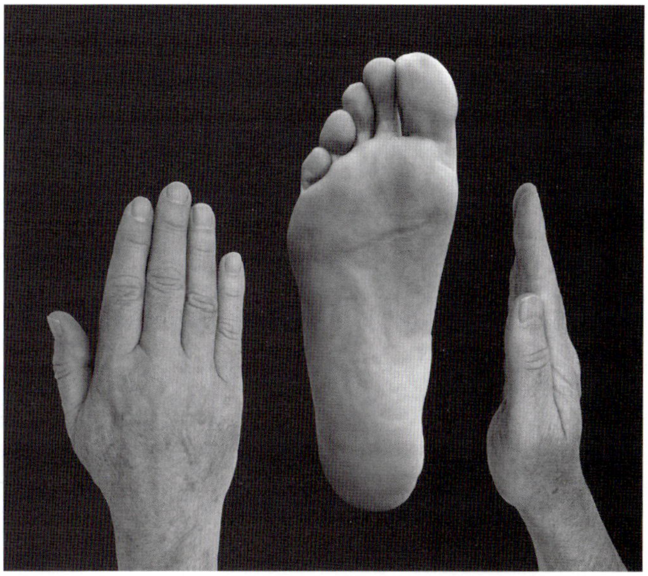

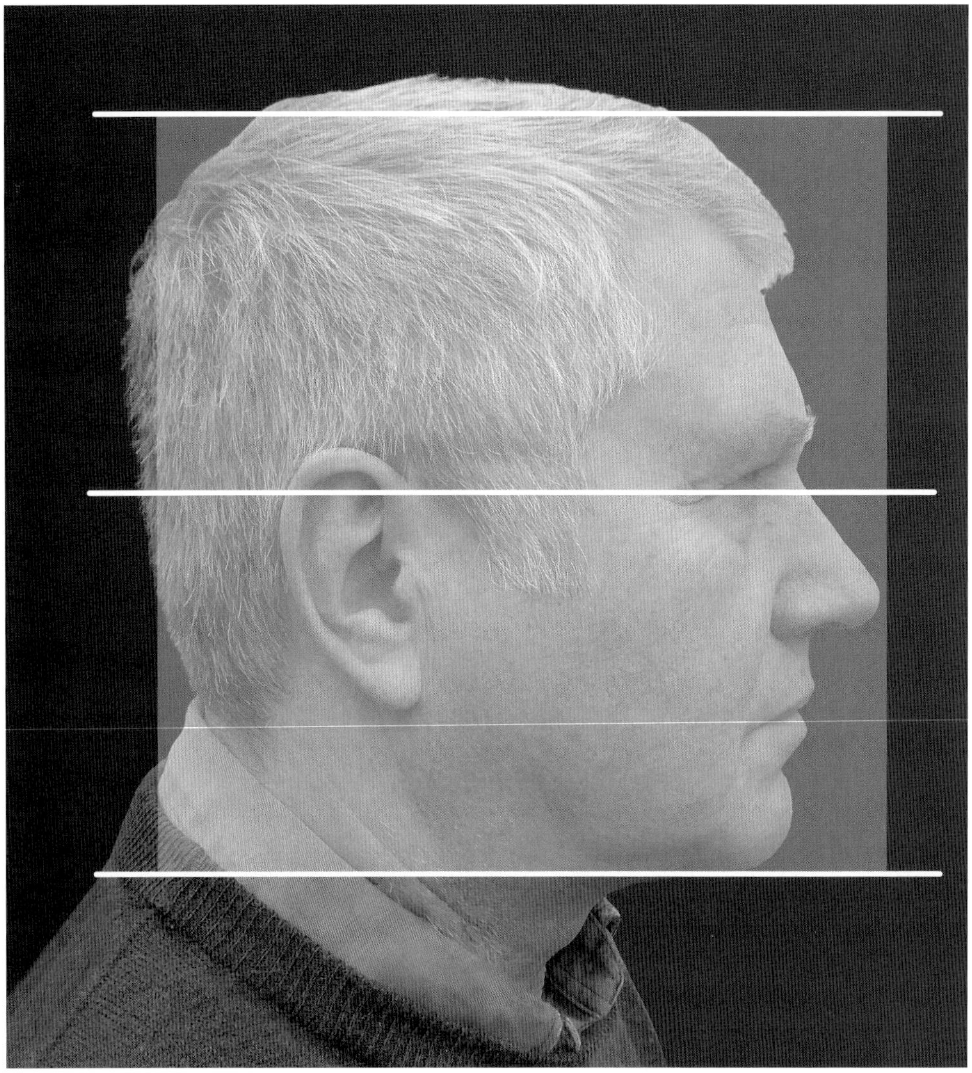

The head fitting within a square with the eyes half way down indicated by the white lines. When drawing within a square, allow for the hair volume, which may be well beyond this area.

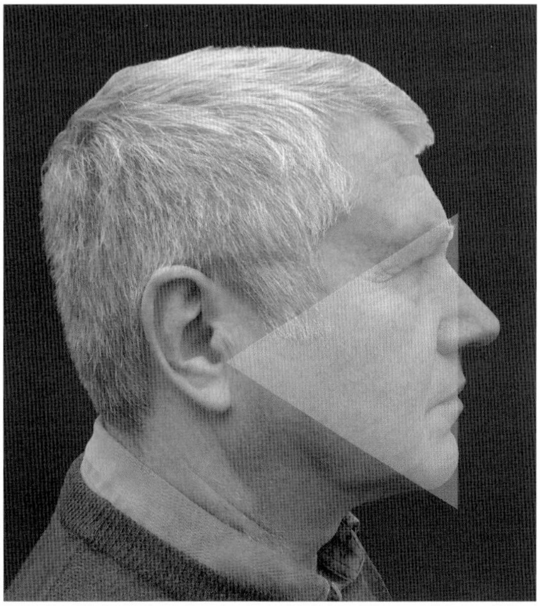

Make a triangle by joining the following three points, for a positional guide joining the eyebrow, chin and the ear. Begin at the point between the eyebrows just above the bridge of the nose; down to the lower frontal protuberance of the jaw (mandible) – being below the mouth; then back across to the head of the mandible just in front of the lower portion of the ear.

The Eyes

The eyes are essentially spheres sitting deep within the orbit of the skull where they are protected. Their movement is controlled by a series of muscles around each eye inside each orbit. These muscles are connected to the eyes above, below and to the sides, allowing for a wide range of movements. Note how far back the eye sits 'as a whole', from the bridge of the nose and mainly hidden within the orbit of the skull: externally, we only see a small portion of the eye. The image below shows the eyes closed for comparison. Eyelids are unique in having the thinnest layer of skin on the body.

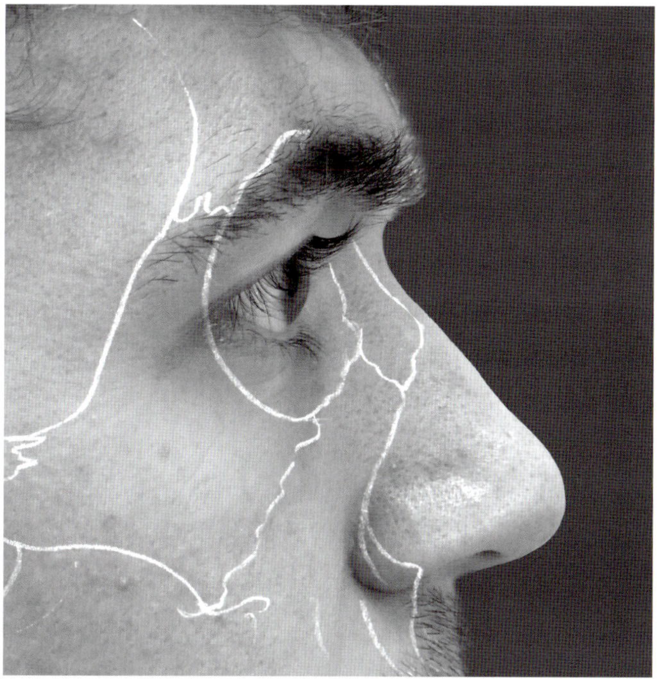

Lateral view of the head with an outline the bony rim of the eye socket.

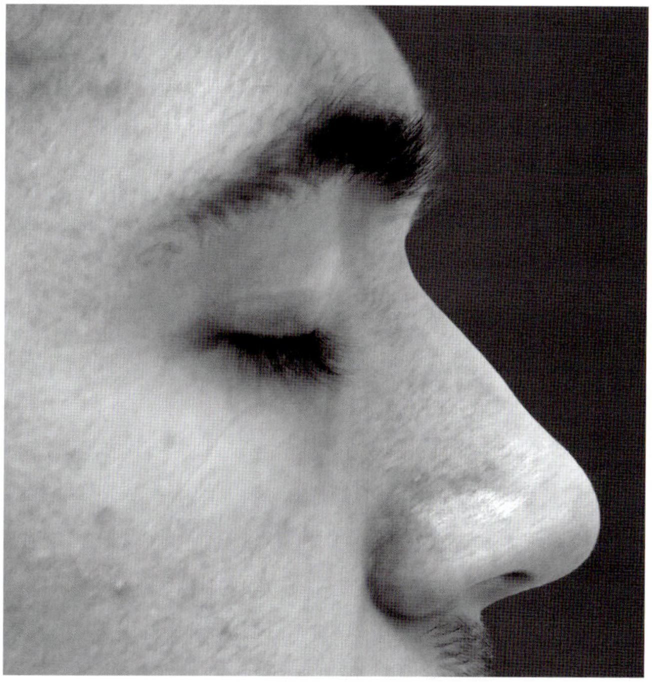

Lateral view with the eye closed for comparison.

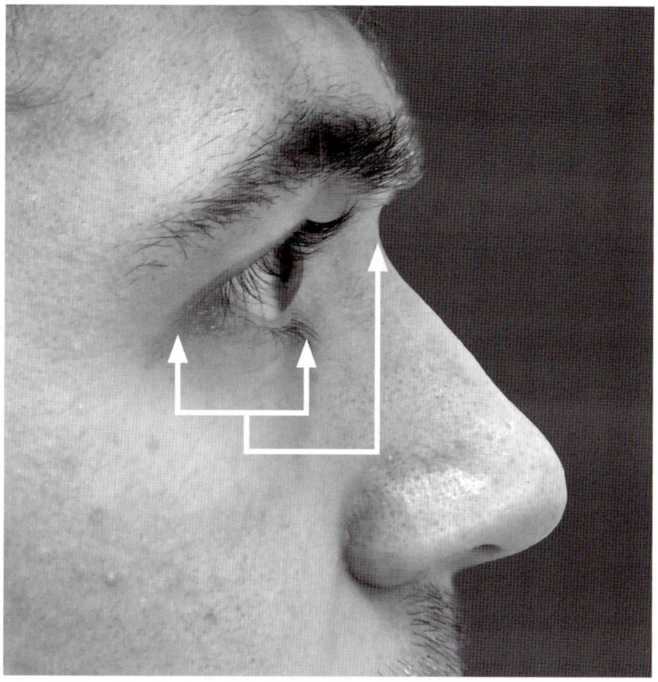

Lateral view with the eye open, with arrows indicating the depth of the eye area seen externally and how far the eye is positioned back anatomically from the bridge of the nose.

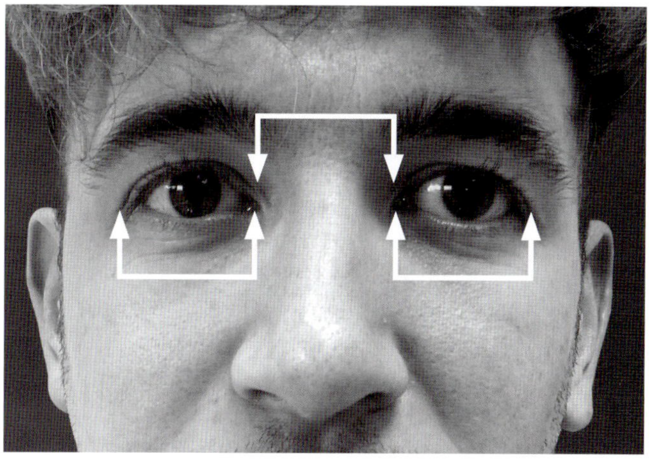

When drawing the face, the total distance between the outside of each eye can usually be divided into thirds. Each eye, as a general rule is one-third of this total distance, leaving the bridge of the nose area creating the middle third. Every face will have its own unique and individual proportions.

The Ears and Nose

Both the ears and the nose are fascinating structures, being formed mainly by strong and flexible cartilage, albeit of slightly different types – the ear is made from elastic cartilage and the nose from hyaline cartilage.

The Ear

The shape and structure of the outer ear, also known as the auricle or pinna, are mainly formed by several thick curved areas of cartilage. The three most distinct areas are the helix (the outer curve of cartilage), the tragus (a small area of cartilage that protrudes and protects the entrance to the ear canal, with an opposing anti-tragus) and the ear lobe, which is non-cartilaginous, soft and fleshy.

There is often a little 'bump' that can be seen along the upper posterior inner curve of the helix. This is considered an inherited condition, presenting as a slight thickening of the helix at that juncture. This is commonly known as the Darwin's or auricular tubercle.

The ear is covered further on pages 122-123.

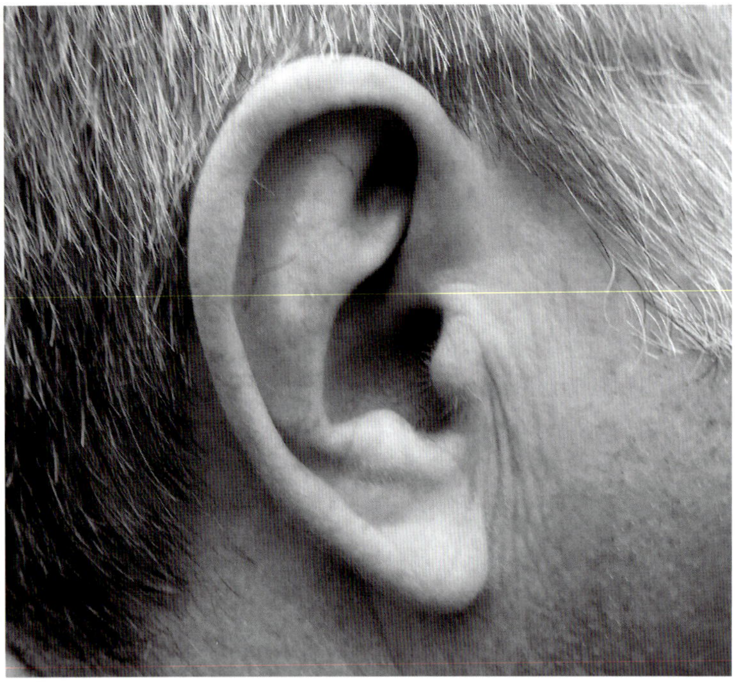

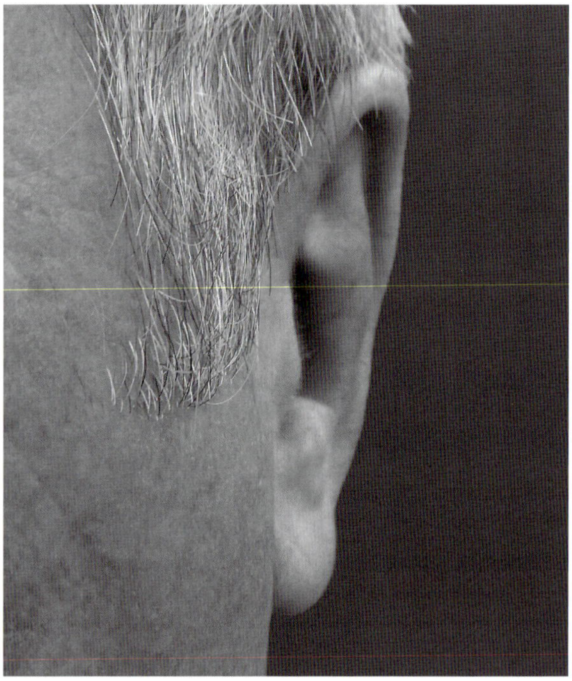

Lateral view of the right ear (above), and anterior view (right).

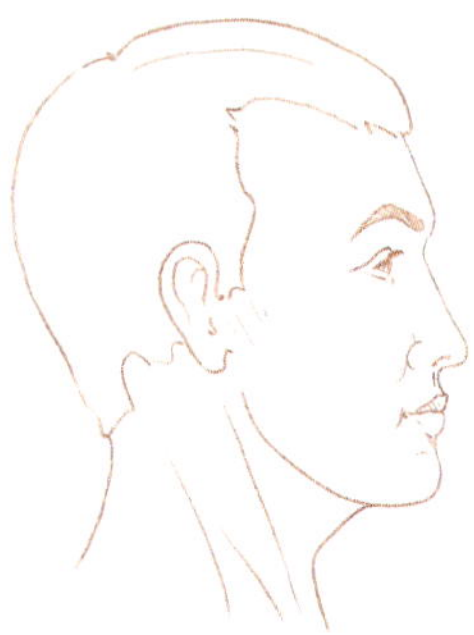

Lateral view of the head, showing the position of the ear (above).

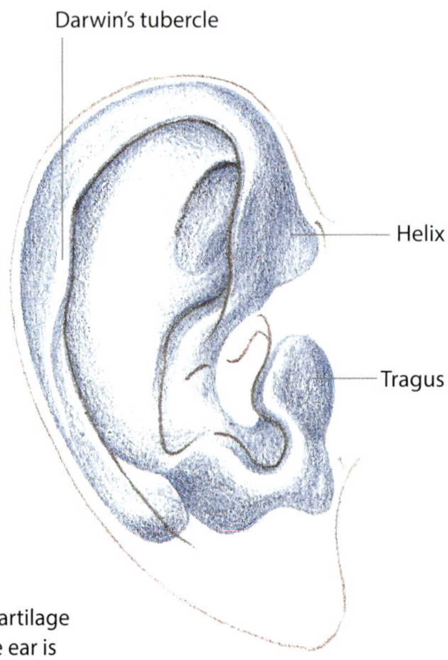

The cartilage of the ear is comprised of two main areas: the helix and the tragus.

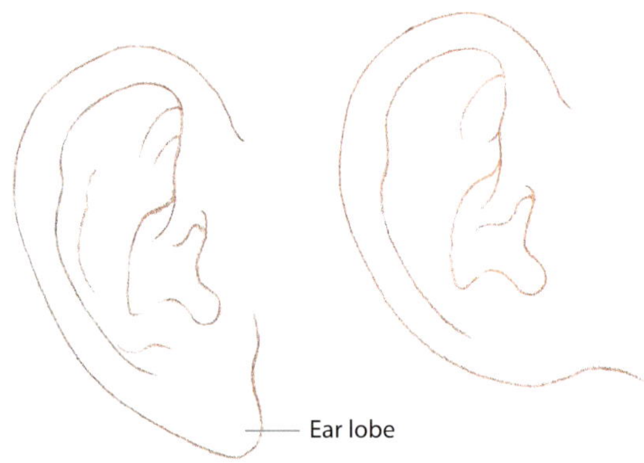

The ear lobe may appear 'free', i.e. with a distinct earlobe hanging down below the attachment area to the head as shown on the left, which is more common; or it may appear 'attached', without a clear and separate lobe as above right. The ear lobe is distinct in having no structural cartilage and can vary significantly in size and shape, especially with age.

The Nose

The nose, through which we primarily breathe, is positioned centrally within the face between the eyes and the mouth. The size, shape and width of the nose varies significantly and can also change as we age.

The nose also has three distinct parts, from the upper nasal bones to the middle areas of cartilage to the apex of the nose where the nostrils are. The nostrils are also known as nares.

You can feel the edges of the nasal bones either side along the upper sides of your nose, from the nasal ridge down to the outside of the nostrils. When looking at the face, this cartilaginous junction on the nasal ridge can often be seen from both the lateral and anterior view. The junction between the bone and cartilage can be especially noticeable if someone has broken their nose, or it may be naturally prominent. You can feel the apex of the cartilage on the ridge of your nose.

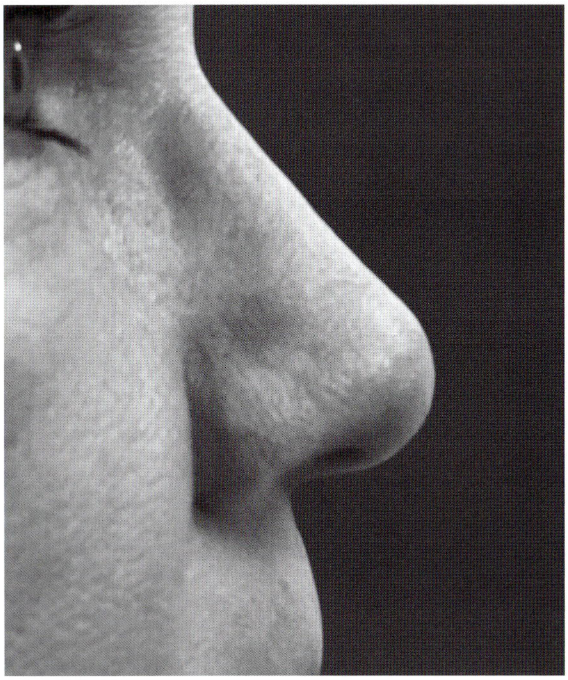

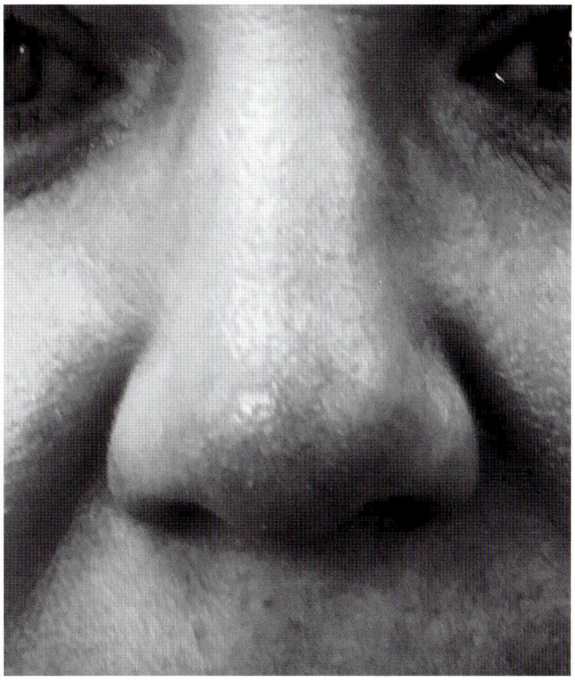

Lateral view of the nose (left), and anterior view (right).

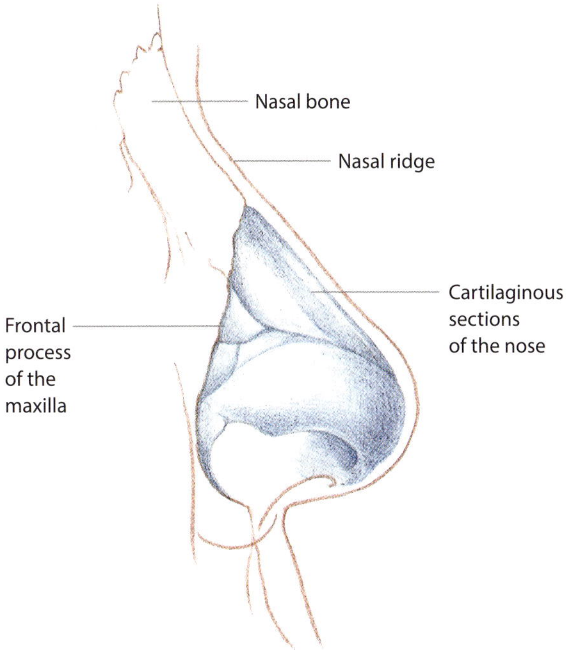

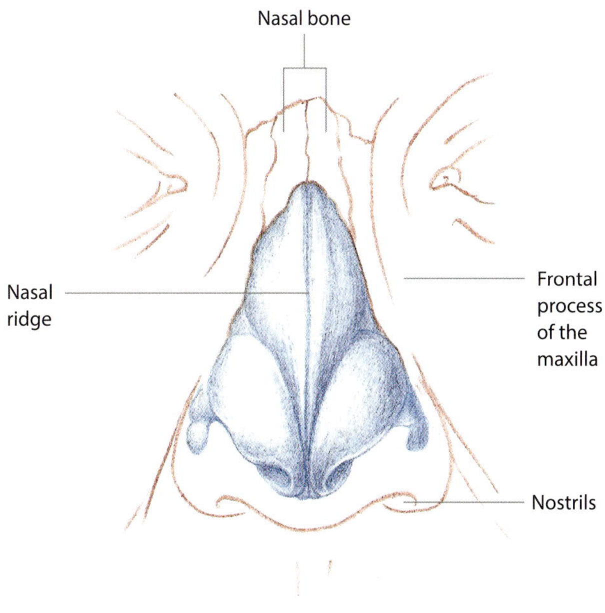

Cartilage and features of the nose. Lateral view (left), anterior view (above).

The Mouth and Lips

Our lips and mouth move and change constantly with our emotions and movements, from talking, smiling and laughing, with each muscle movement giving of us our character and individual facial expressions. The orbicularis oris muscle is the main muscle which circles the mouth, providing shape and structure to the lips, and forming the main muscles for our facial expression.

Our lips usually appear symmetrical. The groove running down between the nose to the upper lip is known as the philtrum, which is considered anatomically as part of the upper lip. The philtrum has a distinct ridge on either side of the groove, forming the 'dip' we see centrally in our upper lips. The border where the philtrum meets the upper lip is commonly known as the 'Cupid's bow'.

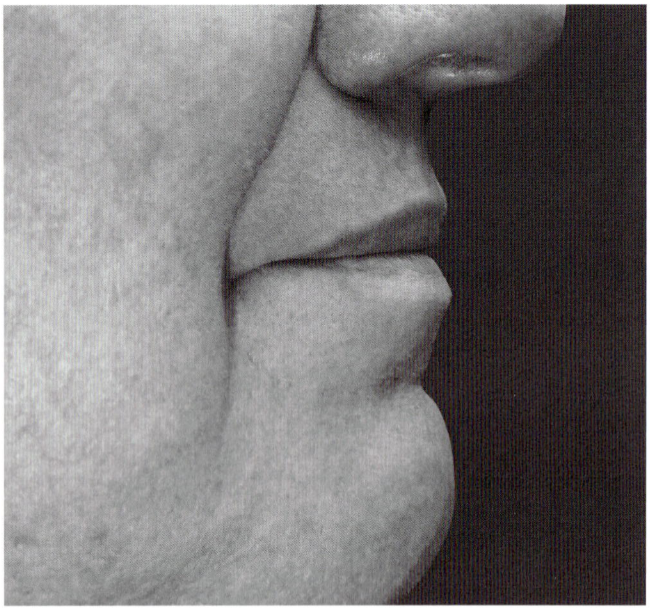

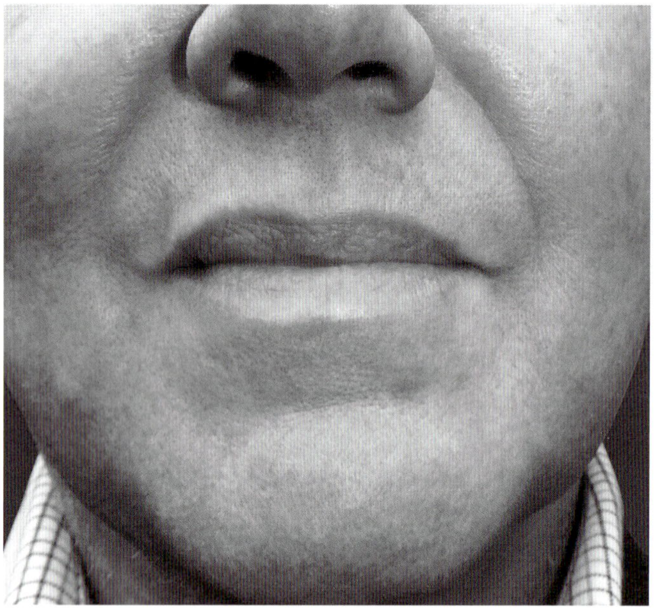

Lateral view of the nose (above), and anterior view (right).

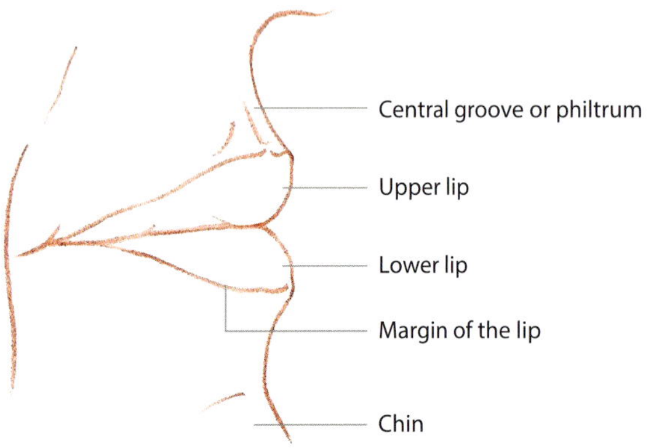

Lateral view of the upper and lower lips. Lips have a clearly defined border in texture and colour known as the margin, distinguishing this from the surrounding facial skin tissue.

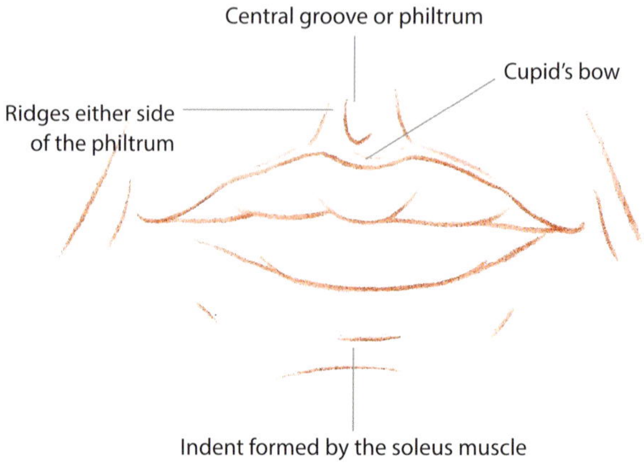

Anterior view of the upper and lower lips. The muscle of the chin, the soleus muscle creates an indent known as the mentolabial sulcus.

PROJECT: SELF-PORTRAITS

Self-portraits are an excellent way to begin drawing and improve your observational drawing for portraiture and understanding the underlying skeletal structure of the skull within the head. First, ensure you are in a comfortable position with a good single light source – multiple light sources may give conflicting shadows, distorting the form. Lighting is further covered in Chapter 6. Begin by drawing your reflection, viewed straight on as a direct portrait, then move on to experiment with three-quarter portrait views, with more dramatic lighting. Placing a lamp or sitting with a stronger light source will reveal more of the structural features of the face, from the raised cheekbones (the zygomatic arch) to the lower edge of the jawbone (the mandible), to the depth and position of the eyes within the orbit of the skull. When you choose a more dramatic pose, the overall shape and features of the head will be emphasised when viewed in perspective. Remember to also spend time concentrating on the hairstyle and colour, which form a distinct part in framing the face.

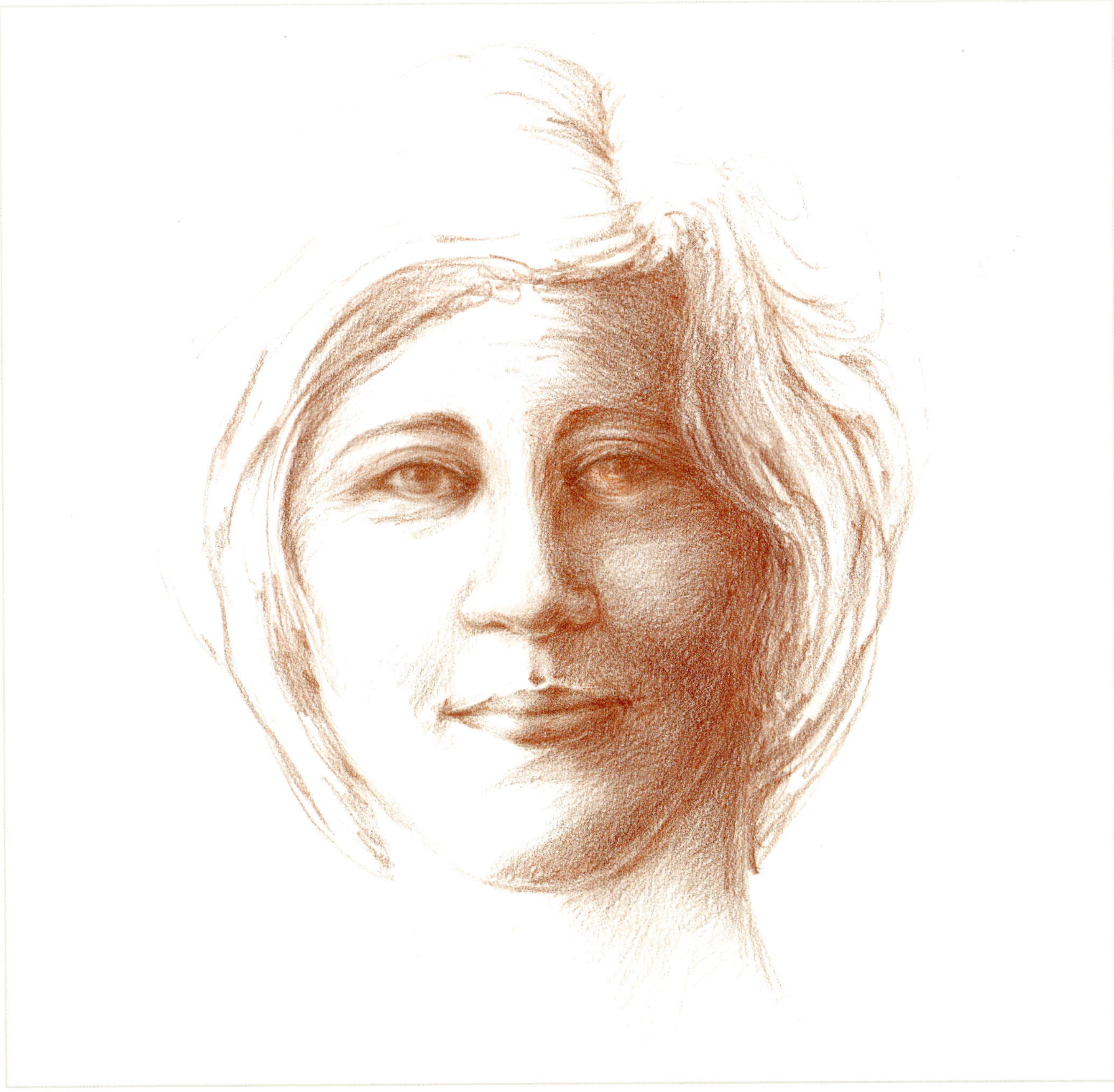

A self-portrait drawn with sanguine-coloured pencil.

BONY LANDMARKS OF THE UPPER BODY

The Sternum, Clavicle and Scapula

These structures provide clear bony landmarks that you can both see and feel below the skin. The clavicles (collarbones) link the sternum to the shoulder bones and anatomical structures of the neck. Run your fingers along the upper edge of your clavicle towards the notch in the centre, called the sternal notch. Centrally, you can then feel the flat, hard, bony surface of the sternum (breastbone) in the middle of your chest; the top portion is called the manubrium. Running your hand down, you will notice a change in the angle of the sternum, called the sternal angle.

The scapula, or shoulder blade, is one of three bones making up the shoulder girdle, including the clavicle and humerus (bone of the upper arm). Visually, the movement of the scapula is often misinterpreted, so understanding the gliding movement is essential. When your arm is at rest by your side, the scapula sits posteriorly and lies flat against the curve of your ribcage. When the arm is raised, however, the scapula glides over the surface of the ribcage downwards and rotates slightly forward.

The spinal process of the scapula form a distinct ridge and the acromion (where the shoulder blade meets the clavicle) can be felt by placing your hand just over your opposite shoulder. Gradually raise this arm forward and rotate it to feel the range of movements of the shoulder girdle.

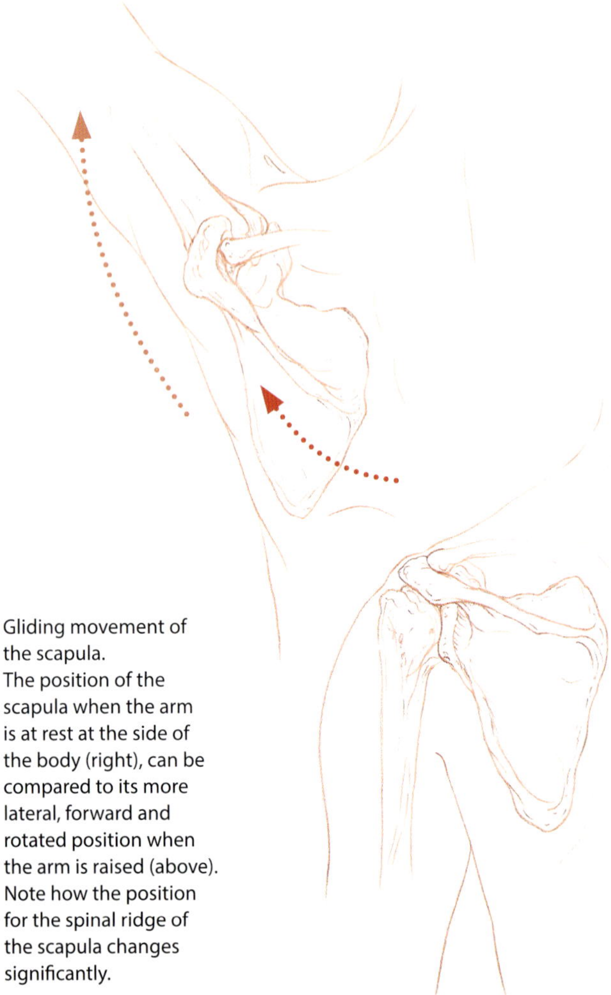

Gliding movement of the scapula. The position of the scapula when the arm is at rest at the side of the body (right), can be compared to its more lateral, forward and rotated position when the arm is raised (above). Note how the position for the spinal ridge of the scapula changes significantly.

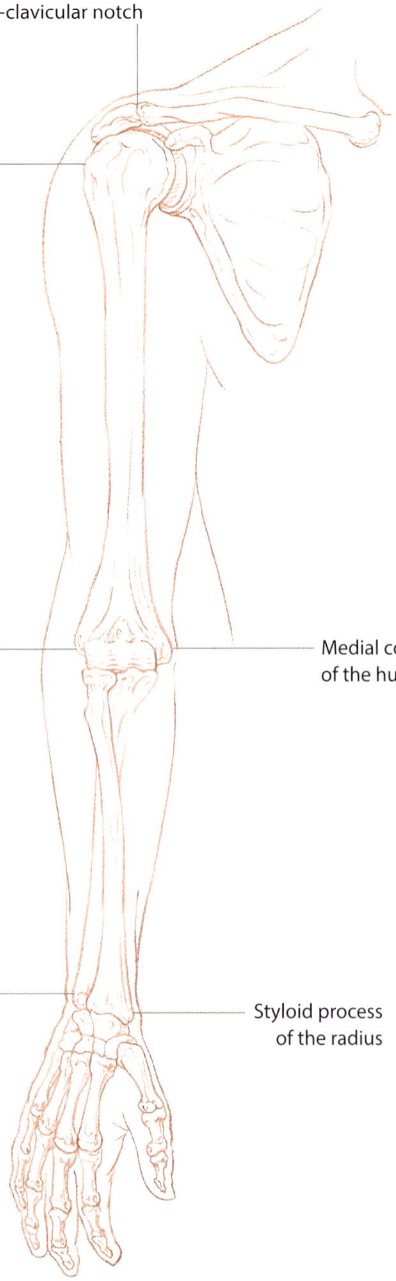

Anterior view of the key bony landmarks of the upper limb, with the forearm and hand shown partially rotated medially.

The Spine

The spine has always been considered harder to draw by artists in terms of the structure and its position due to the main part of each vertebra being set deep within the body and not seen externally. You may be able to feel many of the posterior spinal processes just below the skin on your back, but this is not always the case. They are more likely to be seen when the body and spine are in flexion when leaning forward, for example. The position and curvature of the spine is covered on pages 20-21.

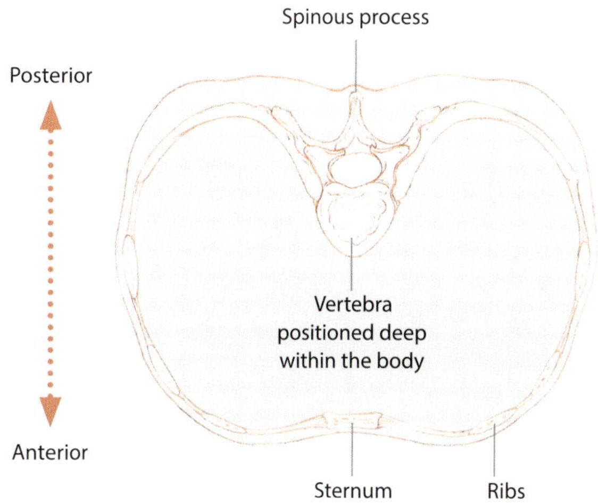

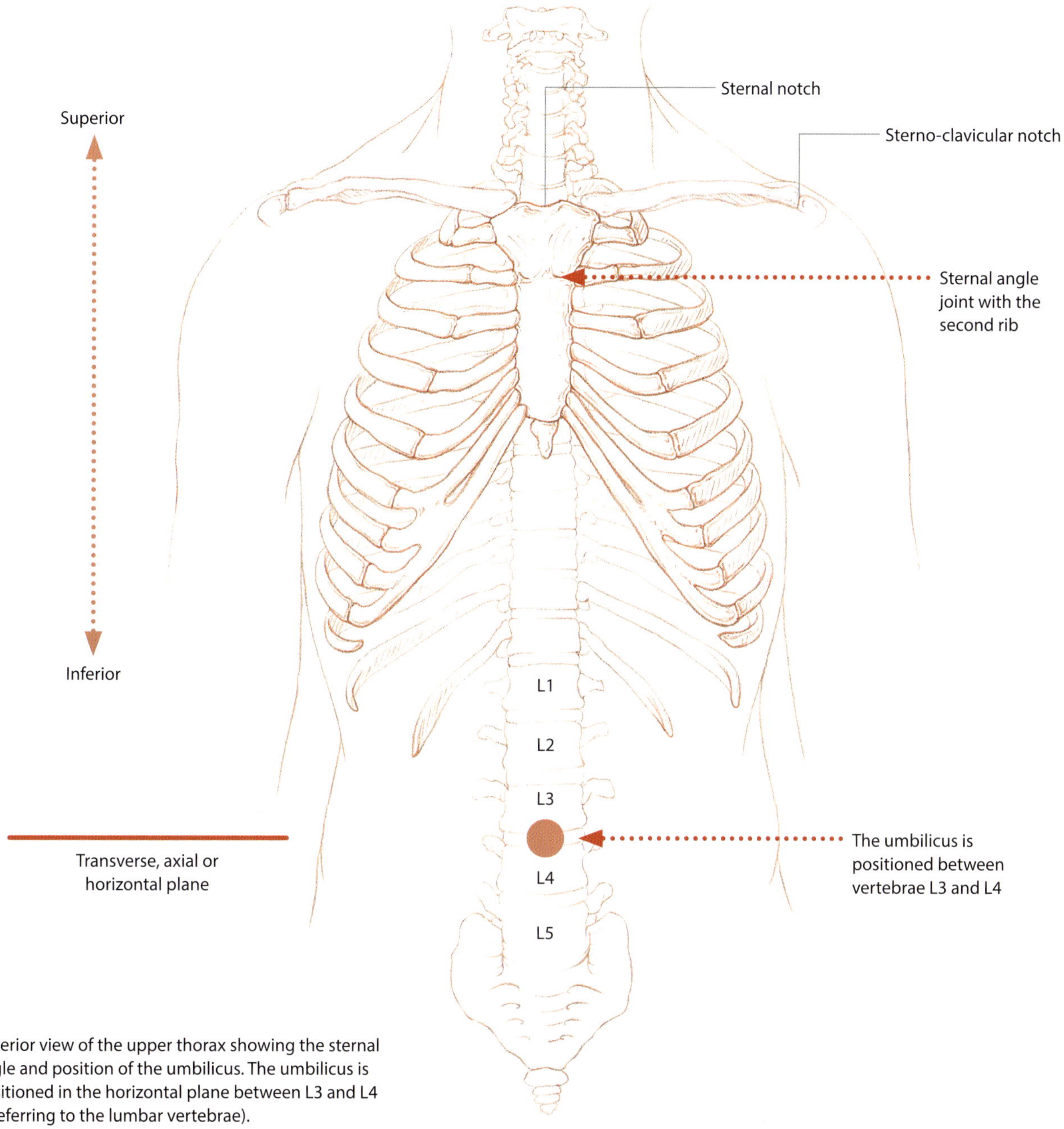

Anterior view of the upper thorax showing the sternal angle and position of the umbilicus. The umbilicus is positioned in the horizontal plane between L3 and L4 (L referring to the lumbar vertebrae).

Arms and Hands

The upper arm bone (humerus) meets the clavicle at the shoulder via a ball and socket joint. The humerus leads down to the elbow, where it meets the bones of the forearm, the radius and the ulna, followed by the fine bones of the hand. For further information covering the bones of the hand and the movement of the thumbs' saddle joint, visit pages 22-23.

The following images include a selection of key bony landmarks for the artist.

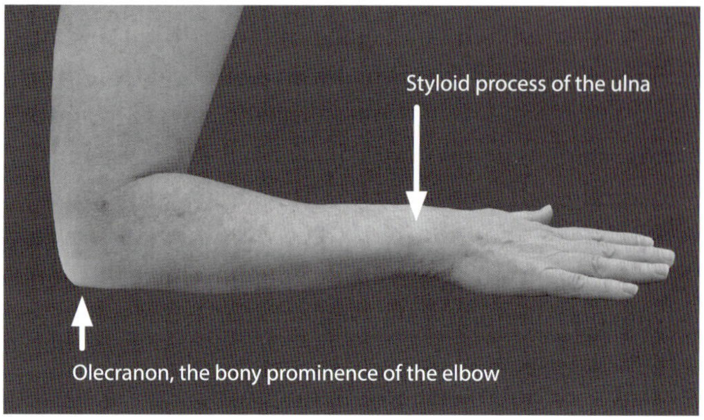

Lateral view of the arm, with the forearm rotated medially and the hand facing downwards. This shows the two key bony prominences, the olecranon of the elbow and the styloid process of the ulna.

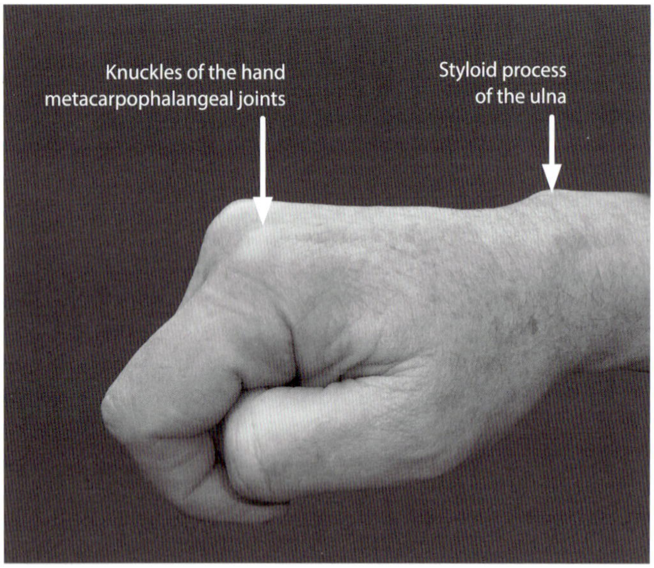

Medial view of the hand, showing the bony prominences of the knuckles and the styloid process of the ulna.

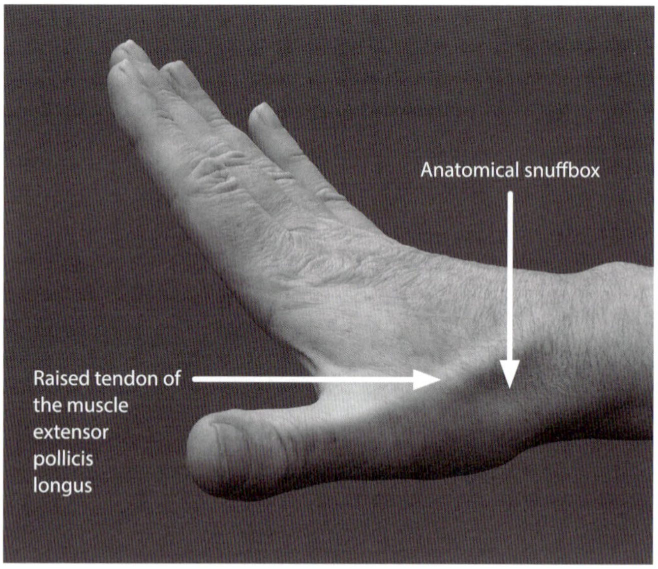

The 'anatomical snuffbox' indent is formed by extension of the thumb using the extensor pollicis longus muscle, which tightens the tendon.

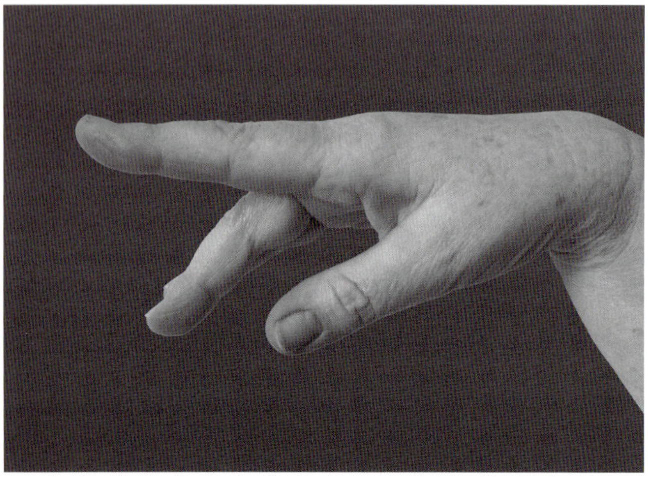

Medial view of the right hand with the first or forefinger extended, often also referred to as the index finger.

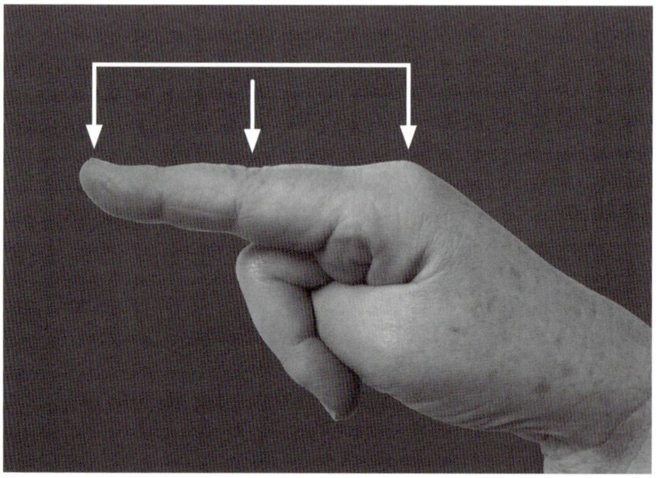

The length of the forefinger, from the knuckle to the fingertip can be divided in half as a drawing guide at the first joint of the finger, with the middle and distal phalanx comprising the second half. This proportional guide only applies to the forefinger and individual hands may vary.

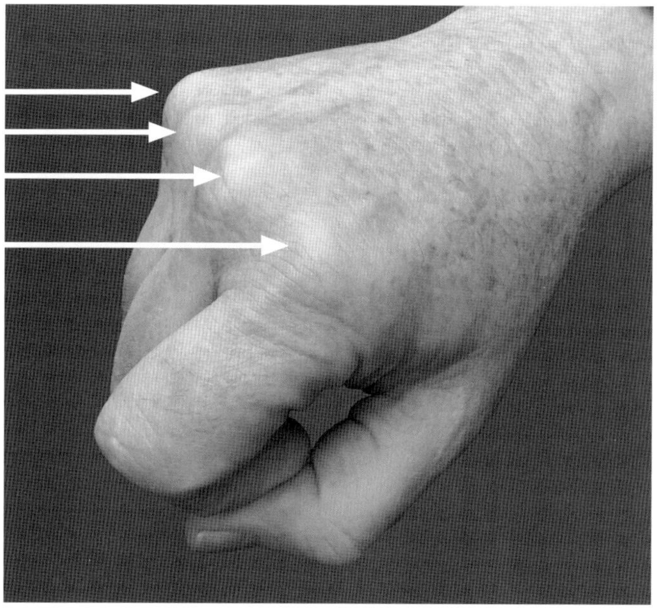

The four knuckles of the hand protrude, which can be seen when you curl your fingers into the palm of your hand. These are called the metacarpophalangeal joints.

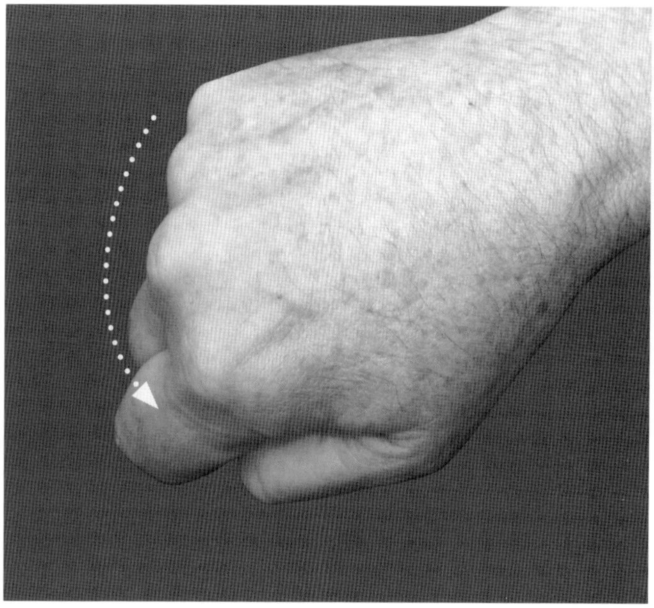

Superior view of a hand, showing the natural curve of the knuckle joints, due to their varying lengths.

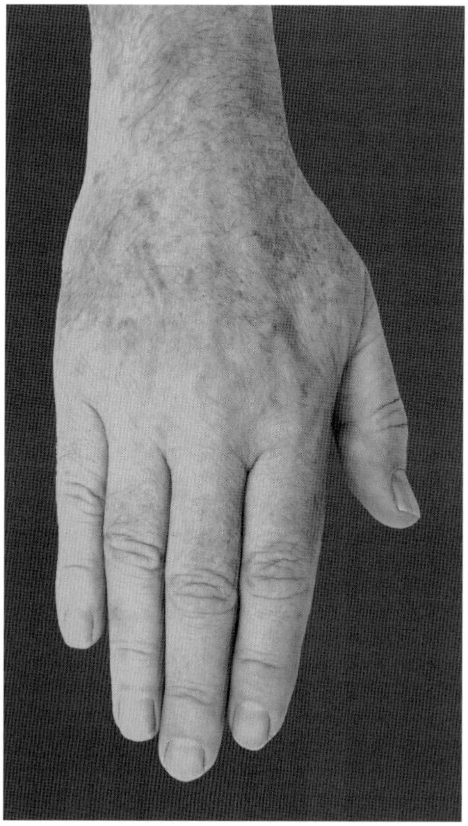

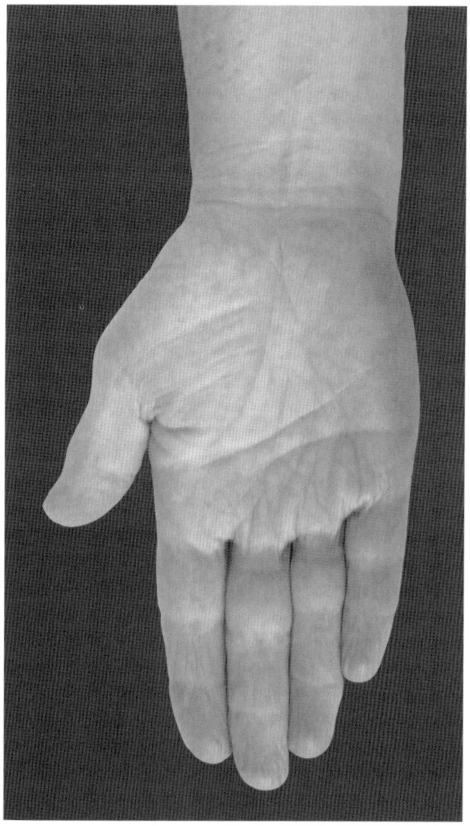

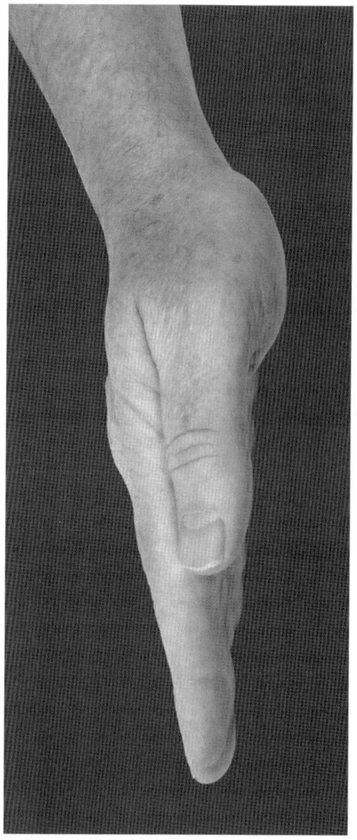

The right hand: Dorsal view (left), palmar view (middle) and lateral view (right).

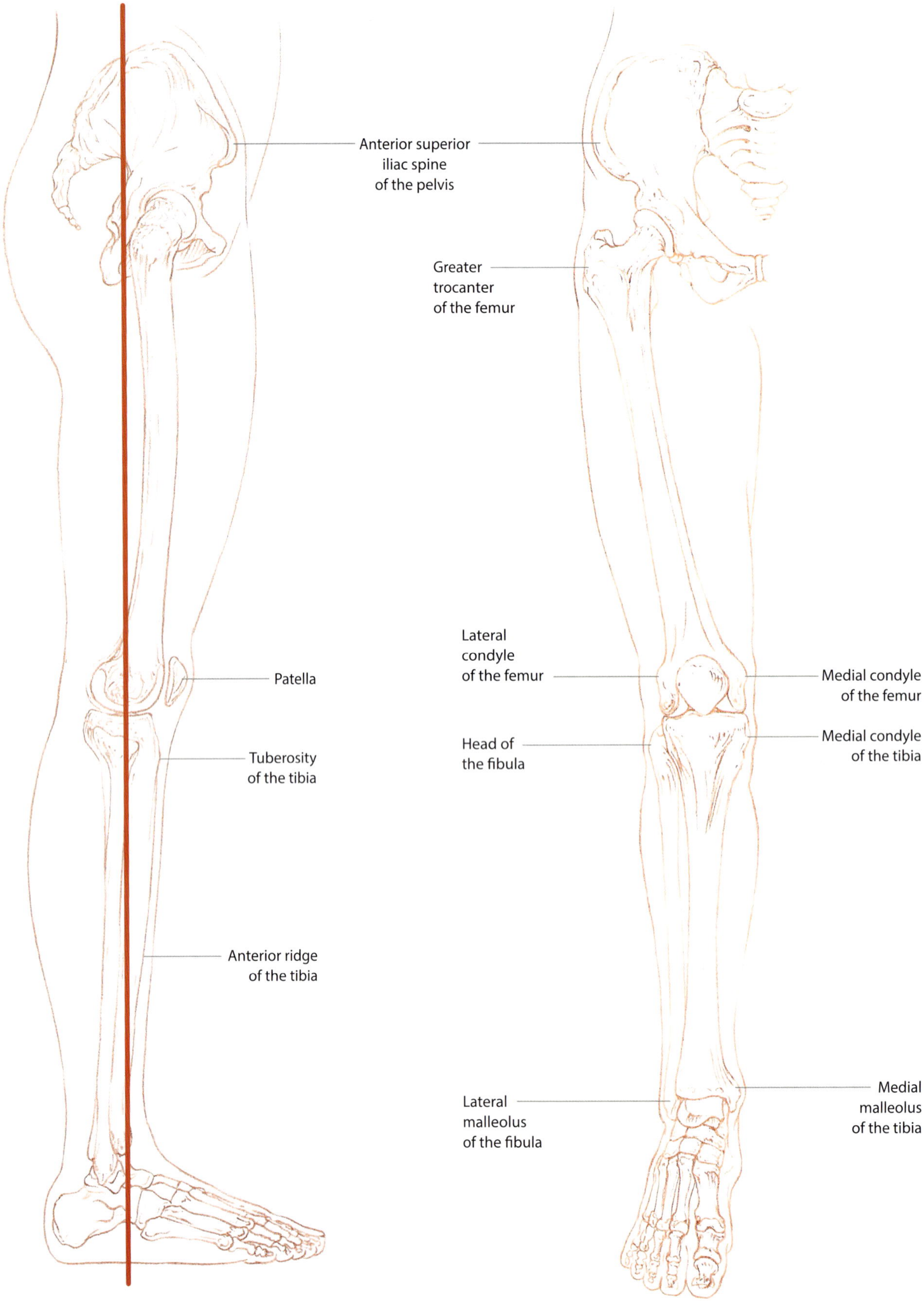

Key bony landmarks of the lower limb: lateral view (above), including the vertical postural line and anterior view (right).

LOWER LIMB

The bones of the leg mirror those in number of the arm but on a larger scale. The femur (thigh bone) attaches to the hip by a ball and socket joint, while the furthest (distal) end forms the knee joint. The two finer bones of the lower leg, the tibia and the fibula, run down from the knee to the ankle joint, where the smaller bones of the feet follow a similar pattern to the bones of the hand.

The lower limb has a number of useful bony landmarks and bony protuberances that are useful for the medical artist to note, with a selection indicated below.
When the human body is in the standing position, a vertical line can be taken running from behind the back of the hip joint and head of the femur, centrally down through the knee joint, to slightly in front of the ankle joint, known as the vertical postural line, as shown in the illustration opposite.

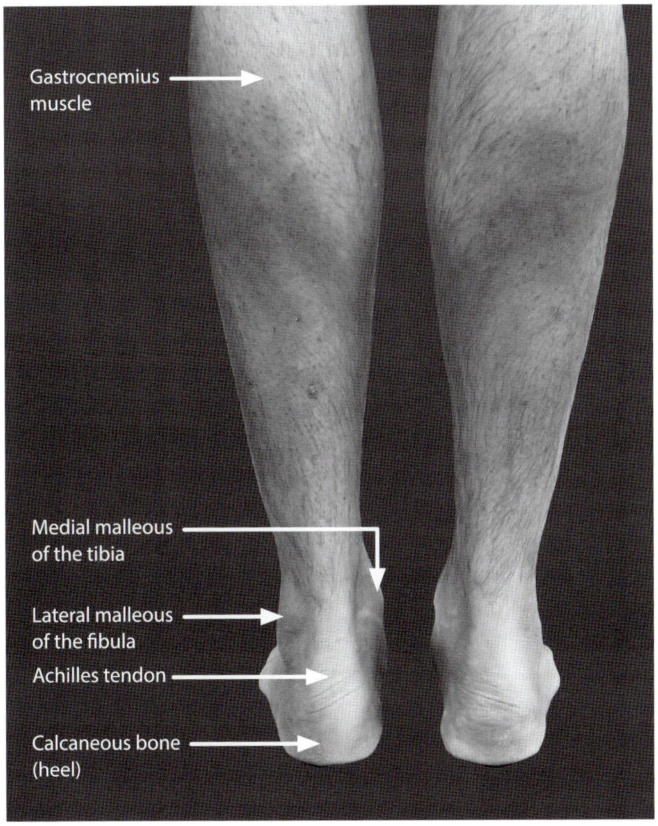

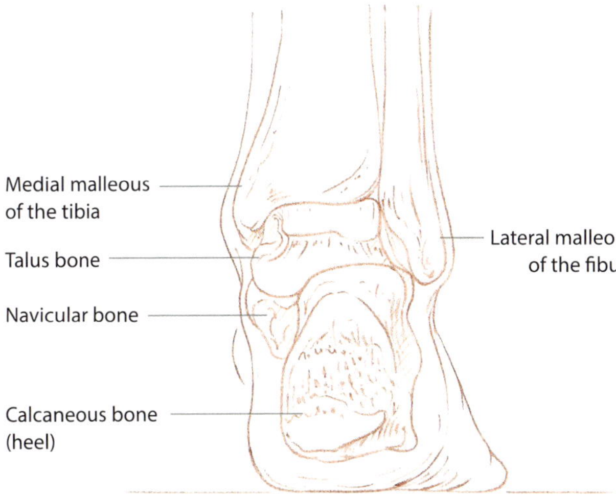

Above. Posterior view of the right ankle joint. The sole of the foot has the thickest layer of skin on the body, acting as a cushion and protective layer against the weight of our whole body when we are standing or moving.

Left. Posterior view of the lower legs showing the key bony landmarks of the ankles: the lateral and medial malleolus and the calf or gastrocnemius muscle. Note the height difference between the medial malleolus of the tibia and the lower lateral malleolus of the fibula.

PROJECT: LIFE DRAWING

To accompany the study of the form and structure of the human body, observing and drawing from life are essential. The importance of sound observational drawing and draughtsmanship skills cannot be underestimated for a medical artist. Artists need to convey the physical presence and form of the body, whether it is moving or stationary, by understanding the collective movement of the bones and muscles in relation to each other.

When drawing directly from life figures, remember they are three-dimensional objects, each within their own space. The light surrounding your model may be soft, creating subtle interpretation of the forms, or bright, forming strong highlights and shadows. Additional areas of reflected light will create form. Further information regarding light and shadows can be found in Chapter 8. Other effects, such as the ambient temperature and the character of the person modelling, will also influence your interpretation.

Observing from life ensures your work feels alive. In contrast, working from photographs, although they are often useful references, is best avoided when building your skills in observation. Photographs are already in a two-dimensional format (i.e. flat) and will undoubtedly have been edited in some way from the source image. Drawing from life will enable you to observe and interpret the subtle nuances in lighting, form and colour, calling on all your observational senses.

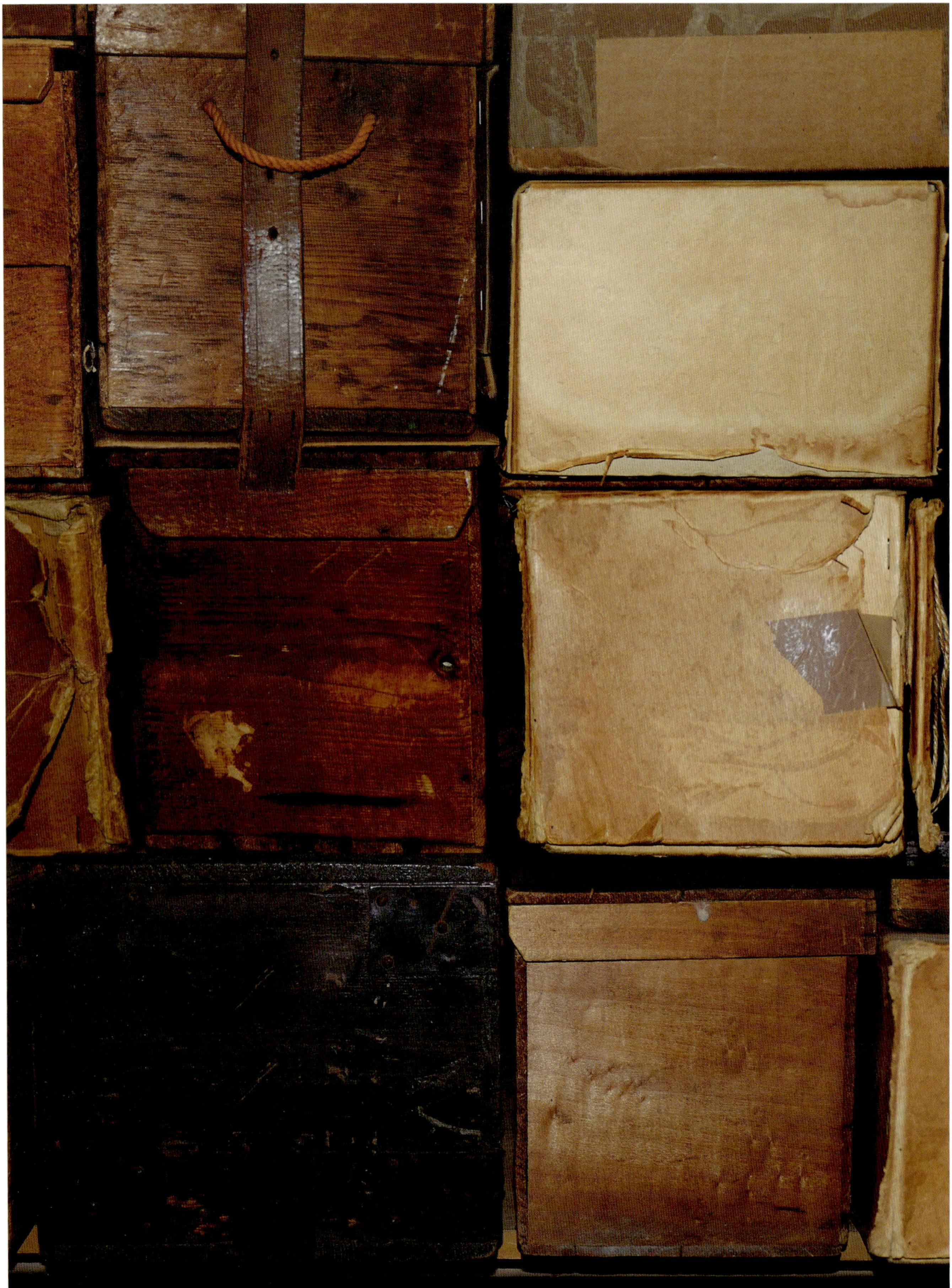

CHAPTER 4

MUSEUM RESOURCES

Museums provide an extensive educational resource, containing billions of specimens worldwide. Medical artists frequently visit collections for study and research to build a collection of observational drawings. If you are planning a career in medical art, it is recommended to build a portfolio from a broad range of subjects, and not necessarily concentrate on human anatomy until you have enrolled on a specialised medical art course. There is an extensive range of material to choose from, especially among natural history subjects in museums with good public access. This section looks at some of these museums and collections, considering content, access and art materials to take with you.

HISTORICAL CONTEXT

There are many excellent anatomical and natural history collections which cover subjects relating to anatomy, medicine, pathology, osteology and archaeology, with related artefacts and often holding regular exhibitions open to the public. Many of these collections are now considered historically important. However, it is important to note,that many of these collections need to be viewed in the context of the era in which they were created, by whom and why – for example, whether they were created for a comparative collection, following on from archaeological explorations, or for the evolving medical and scientific discoveries of their time. Most of these collections were assembled long before the current regulations came into being. The context and culture that prevailed at the time may differ substantially from modern practices, especially in relation to current collecting methods, education, access, display and ethical considerations. Behind the scenes, collections are constantly researched, updated, and prepared for displays and themed exhibitions. Today's museums provide unapparalleled access to these incredible educational resources for a worldwide audience, whether researching online or visiting in person.

HUMAN TISSUE REGULATION

Within the United Kingdom, access to human remains and related specimens is restricted and rightly so. Today, all human tissue specimens are protected by law, which regulates the preparation, use, storage, removal, display, moving and disposal of human remains. This includes everything, including tissue, organs and bones. The regulation also covers the organisations that hold the material, whether being used for teaching within a university, a training hospital, or for public display in either a small independent or a large national museum, with many millions of specimens to care for. Each museum collection is looked after by a museum team, including the museum curator and specialist conservators, who are responsible for restoration, displaying and keeping the content relevant for today's audience for both study and education.

Selecting a Specimen

With so many accessible specimens to choose from, it is strongly recommended to avoid subjects and materials that could be potentially sensitive or controversial, especially with regard to human material. Human remains, whether bone or soft tissue, need to be treated with respect. Create every artwork with thoughtful consideration to avoid sensationalism. Always refer to each collection or museum guidelines for their own protocols and further information.

Human bone collections have historically been stored in either wooden or cardboard boxes.

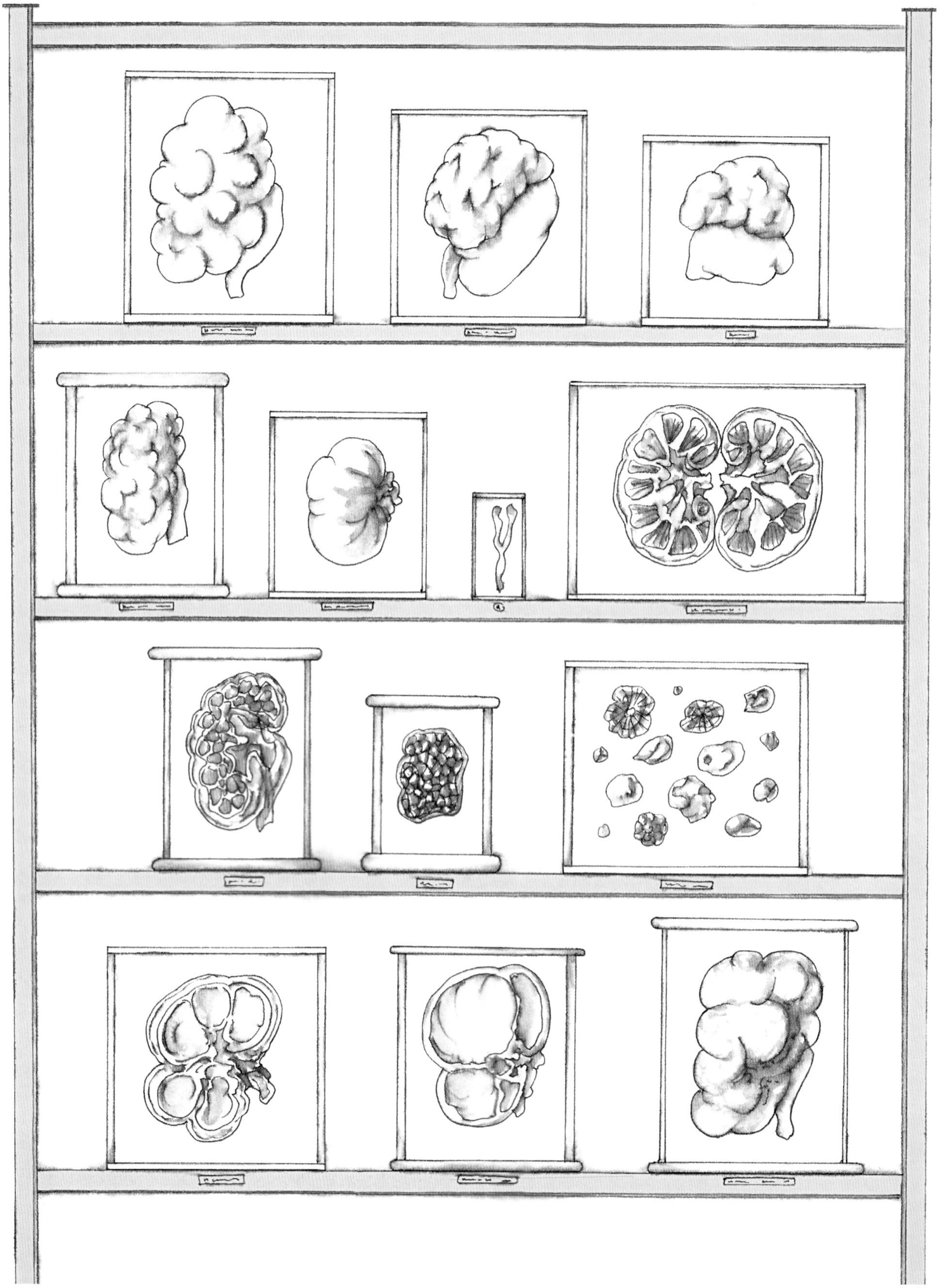

Representational museum specimen display, portraying a variety of kidney pathologies in round or square sealed glass pots. Pen and wash.

FINDING WHAT YOU NEED

Museum collections are extensive and are an amazing resource for medical artists, not just for medical-related subjects but also for comparative anatomy, natural history and botany. Available resources cover human anatomy, osteology, pathology, forensics, surgical instruments, worldwide health, microscopic slide collections, zoology, odonatological collections, design, patient leaflets, books, historical to contemporary artworks, artefacts, ephemera and so much more.

Within the London area, for example, there are many excellent medical museums to visit, including the recently refurbished Hunterian Museum at Lincoln's Inn Fields, the oldest hospital museum in the world – St Bartholomew's Hospital Museum and the Old Operating Theatre and Herb Garret, the oldest surviving operating theatre in Europe, near Guy's Hospital.

Across the country, there are hundreds of smaller collections holding millions of accessible items held at universities, local museums and country houses, as well as the larger national museums. Locating what you need among the vast number of collections may appear overwhelming at first, so looking across the range of collections will help you to start narrowing it down. A list of museums that are a good starting point for research is given in Appendix III.

Online Collections

Before travelling to visit a museum, it is recommended to first search its online databases; you may find there what you are looking for, and then be able to refer to the database reference number. Currently, there is not a comprehensive list of all museums and their collections available to the public. However, museums are increasingly listing many of their specimens online, alongside recorded lectures, talks, library catalogues, accessible reading rooms and exhibition information.

BEFORE VISITING THE MUSEUM

Although most museums are open to the public, a small selection of specialist collections may have restricted access. Always check before travelling whether the museum will be open, what their opening times are and if pre-registration or booking are required; while many establishments are free to enter, some now require bookings to be made online in advance. You may not be given access on the day without having pre-booked.

If you are planning to visit for research or drawing from specimens in the museum, whether in the public galleries or from a specific specimen, always contact the museum curator beforehand and give as much notice as possible when making your request. Allow time for the staff to reply, as they often receive multiple enquiries each day or maybe busy with events and unable to respond immediately.

When enquiring, try and be as specific as possible about what you are looking for in terms of the specimens you wish to draw. For example, if you wish to draw a human skull, specify whether you require a male or female skull, an adult or juvenile, part of an articulated skeleton or just a single item. Always check their online catalogues in advance, where you may be able to identify a specimen to request. By being as specific as possible, you are more likely to be directed to the most suitable specimen. If you have a particular one in mind, the museum can let you know whether it is available, as it may be withdrawn for conservation or out on loan to another museum.

Each museum or establishment will have its own policies covering rules and regulations for visitor access, which may differ from country to country; this is particularly important in relation to human remains. Ensure you have read any documents relating to your area of study before you visit. Each country will also have its own regulatory authorities, whose rules and regulations must be observed. If you are seeking access to material abroad, always gain approval from the museum or establishment before you travelling. The last thing you want is to undertake a long, expensive journey only to be denied access on arrival.

Registering with a Museum

Many museums and collections now require for you to register online prior to your visit. By becoming a member of their institution, you will then be able to have access to their collections or pre-book a visit. You may need to be over eighteen to register due to the nature of some of the collections. Registration is usually free, confirmed on your first visit, when you take a form of ID with your address with you, whereupon a museum or library card will be issued. Once registered, although visiting is normally free, there may be nominal charges for image or text downloads, for example, or for requesting specific resources and images. Each museum will be able to supply you with details of any applicable fees in advance.

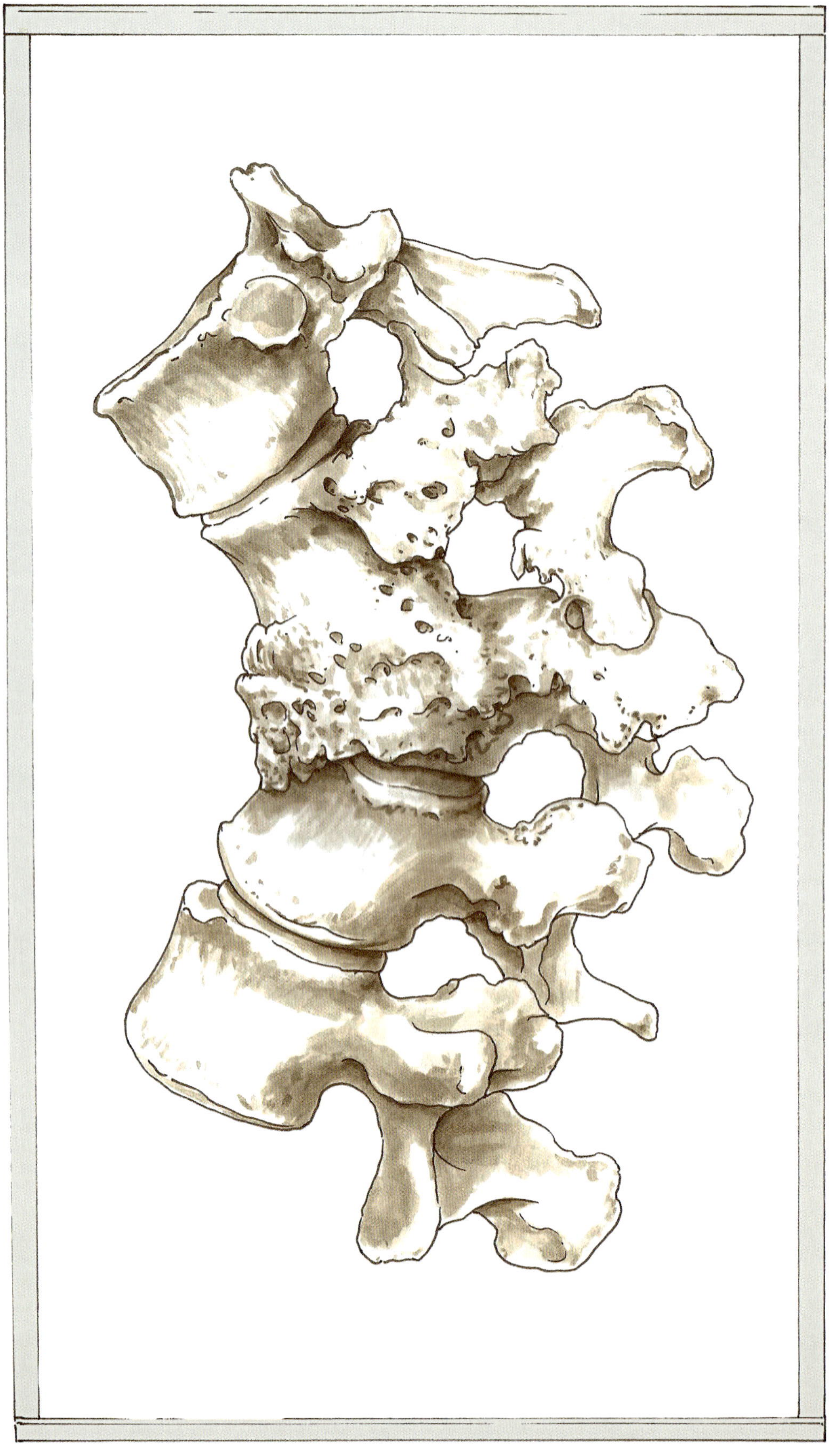

A pathological specimen of the spine, displaying five vertebrae. Several vertebrae shown above are extensively damaged and ossified. Pen and wash.

CHECKLIST FOR DRAWING IN A PUBLIC MUSEUM

1. Research potential specimen/s through online resources
2. Check opening hours of the museum and any restrictions
3. Contact the museum curator
4. Confirm access time and arrangements
5. Confirm permission to draw
6. Complete all access and permission forms in advance
7. Always follow the museum's code of conduct
8. If you have access to specimens, the museum staff will move anything you need repositioned. Only move specimens yourself, if you have been given prior permission. Specimens are frequently either fragile, historical, or often heavy
9. Always follow instructions given by the museum staff

When you have Finished

10. If you have had access to specimens, ensure they are placed back in the correct box or location
11. Take all your personal items home with you
12. Leave the area clean and tidy, as if you have not been there
13. Send a thank you message to the museum curator and the staff who have helped you – you may wish to visit again
14. Send a copy of your artworks and/or images to the museum for their records

TYPES OF MUSEUM COLLECTIONS

Museum collections hold a broad range of specimens, varying in subject, specialisation, or the type of material and how they have been prepared. Whether they specialise in human material, natural history or archaeological finds, collections are important as earning resources for students, artists, researchers, anatomists and physicians.

Natural History Collections

Natural history collections cover a broad spectrum, including human collections as well as zoology (animals), ornithology (birds), entomology (insects), palaeontology (fossils) and botany (plants).

Osteological Collections

Osteology refers to the study and function of the skeletal system, whether human or animal. Museums will often have multiple examples of the same osteological specimen. In Greek, *osteo* means bones and *logos* means to study.

Pathology Collections

Anatomical pathology collections are concerned with the preservation and study of tissues and organs affected by a cause or disease, for example a kidney stone or a tumour, which will directly affect the shape, structure and function of the kidney.

'DRY' AND 'WET' SPECIMENS

Today, specimens are classified as either 'dry' or 'wet' specimens. Dry specimens refer primarily to bones that have been dried, varnished or mummified.

Wet, or potted, specimens appeared from the seventeenth century onwards, when new techniques for preserving anatomical or pathological specimens in clear liquid were developed. Initially alcohol was used, then later formaldehyde and each specimen was suspended in a bottle or jar for study. From the nineteenth century, formalin was introduced as the primary preserving liquid, allowing organs and soft tissues to be preserved and stored safely and displayed in a museum collection for educational purposes.

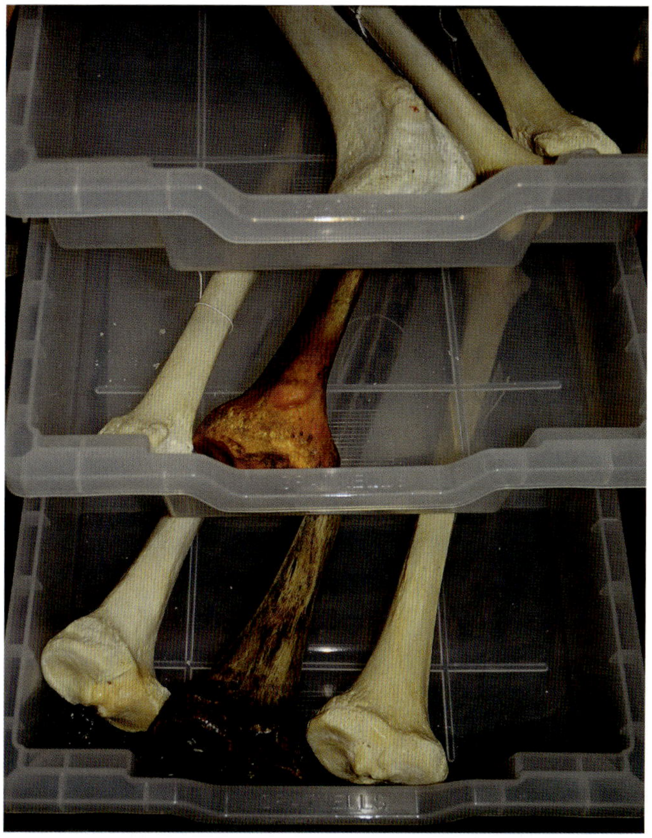

A femur bone collection, stored for comparative study. Note the differences in colour, which may be caused by many factors, from their age to how they were prepared or stored.

Round glass jars often distort the specimen when viewed through the circular glass; square storage pots were introduced to reduce this.

In most museums and collections, you will find a combination of round and square pots on display.

Corrosion Casts

This is an advanced preservation technique, which involves injecting blood vessels or cavities with resin. Once the resin has set, the soft tissues are removed, revealing anatomical intricacies that would not have been otherwise seen, such as the smallest of blood vessels.

Plastination

Plastination is a relatively new preservation technique in which anatomical specimens are realistically preserved using silicone and other solutions to replace the fat and water content, which prevent tissue decomposition and retain their structure and colour.

DRAWING IN A MUSEUM SETTING

Visiting a museum to make a few quick sketches in a notebook while standing should not cause any problems, but arriving with a stool, sketchbooks and art materials and setting up to draw for maybe an hour or more is another matter, so do always check in advance that the staff are happy for you to be there. For example, if your specimen is on a narrow corridor, access for the public could be restricted, or there may be a large school party scheduled to visit that gallery of the museum; staff may suggest a quieter day to visit or even have a specific specimen placed aside in room where you can sit and draw.

Due to the delicate nature of many specimens, lighting in museums if often kept intentionally low to avoid damage by bright lights. You should still be able to see the specimen clearly, however, do be aware of lighting considerations for drawing.

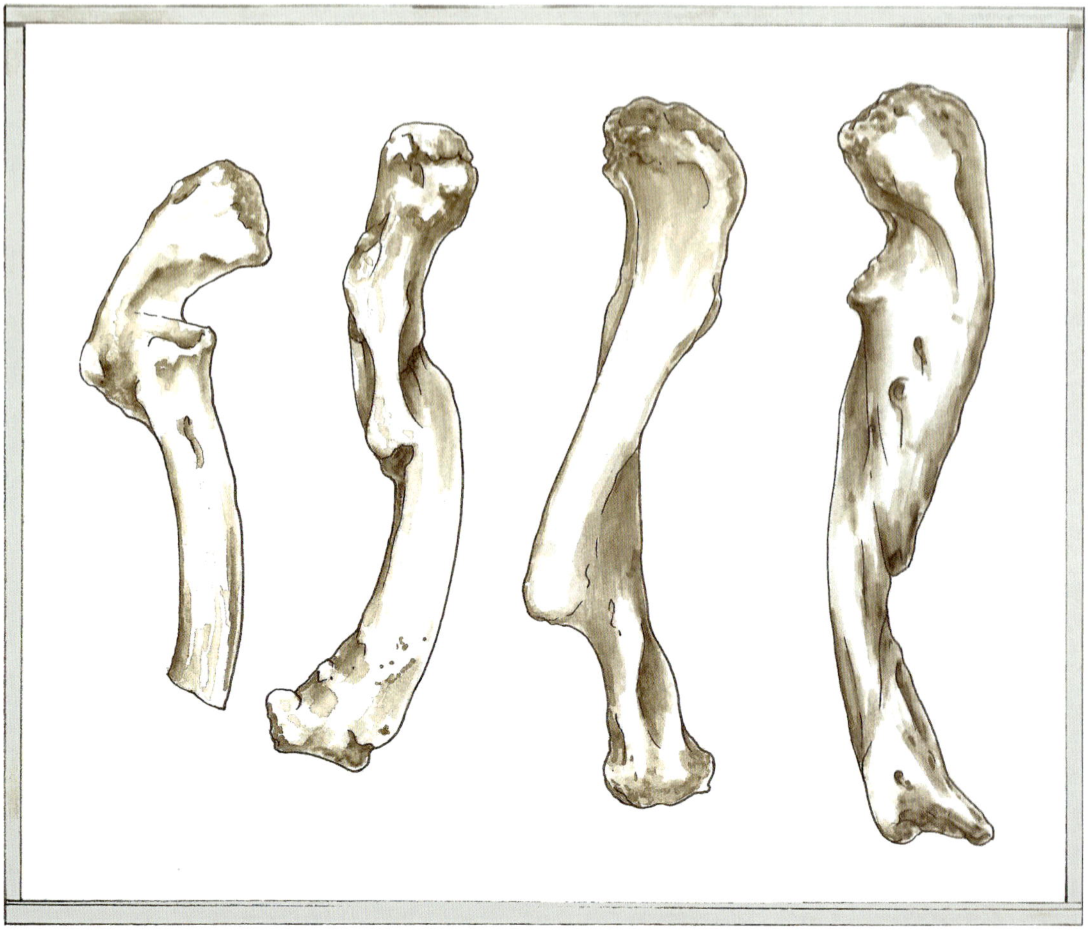

Four clavicles (collar bones) displayed showing healed fractures. The clavicles and shoulder girdle can continue to function effectively despite the clavicles having been displaced following the fracture and subsequently healing in a different alignment. Pen and wash.

DRAWING MATERIALS TO TAKE INTO A MUSEUM

- A spiral-bound sketchbook with a hard back for support
- Tracing paper
- Putty rubber and/or rubber
- Paper blending tool
- Graphite pencils – a range from 2H to 4B. Consider clutch pencils. If you prefer a conventional pencil, always take an enclosed pencil sharpener case to catch all the sharpenings
- Coloured pencils – primarily red, yellow and blue. A range of colours will be useful
- Small folding stool – contact the museum in advance whether they have stools available or you need to bring your own
- If you require a table, contact the museum in advance

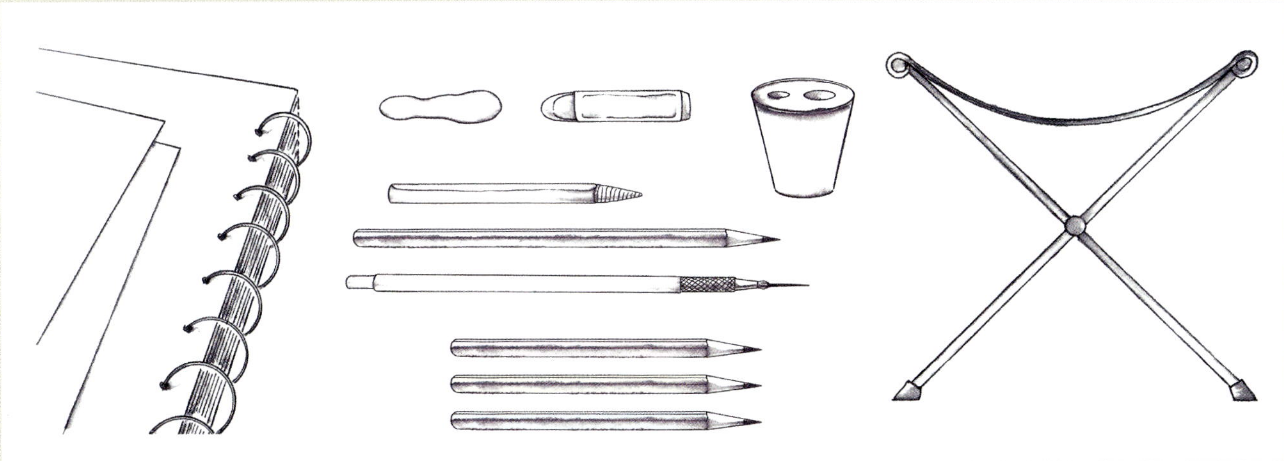

PHOTOGRAPHY

Human anatomical collections have a 'no photography or filming' rule out of respect to the human remains. There are strict rules governing specimens, and each museum will have a code of conduct for visitors. Photographs are occasionally allowed for research, educational purposes or personal study, depending on the subject or specimen. Discretion should always be used even with those subjects that are familiar to you, as others may not view these in the same way and may find images and artworks upsetting. Always refer to each museum's guidelines for further information on their own protocols.

Before visiting a museum, check with the museum curator or a member of staff to confirm access arrangements and relevant permissions before attending; always ask in advance if you are unsure about any aspect of your visit. If you have been granted permission to take photographs, do not share these images on social media or with anyone else, who may then share them further beyond your control.

Many museums allow visitors to prepare drawings, and a photography request may also be granted if it is for your scientific research, educational purpose, or study – that is, not for commercial use. Consider also that some specimens may be vulnerable to strong light such as camera/phone flashes and tripods will not be allowed under any circumstances. Ask a member of staff or look for signs regarding photography. It is the artist's responsibility to follow each venue's specific regulations.

COPYRIGHT

Each museum or collection will have copyright assigned to its own images. Always check their policy in relation to their use.

Whether permission to use copyrighted material will be granted by the museum will depend entirely on the planned use of your artwork: for example, will it be purely for your own personal use and study or is it for a commissioned project or publication? Steering clear of potentially ethically contentious subjects will make things easier.

Offer to send the museum a copy of all drawings you create from its specimens. The museum will usually require a copy of any works you create for its records.

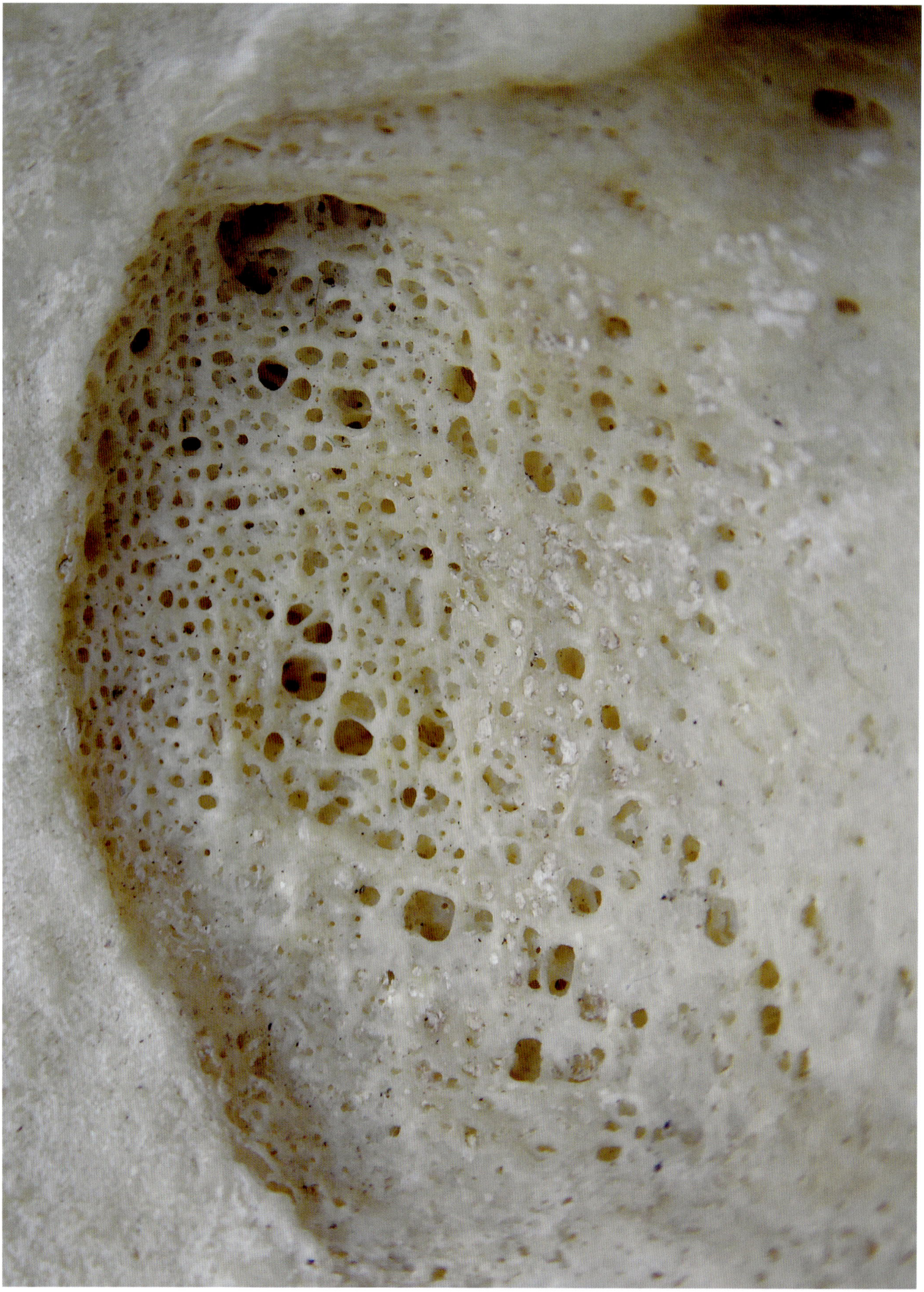

CHAPTER 5

STUDYING BONES

Osteology is the study, structure and function of the skeleton's bony parts. Our human skeletal system is made up of 206 individual bones and these form the internal framework and define our body's shape and structure. Bones can be easily studied by artists, as by their nature they are dry specimens and therefore very accessible. This chapter will look at a variety of bones, highlighting points to consider when selecting specimens to draw.

THE PURPOSE OF BONES

The spine is the most important central structure within the body. From the skull at the top, it runs down to the ribcage that forms the chest (thorax), to which our shoulder girdles also attach. The shoulder girdle comprises the scapulae (shoulder blades) and clavicles (collarbones), each leading to the upper limbs, the arms and hands. At the base of the spine, the pelvis connects to the lower limbs, the legs and feet. With the muscles, tendons and ligaments all functioning together, these bones allow the body to move.

Bones are the body's scaffolding, supporting and connecting the overlying muscle, fat and tissues, and are very strong. Through close observation, you will see our bones, just like our body shape, are all broadly similar yet individually different. The average body has 206 bones, but it can be up to 213 bones – for example, an individual may have extra vertebrae, ribs or digits (fingers or toes). We begin our life with up to 300 bone segments, many of which fuse together as we grow. These are seen as cartilaginous plates on bone cross-sections, ultimately becoming one single bone.

Specialist stem cells are created within the inner bone marrow, through a process called haemopoiesis, a developmental stage for our blood cells. Bones also store minerals, primarily calcium. The cross-section of the head of a femur (thigh bone) shows both the inner trabeculae structure, remains of the former epiphyseal cartilaginous plate and the inner shaft of the bone: the bone marrow cavity.

Both cast resin bones are readily available within collections, however there is no substitute for studying a real bone specimen to observe its specific features, characteristics and intricacies. It is recommended to observe bone specimens in conjunction with one or more good-quality anatomical textbooks.

STUDYING BONES IN A MUSEUM SETTING

Once you have arranged museum access with the correct permissions, you will be able to view their collection. Each collection usually has more than one example of each bone, so careful selection for your needs may be required.

Once you have sourced a specimen to draw, first spend time closely observing and looking at each bone, either on its own or comparing it with other examples of the same type. If you can hold the specimen, then feel the weight, as bones vary considerably in how heavy they are. The femur, for example, is extremely heavy because it has to be exceptionally strong, whereas others are very light. Study the bone from every angle, observing the varying surface textures. Explore each specimen with both your eyes and hands.

Bone: foramina in the area of attachment for the strong internal ligaments connecting the pelvis and femur – ball and socket joint.

Generally, the rule of thumb is to illustrate an accepted average unless your requirement is to draw a specific specimen to show a particular feature. If you are unsure, the museum curator will always be able to give you guidance, and you will soon become familiar and comfortable with handling and observing the features of each bony specimen.

Looking at the clavicles shown below, you will see they are very different in size and proportion although both are examples of adult clavicles. The upper example is fine-boned with little definition, and the lower example is broader and longer, with areas where muscles and tendons would have attached to the bone from a strong individual. The two sacrum examples (the rear section of the pelvis) also demonstrate how varied the sizes and proportions of specimens may be.

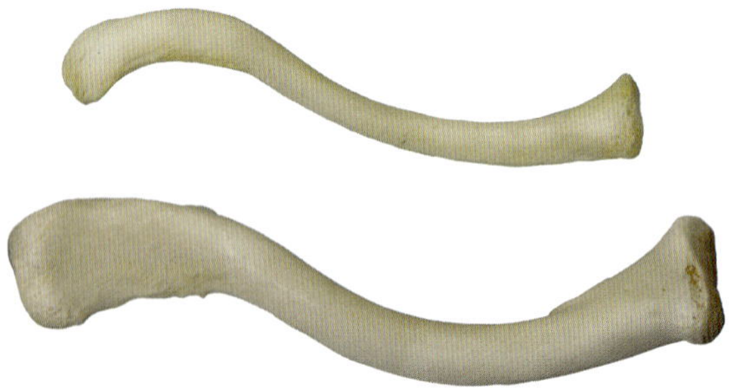

Note the overall differences in size and proportion between these two clavicle specimens; the areas for the muscle and ligament attachments are more pronounced and developed on the lower specimen.

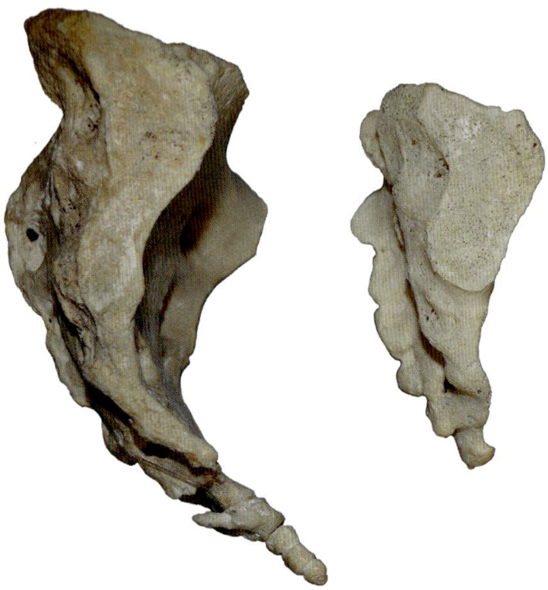

These two images of a sacrum, show how varied specimens can be. Left: note a wire will be holding the sacrum and the coccyx together in position. Right: note the coccyx is missing from this specimen.

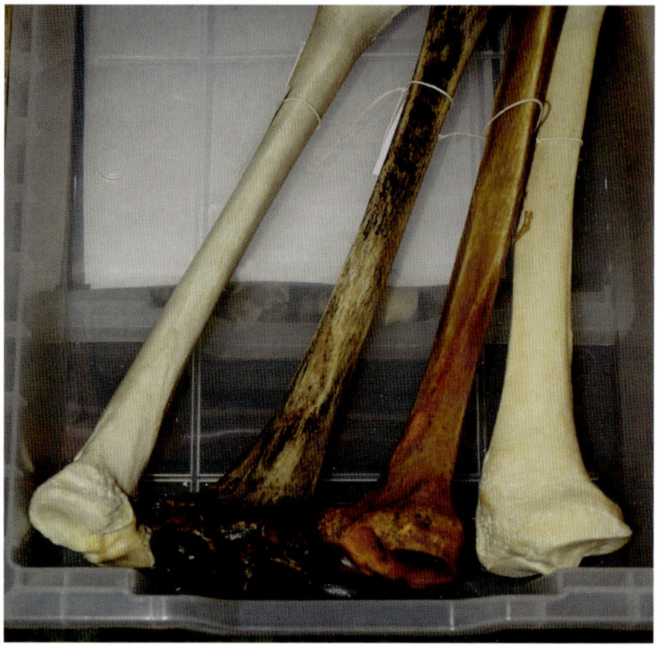

Museum bone collections are carefully prepared, stored and archived. Each specimen will have its own specific reference and a numbered label for cataloguing purposes. Enusre you keep the correct label attached to its relative specimen. Here a selection of four femur bones can be seen in a storage tray, showing the colour variations that can occur.

BONE STRUCTURE

Bones can be classified into three categories:

- Long bones, those with a long shaft – for example, the femur (thigh) and humerus (upper arm)
- Flat bones – for example, the scapula (shoulder blade) and many bones of the skull
- Irregular or short bones – for example, the vertebrae (spine) and the wrist and ankle

Surface Texture

All our bones have an outer membranous layer called the periosteum which supports the blood supply through the arteries as they enter the bone. The periosteum covers all the surface of the bone except where the joint articular cartilages attach. On a dried bony specimen, the surface evidence from the periosteum and any attachments for muscles, joint capsules and ligaments can still be seen, each feature giving the bone its distinctive texture relating to each element.

Male or Female?

Each specimen may have distinct features on each specimen to indicate whether a specimen is male or female. For example, there is a clear difference in size and shape between a male and female pelvis (see opposite) – the female pelvis is broader to accommodate giving birth.

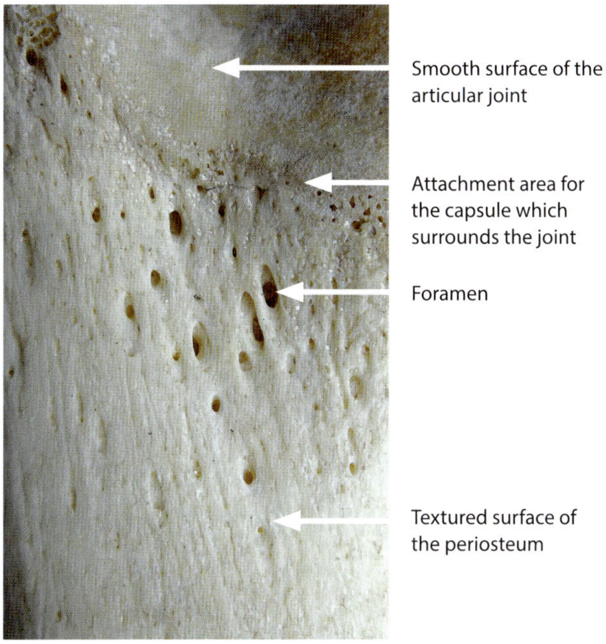

Bone surface of the head of a femur, showing the distinct differences between the external surface (where the bone's outer tissue layer attaches, called the periosteum) and the foramina, through which vessels pass into and out of the bone's core. Note the rougher appearance of the line where the joint capsule would have attached to the bone, compared to the smoother articular surface seen in the upper right section of the image.

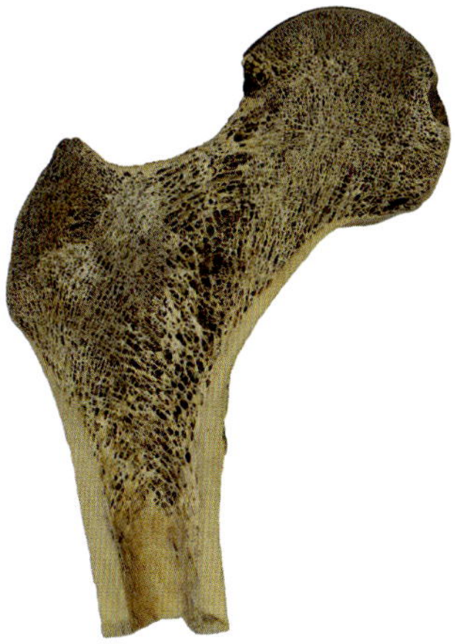

Femur cross-section (thigh bone), revealing the intricate inner trabeculae network. This closely interlinking bony structure gives the femur its incredible strength.

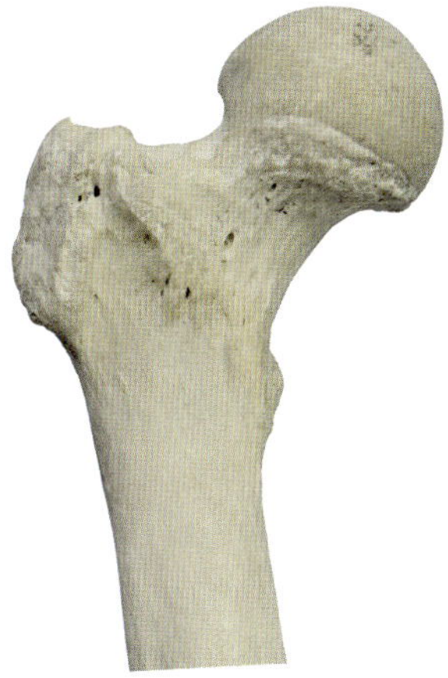

Femur external surface of the head of a femur; compare this exterior view with the image of the cross-section.

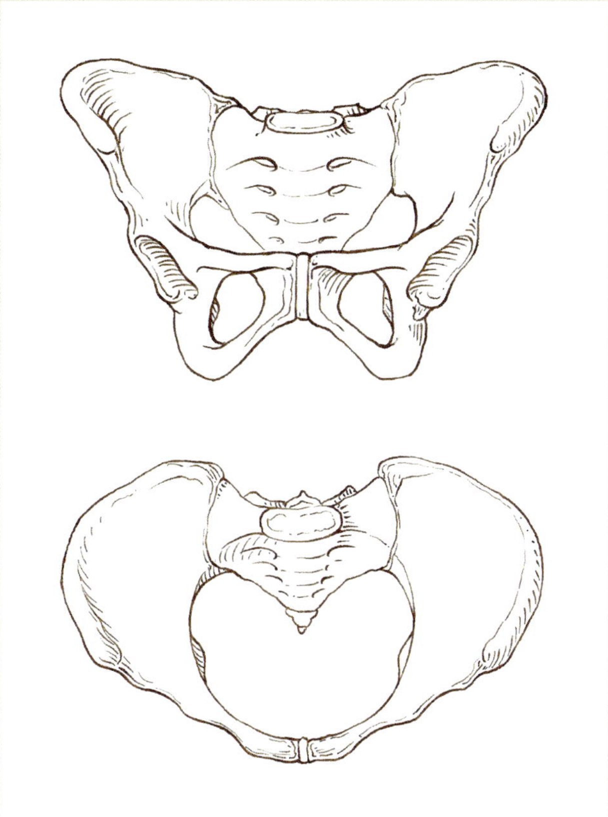

Female pelvis. Top: anterior view. Bottom: superior view.

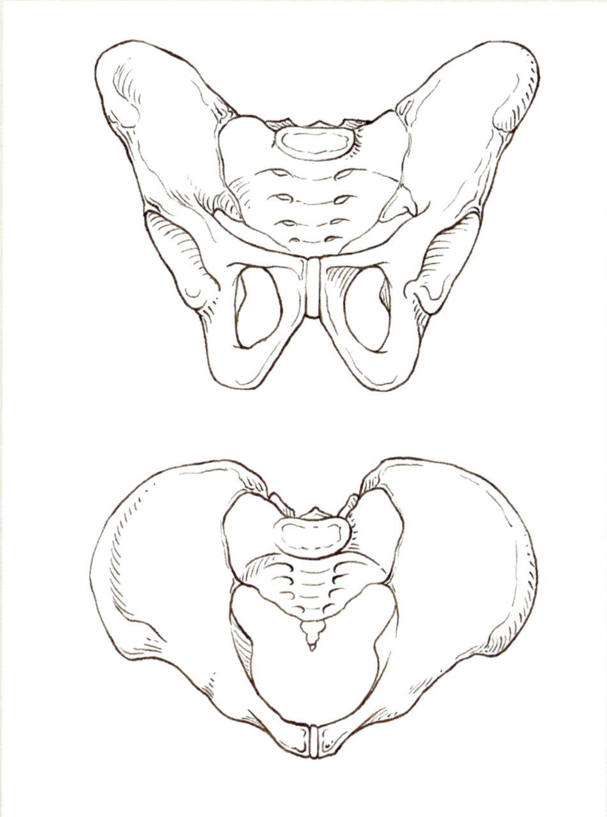

Male pelvis. Top: anterior view. Bottom: superior view.

Foramina and Other Holes

Bones have many holes called foramina, often where blood vessels or nerves enter or exit the bone. Larger foramina may correspond to key structures such as ligaments, for example the cruciate ligament attachments (see right), formed within the fossa of the bone and shows the area of these strong ligaments. Alongside with other naturally occuring examples, such as the perforated seen in the sternum specimens (below right).

You may observe other non-natural holes on the specimen, such as drilled man-made holes for articulated skeletons (see below). These have been drilled specifically for wires to pass through and hold a spinal specimen or full skeleton together for display. Drilled holes are usually quite obvious due to their uniform, neat, deep appearance, invariably passing all the way through the bone. A foramen, in comparison, has a more natural look, with smooth sides and often presenting at an angle.

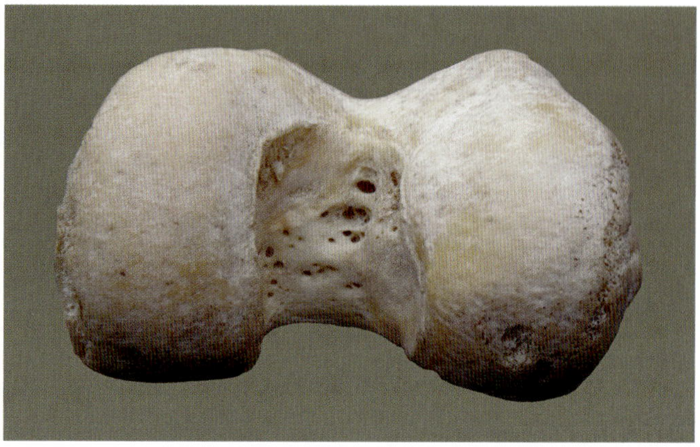

Within the inner arch of the distal end of the femur (above), called the condylar fossa, large distinct foramina are visible. These natural foramen support the attachement for these strong cruciate ligaments, which in turn support and stabilise of the knee joint. An enlarged view of the foramina of the cruciate ligament can be seen below.

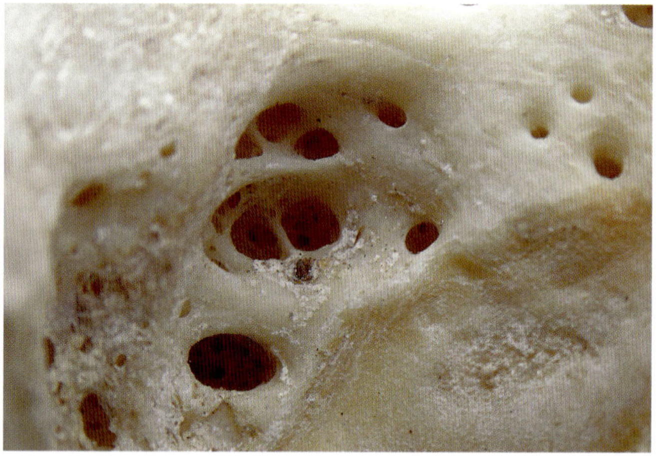

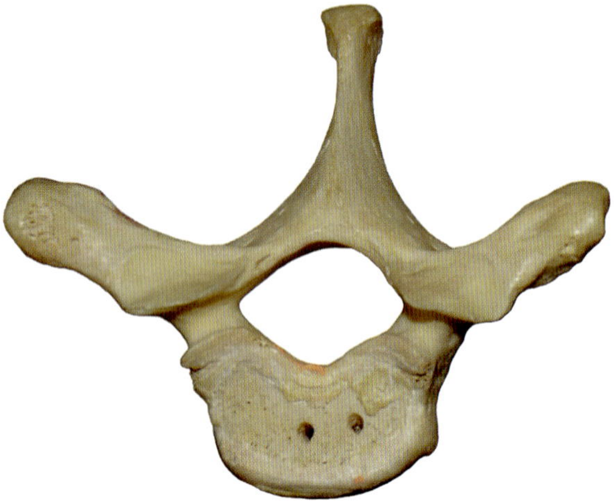

Two drilled holes can be seen centrally on the body of the vertebra (above) and on the sacrum (below). These drilled holes were made to articulate the whole spine together in the anatomical position with wires.

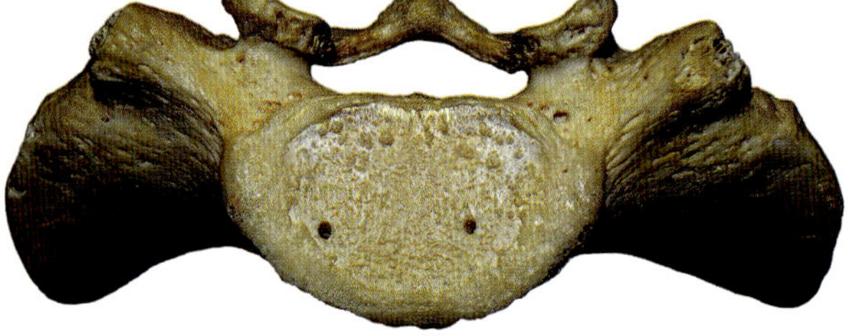

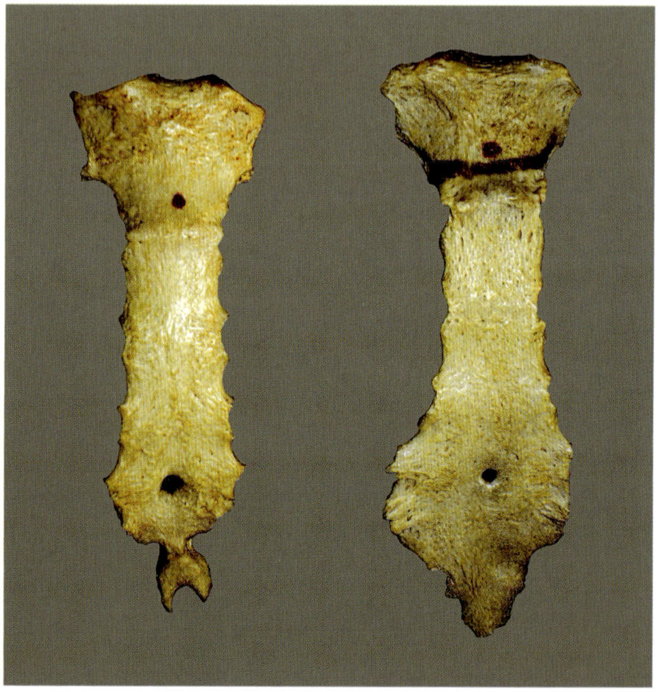

The two sternums above, each have a naturally occurring foramen. This is known as a perforated sternum and occurs when the sternum has not fully fused together during development, leaving a residual foramen or hole.

BONE DAMAGE

Scapulae, for example, have very thin, fragile areas across the body (or fossa) of the bone, and these often show broken areas of damage, perhaps caused by poor storage or handling. These damaged areas will have sharp, angular edges. The infraspinous surface of the scapula here shows an example of hole damage, leaving jagged edges. The specimen below has also darkened with age, and pencil lines are visible where students have marked areas of muscle attachment.

Bone specimens may become damaged over time, where areas become brittle and pieces break away. Seen on the femur shown here, are clear areas of damage to the outer surface, revealing the inner bony structure. Be aware of fractures and pathologies, for example a bone break, arthritis or other diseases causing bone deformities that will differentiate a specimen from a 'normal' one.

Generally, unless an area of bone damage was considered of pathological or archaeological importance, it is recommended to edit these variations from your final drawing. As a medical artist, you would usually be expected to revise and edit any areas of unrelated damage unless it appears on a particular specimen and is being specifically recorded.

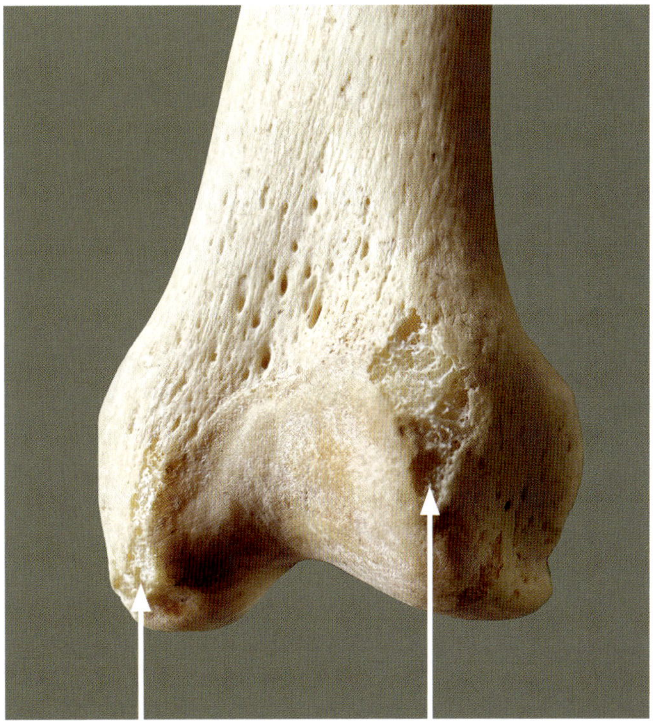

Superficial surface damage can be seen on several areas, on the distal end of the femur above. The inner intricate trabeculae network is clearly visible on both the anterior and lateral anterior surfaces.

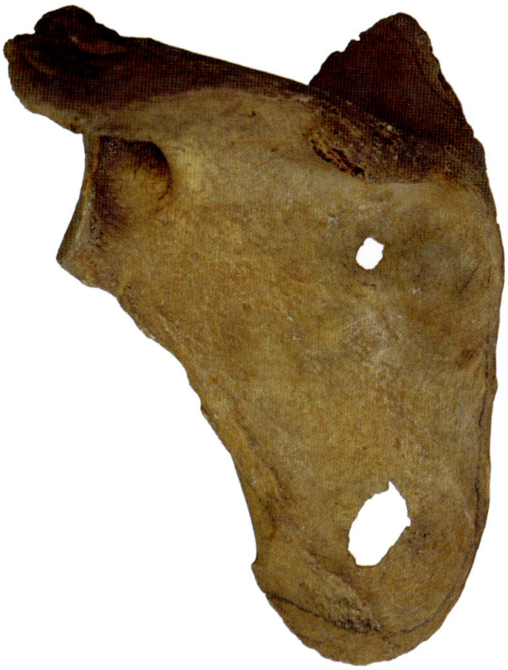

Two large areas of damage in the central infraspinous fossa of the scapula, have left ragged holes. This area of the bone is very thin and fragile, older specimens may often be seen damaged in this way.

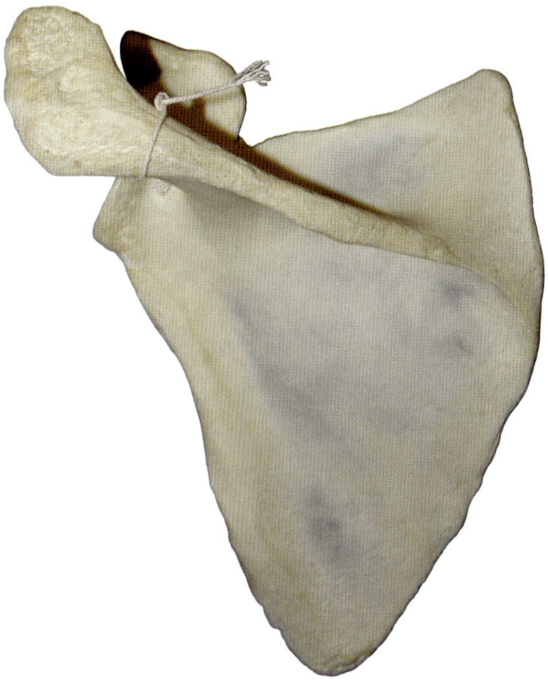

This scapula shows no damage. Occasionally scapulae may have naturally occurring foramina.

JOINTS

The skeleton has a range of joints, which were covered previously. The skull comprises 22 fused bones and has specialised interlocking suture joints, which create a strong bond to lock the bones together. Interestingly, the skull is relatively light, considering the important role it plays in encasing and protecting the brain.

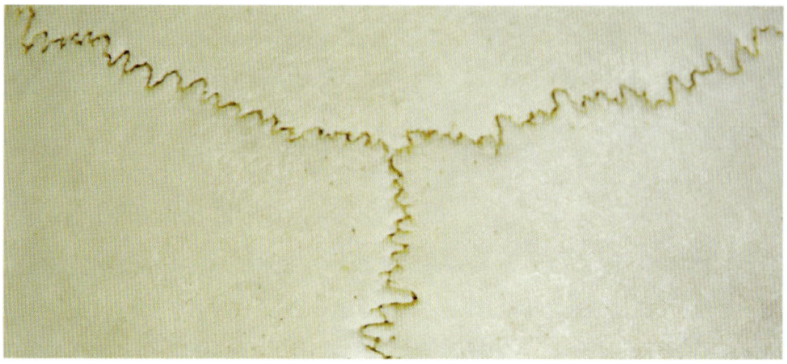

Interlinking sutures of the skull, showing how the bones developed and fused together, forming a tightly knit and strong structure.

REAL VERSUS CAST SPECIMENS

The skull example (below left) shows the advantage of studying from a real specimen. Resin casts can very useful, however, where it is not possible to obtain a real specimen to draw from. Whole-cast skeletons are widely available to purchase, as are separate limbs, such as a single hand or foot. A high-quality cast can show you the shape, form and structures of each bone. On a real specimen, you will be able to see much more detail, for example the foramina, attachments, sutures etc – as well as local colour changes in the bone, where the bone is thinner and almost see-through, or thicker, dense and more solid. If you are building a portfolio as a medical artist, it is highly recommended to work from real specimens whenever possible.

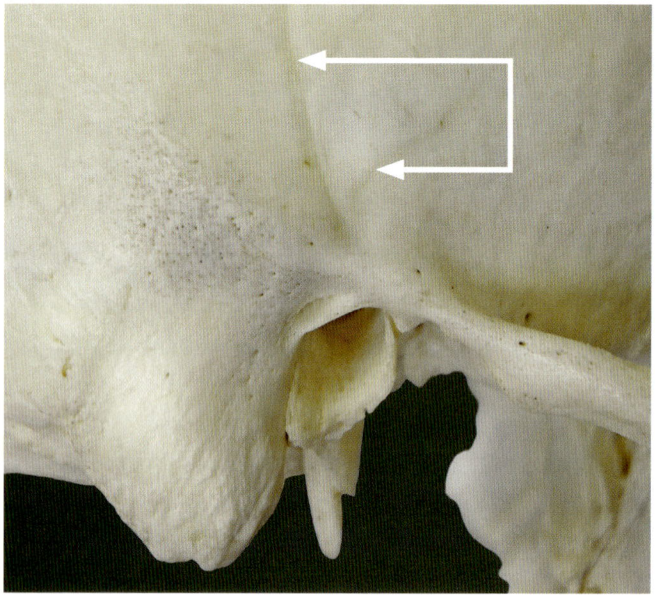

Observe where larger blood vessels passing over the surface of the skull have left indentations.

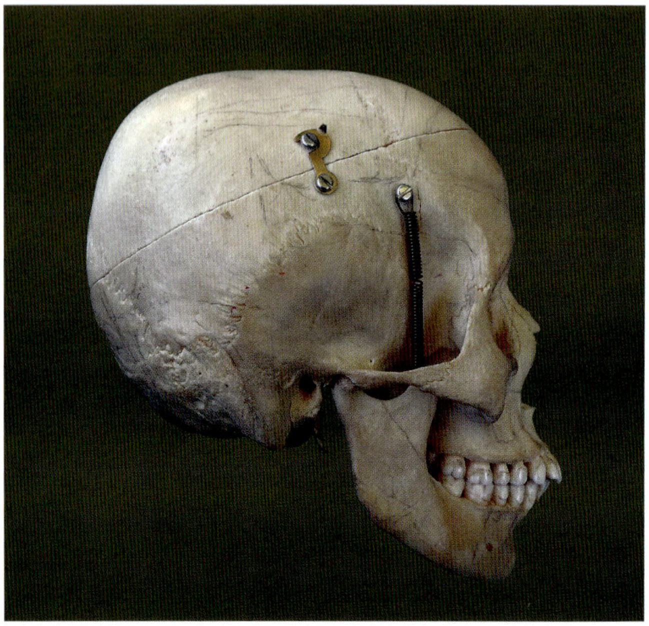

A real skull specimenx. You will often find these have been well studied by students before you, leaving the occasional pencil or pen mark on the skull, for example to demarcate muscle attachments.

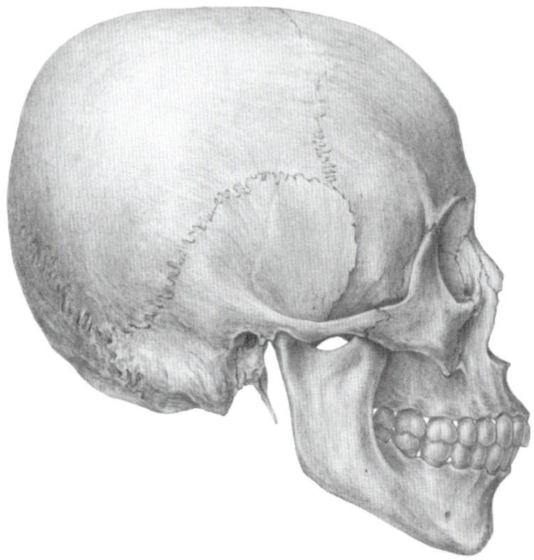

Drawing from real specimens will enable you to see and interpret all the intricate details of the bone structure and its form accurately. While learning to remove any unnecessary information such as the hooks etc.

COMPARATIVE ANATOMY

Another good approach to widening your medical art skills is to look at specimens from different species, for example comparing a human hip joint to a sheep's hip joint (right), both being ball and socket joints.

Articulated Skeletons

Articulated skeletons or limbs are those which have been placed together with supporting wires, screws, hooks, and/or on a metal frame. However, be aware that skeletons presented in this way may show the joints articulated further away from their actual anatomical position, compared to the placement in a living person, as can be seen on the shoulder joint below. This type of articulation allows for the study and movement of the shoulder joint from all angles.

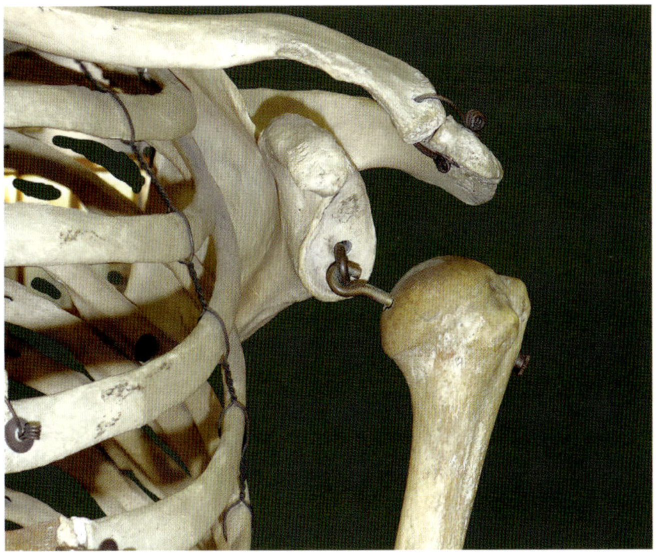

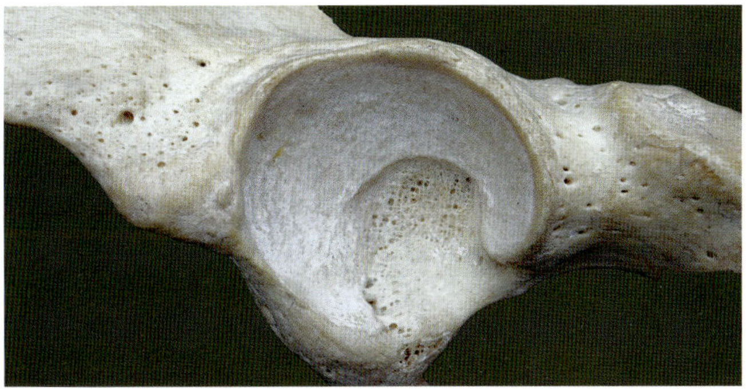

The smooth internal articular surface of a human hip joint socket.

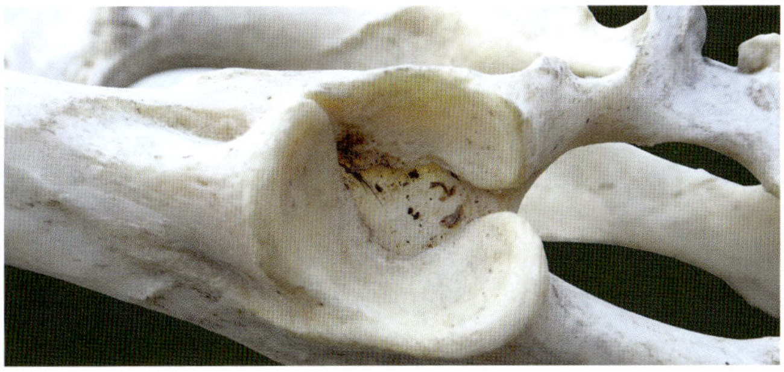

The comparative anatomy of a sheep's hip joint.

BOOK REFERENCES

There are many excellent anatomy books available to purchase for illustrated and photographic reference alongside online resources. Wherever possible, buy the most recent printed edition, which will be up to date with anatomical terminology. However many older or out-of-print texts include some fabulous illustrations. Many bargains can be found in second-hand bookshops or online. Medical artists tend to acquire numerous textbooks and need sturdy bookcases!

A selection of anatomical textbooks are listed in Appendix III. Texts are essential for studying and understanding anatomical details, so allow time to read and absorb the information.

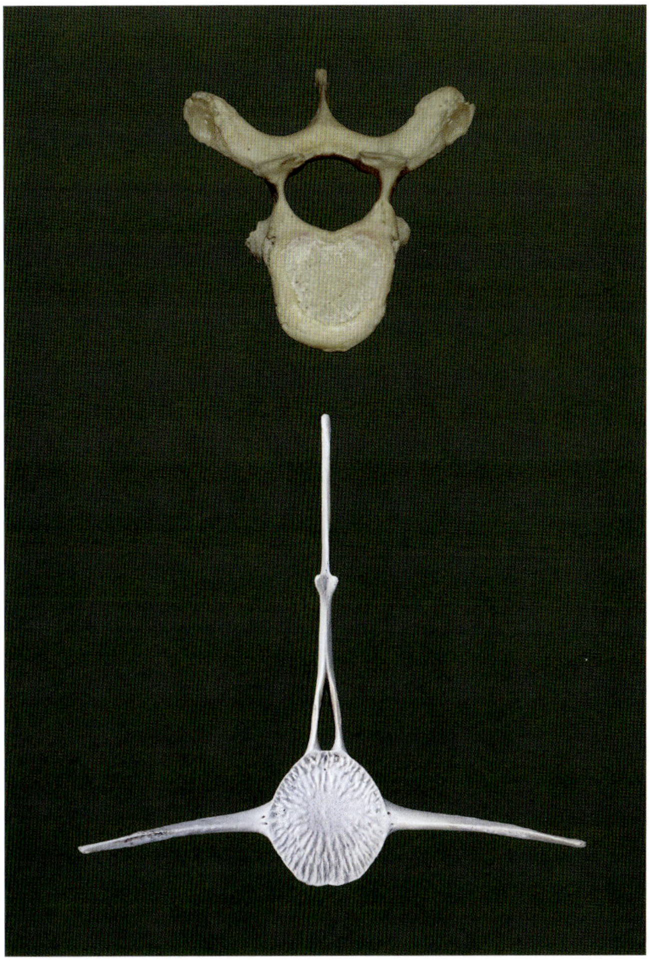

A human vertebra (above). Compare the bony elements in shape, form and size to the vertebra from a sea mammal (below), possibly a dolphin from the cetacean family. Note how pale this bone is, having been bleached by the sun on the beach.

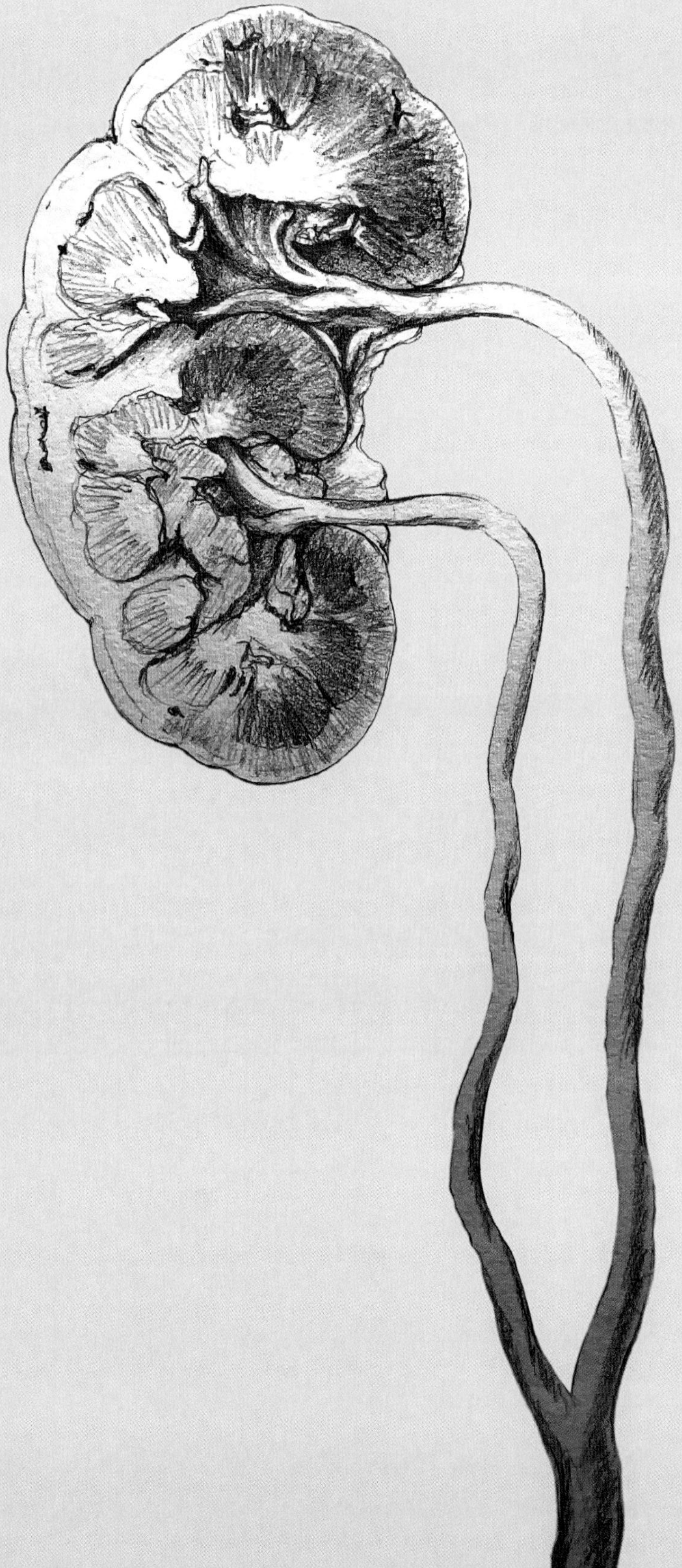

CHAPTER 6

STUDIO AND EQUIPMENT

An artist's studio or work area is important, becoming your own personal and creative space. The subsequent choice of equipment and materials as you develop your style is equally so. The following section covers how to select helpful studio items for setting up your studio, for example lighting considerations, papers and measuring callipers to a lightbox. Pencils, inks and watercolour materials will be covered in the following chapters.

THE STUDIO WORKSPACE

Setting up your studio or workspace to become a comfortable and creative area, whether at home or work is essential. There are many items to consider, from the type of lighting and equipment to your reference materials, such as books, which are always an essential source of information and inspiration for medical artists.

The position of your work area or table will be primarily dictated by the direction of the light source – usually this will be the direction from which daylight comes into the room. The position you choose for your artboard or table will be further influenced by whether you are right- or left-handed. If you are right-handed, then consider positioning your desk with the light or window on your left-hand side, or vice versa if you are left-handed. This will allow light to fall freely onto your work area and means you won't be drawing in the shadow of your hand or any other obstacle.

DESK LAMP WITH A DAYLIGHT BULB

Select a good adjustable desk lamp and select a daylight bulb. Daylight bulbs are designed to produce a clean bright light, in comparison to most household light bulbs, which can produce a yellow or blue hue, which may affect how you view the colours of your artwork and affect the subsequent choice of colour. Even with an excellent daylight source from a window, the light will change constantly throughout the day, collectively depending on the time of day, the season and the weather, which will all affect your work. Having a good daylight lamp will allow you to continue working even if the outside daylight may not be ideal or as you would wish, and this will help ensure consistency of lighting through the day while you work.

Studio lamps are also available with an incorporated magnifying lens, which are ideal for working on detailed anatomical artworks. Position your art materials, paper, sketchbooks and references close to hand. Gradually, you will decide where you like everything to be placed and create a comfortable studio space that works for you.

Kidney cross-section with a double ureter. Graphite pencil sketch.

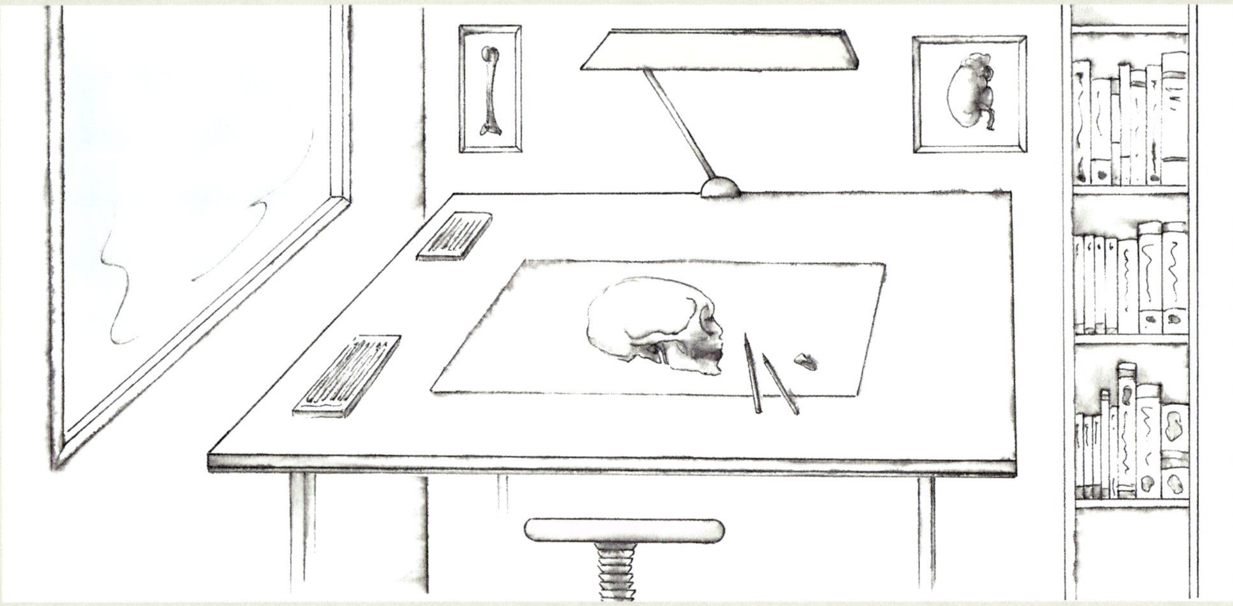

A studio arrangement with the window on the left and a daylight lamp on the front of the desk if you are right-handed. If you are left-handed, reverse the studio arrangement so the window is on your right-hand side.

PAPER

For any artist, the paper on which they choose to work is of paramount and selecting the right paper for the right job is essential. There are papers designed for every requirement, from thin layout paper for preparatory work to cartridge drawing papers, watercolour and painting papers and boards, printing papers and more. Many will also come in varying weights and sizes and different grades of quality: for example, cartridge drawing paper may be classified as student's or artist's quality and range in weight from 100gms to more than 350gms. The paper you choose for quick preparatory drawings or sketches may be completely different from the high-quality paper you choose for the final artwork.

Paper weights are given in grams (gms), with a high-quality watercolour paper typically falling in the range of 300–450gms, whereas for a drawing cartridge paper, 150gms would be more appropriate for its designed use.

Many papers can also be purchased as individual sheets in a wide variety of sizes, textures and colours. This particularly applies to handmade papers, for example specialist watercolour papers. Sizes for these may also vary between manufacturers, or even (slightly) within each handmade batch.

Paper Sizes

Paper is measured and supplied in sizes and weights, with the most frequent size and accepted standard being the rectangular 'A' format – where each size is half the size of the preceding size – which has become the accepted measurement for paper across Europe and the USA. Historically many other paper sizes have been used with names that may still be familiar today, such as atlas, foolscap and elephant sizes. We commonly see A sizes as small as A6, however, there are even smaller sizes available, progressively reducing down to A7, A8, A9 and A10. An A10 size is only 2.6 × 3.7cm (1 × 1.5in). The most frequently used sizes are listed below for reference.

A0 – 84.1 × 11.9cm (33.1 × 46.8in)
A1 – 59.4 × 84.1cm (23.4 × 33.1in)
A2 – 42 × 59.4cm (16.5 × 23.4in)
A3 – 29.7 × 42cm (11.7 × 16.5in)
A4 – 21 × 29.7cm (8.3 × 11.7in)
A5 – 18.8 × 21cm (5.8 × 8.3in)
A6 – 10.5 × 14.8cm (4.1 × 5.8in)

If you are planning artwork for printing, there will often be a 'bleed' area beyond your artwork; this extra size allows for the image and paper to be trimmed after printing.

ADDITIONAL STUDIO ITEMS

Measuring Devices

For simpler or larger objects, artists will be familiar with measuring by the traditional 'thumb and pencil' technique. Hold your pencil up in front of you, either vertically or horizontally. This is best done with one eye closed to keep a single fixed viewpoint. Position your thumb along the pencil shaft to select the area or size being measured. The measurements can then be transferred proportionally onto your paper. The image can subsequently scaled up or down in size.

Medical artists, however, frequently require measuring devices to create accurate artwork. Callipers will help you measure size, width, depth and detail with precision and accuracy. Measuring callipers, such as those used by sculptors, come in a range of styles and sizes and are good for larger objects such as portraits. Scale calliper dividers are useful if you wish to scale the size of your subject up or down. Specific measuring callipers are for fine measurements and will be needed where detailed anatomical measurements are required.

Becoming familiar with each measuring method, style and use will enable medical artists to select the most relevant method or device.

Some measuring devices and dividers have a locking option, to 'hold' and lock the device in position while the measurement is being taken. A variety of measuring devices are shown here. In addition, there are callipers on the market replicating the 'golden ratio', a mathematical division of symmetry designed especially for artists.

Lightbox for Tracing

A lightbox is a perfect studio addition for tracing your drawings from one surface onto another, for example, to complete the final stage of an artwork. An A3 size is ideal, but even an A4 size lightbox is good if you are limited on space. There are also slimline portable lightboxes available, some with adjustable brightness options, similar to a home dimmer switch.

There are also other tracing options available, such as graphite transfer paper. However, if you are using delicate paper, it is advisable to reduce the number of stages and stresses the paper may go through to complete your artwork. A single image transfer via a lightbox is preferable in many instances.

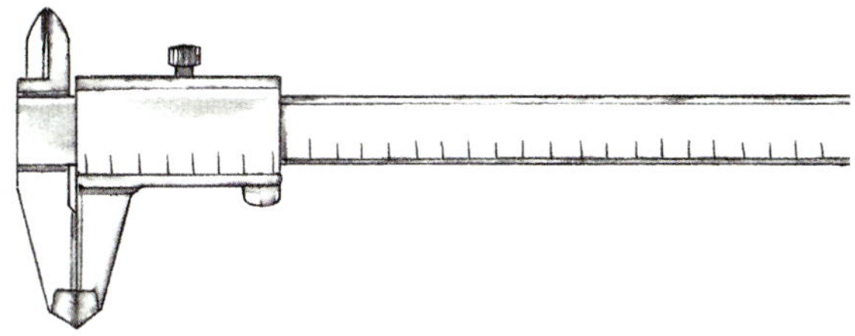

Precision style measuring callipers, shown here in a closed position. Callipers may have an optional digital display screen for viewing the measurement.

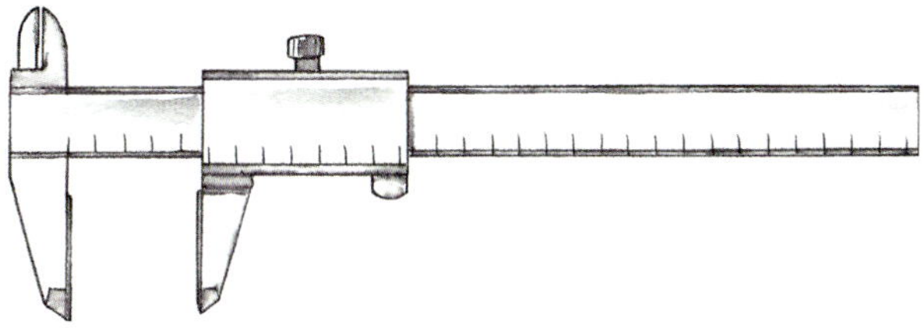

Callipers shown with the measuring slide ruler bar in the open position. There will be a screw locking nut on the top of the device to hold the callipers fixed in place once the measurement has been taken.

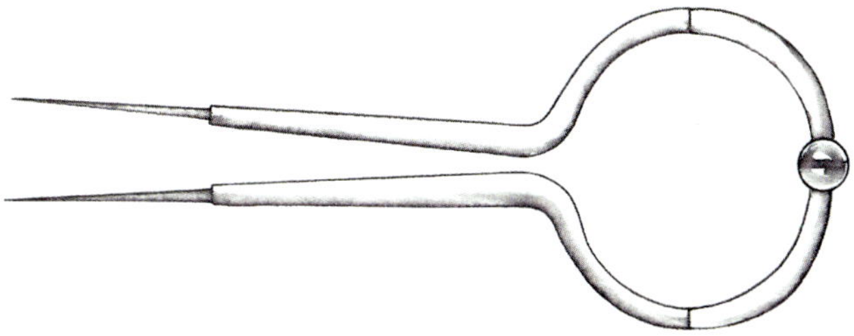

This style of measuring calliper has a much wider reach, being able to measure between the two points. The final measurements can be taken against an accompanying ruler as required.

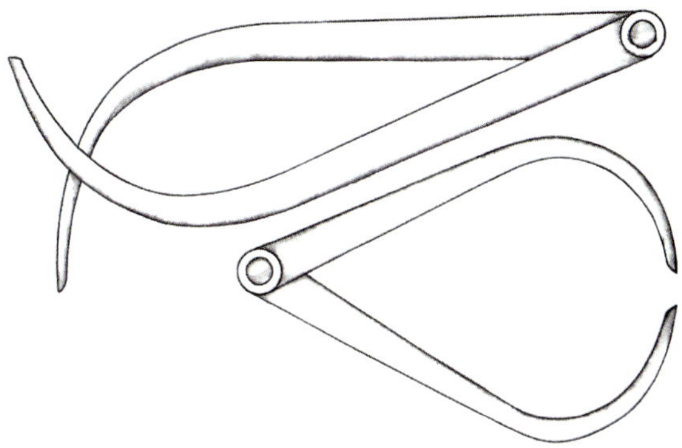

Sculptors frequently use these 'bent leg' style callipers, which come in a variety of sizes and are useful for measuring large objects, because they can fit and measure around the subject.

Magnifying Glass

A hand-held lens is ideal for your studio and being small also easily portable. Keep your lens in a soft cloth case to protect the surface from becoming scratched.
A hand-held lens in conjunction with a studio lamp with an incorporated magnifying lens is an ideal combination for detailed artwork.

Reducing Lens

A reducing lens produces the opposite effect of a magnifying glass, so instead of seeing an enlarged image, you will see a reduced image. This is ideal for quickly reviewing an artwork that will be reduced for printing. For example, an artwork may initially be prepared to a larger size, say 125, 150 or 200 per cent. Once resized and reduced for printing, the image will become sharper. A reducing lens allows you to review your artwork to check how a reduction could look. This will also help you to see if any areas need to be darkened or lightened while you work on your drawing or artwork.

Mirror

A good-sized wall-mounted mirror in conjunction with a smaller hand-held or small table-standing mirror, makes a useful studio set-up. Mirrors have many uses for an artist. For self-portraits, a mirror is essential. Artists throughout history have created self-portraits as a method of study. You may also need to draw your own hands and feet, for example, and having a mirror will help you see all angles.

Mirrors are also useful for viewing your own work. Hold your work up to the mirror to see the image in reverse, often highlighting areas that require further attention, such as form and lighting.

Camera Lucida

This optical device used to be frequently used by artists as a method for directly tracing the object they saw through a lens, mapping out an impression of the image onto paper. It can be a useful optical aid; however, it may be limiting in only aiding you to create an initial 'tracing' of the image, from which you can then develop your drawing through observational drawing and measurements. If you wish to try this optical technique yourself, why not experiment with your own simple camera lucida by following one of the many online tutorials available.

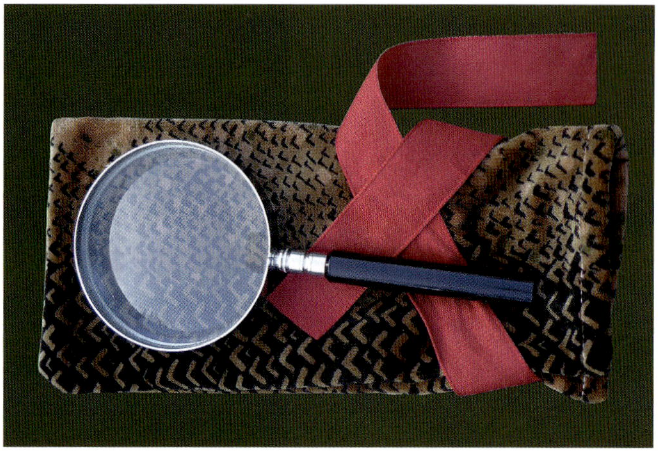

A hand-held magnifying glass with a soft protective case. This homemade example has a tie handle to keep the glass securely inside when not in use.

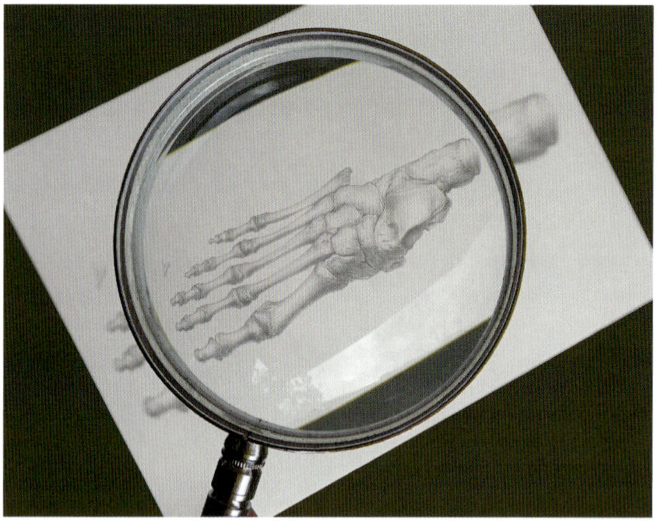

A hand-held reducing lens works in the opposite way to a magnifying glass. Looking through the reducing lens will show how your image will appear when reduced in size. Move the lens closer towards or further away from your artwork to achieve the scale and reduction visually required, in order to assess whether your artwork will reduce effectively when printed.

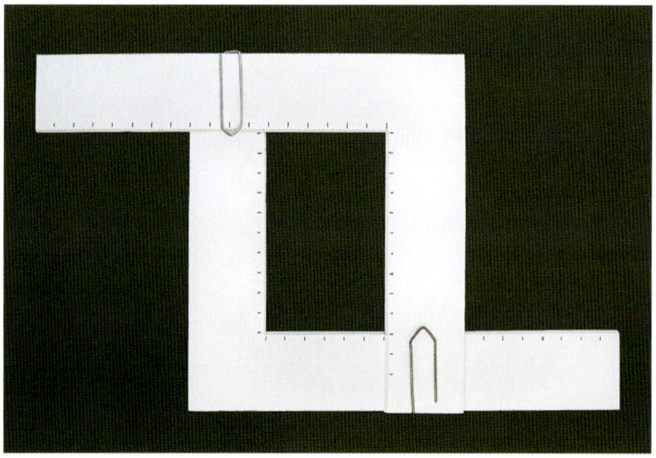

Making a viewfinder. Cut card into two L shapes, forming the viewfinder's two 90-degree corners, overlapping to become a viewfinder. Mark evenly spaced measurements along the inside edges with a pen.
Two paperclips placed either side of the square will hold the card in place.

Viewfinder

Making your own viewfinder, or indeed having several in varying sizes is very useful for planning your artwork layout and design and also for considering framing proportions of your final artwork. Often, medical artists work to specific pre-set publication sizes and proportions, so they frequently need to select the best proportional arrangement for their artwork within an allocated space. A viewfinder will help you focus your image within a limited area through the viewfinder, allowing you to concentrate on the subject alone without being distracted by unnecessary areas or items beyond the view. This is a very useful additional tool for everything from life drawing to landscapes and may be purchased from art suppliers or homemade. Viewfinders are very easy to make by creating two L-shaped corners of the card and holding them in position with clips or tape.

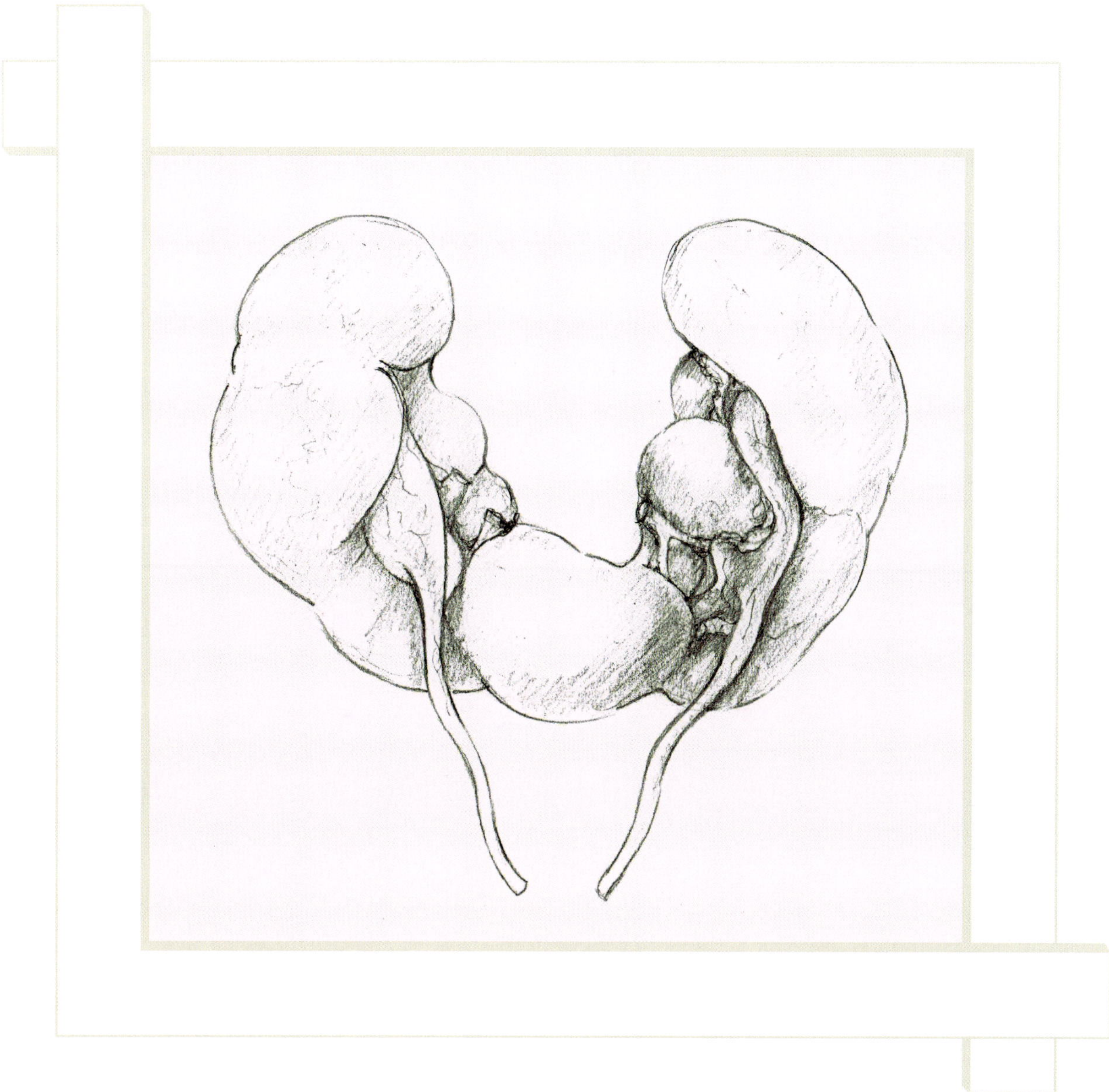

Double kidney drawing shown within a viewfinder. Graphite pencil sketch.

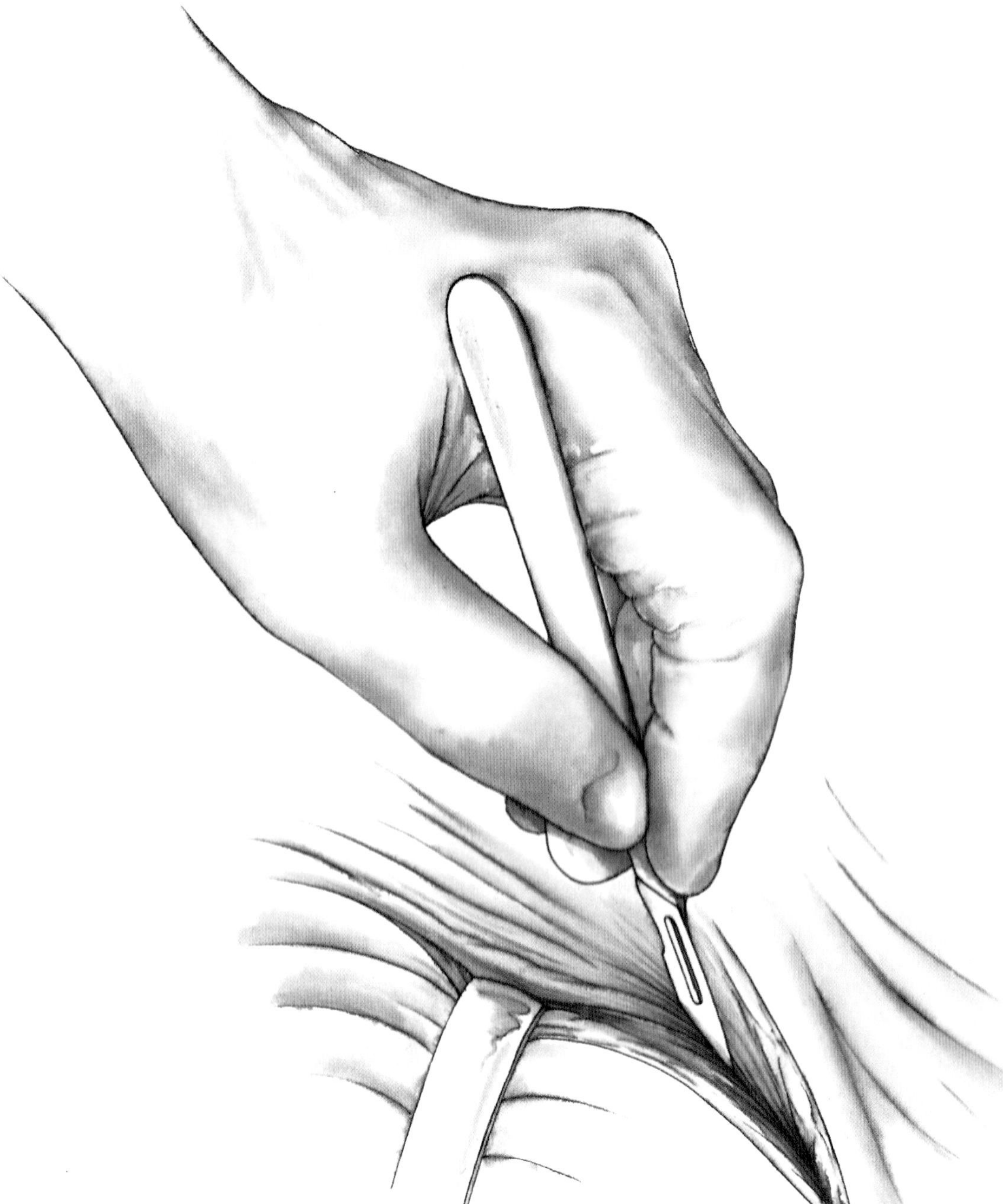

CHAPTER 7

PERSPECTIVE

Medical art requires elements of technical drawing, from surgical instruments to clinical equipment and patient positioning. Mastering the basic rules of perspective will enable you to create realistic and relatable drawings. To create the illusion of three-dimensional depth within the subject you are drawing on flat two-dimensional paper requires the ability to interpret what we see into a three-dimensional image. The following guides and projects introduce the basic principles of perspective, and explain how to create expressive lines, curves and tonal values to produce an artwork that looks as though you could pick it up from the page.

FORMS OF PERSPECTIVE

Drawings may not necessarily need the complexity of a detailed construction design, however understanding how to translate your images using either simple one-, two- or three-point perspective is essential.

One-point perspective All the lines converge towards a single vanishing point.
Two-point perspective The lines converge towards two vanishing points, and all the vertical lines remain vertical.
Three-point perspective The vanishing point is not on the same level as the eye-level/horizon line, so you are either looking up or down at an object.

In medical art, we are often called upon to prepare technical elements within our drawings, for example surgical instruments, anatomical or surgical sequences drawn realistically in perspective, or a scalpel blade being positioned at the correct angle in relation to the anatomy, as if in the hands of a surgeon.

The first step is to identify your horizon line or eye-level; the horizon line is the line that is on the same level as your eye. You can easily see how this can change by looking across your room, first sitting on the floor, then on a chair, then standing up. Your eye level and how you view each item will change significantly.

Now, imagine you are preparing a drawing of a nurse taking a patient's blood pressure. Are you on the same level – that is, sitting at the same level as the nurse? Or are you positioned slightly higher, looking down? It will be necessary to consider what is the best angle to show the action and the anatomy you wish to illustrate.

In the following diagrams, your position and eye-level in relation to the object is represented by the central red dot. This position will then determine the angle from which you view the object in front of you. Where objects recede away from your eye-line, they will become smaller, thereby appearing to reduce in size into the distance. The lines from each corner or edge of an object converge towards the vanishing point/s.

Gloved hand holding a scalpel. Pen and wash.

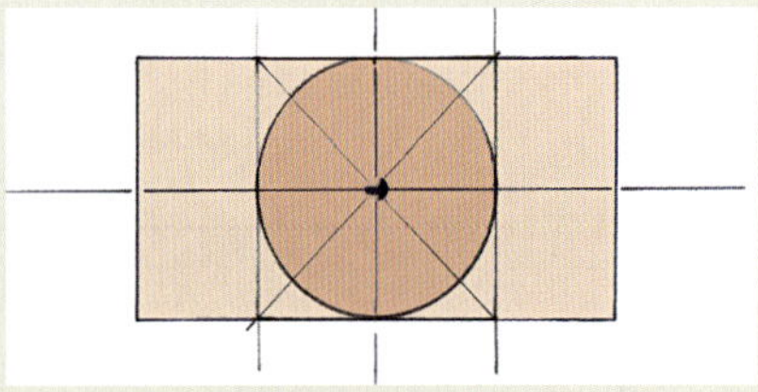

Drawing an object 'flat' is referred to as a plan i.e. not seen in perspective.

Two-point perspective. Your eye-level is in line with the horizontal line and your body position is interpreted by the vertical line. Taking your visual angle out towards the horizon line will give you your vanishing points. As the lines converge on the two outer vanishing points, the box sides converge towards these points and create the impression of receding into the distance.

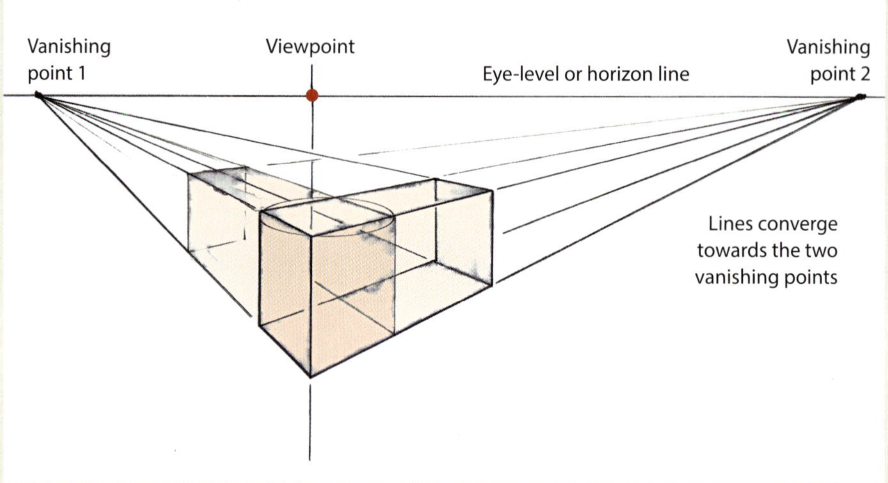

A simple rectangular box drawn to demonstrate two-point perspective.

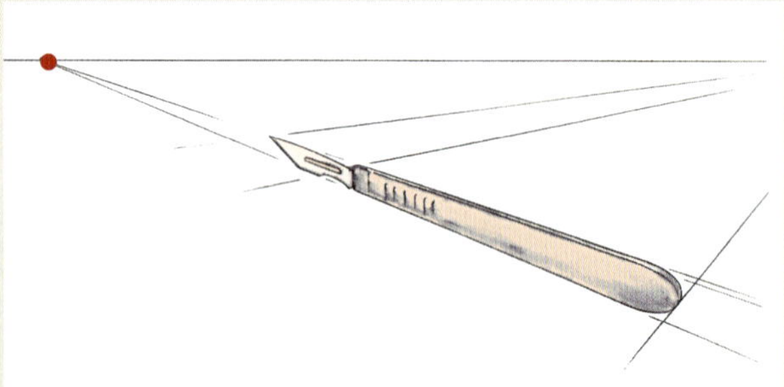

A scalpel shown within perspective guides.

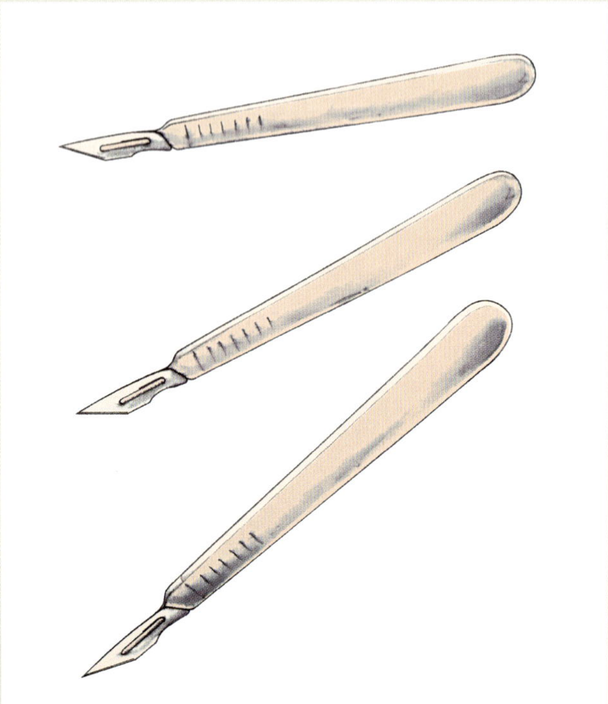

A scalpel viewed from three different angles. This can be a tricky instrument to interpret into perspective. Keep a spare scalpel or two for drawing reference. These will be a useful resource in your sketchbook when you come to prepare clinical or surgical artworks.

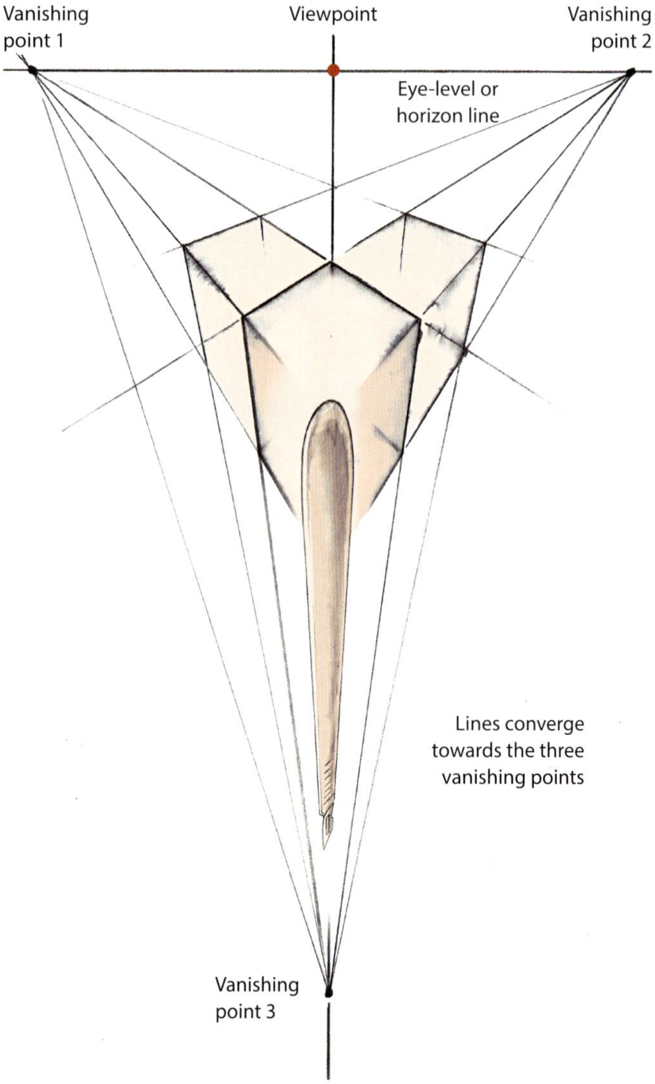

Three-point perspective. Your position in front of the object creates the vertical line and your eye-level creates the horizontal line. The closer the vanishing points, the greater the perspective. However, if you draw the vanishing points too close together, your image may appear distorted.

CIRCLES IN PERSPECTIVE

A circle in perspective becomes an ellipse. As a circle decreases in depth to become an ellipse, the tight curved 'corners', i.e. those seen to the right and left-hand sides become narrower. The most common mistake is to draw the curves to the sides of the ellipse 'pointy' instead of keeping the outer edge of the ellipse curved.

The diagram below shows how a circle becomes an ellipse from a one-point perspective i.e. receding towards a single vanishing point, showing the recession and the change in depth of the ellipse as the circle recedes towards the vanishing point.

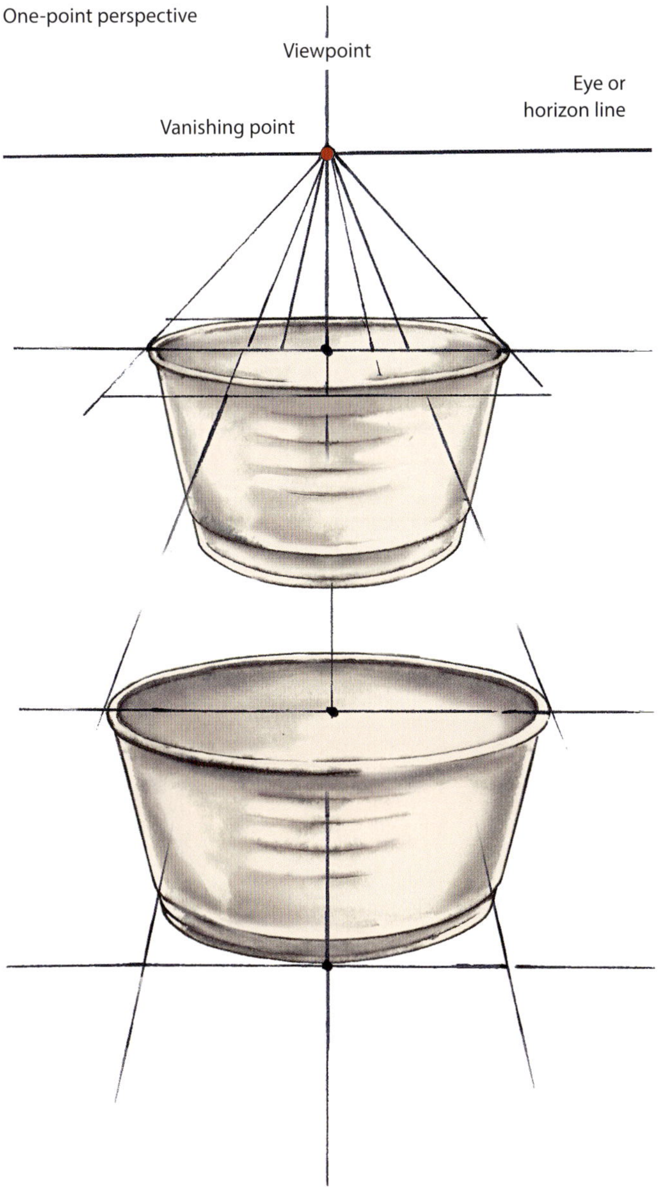

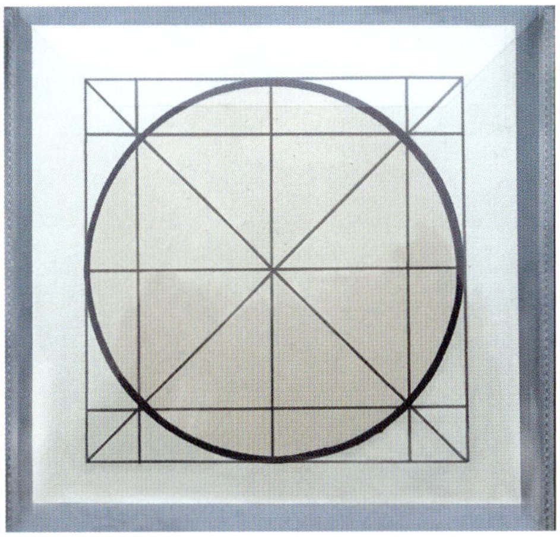

Create your own ellipse aid on a piece of card, by drawing a circle within a square, adding accompanying guidelines and keep stored in a clear sleeve.

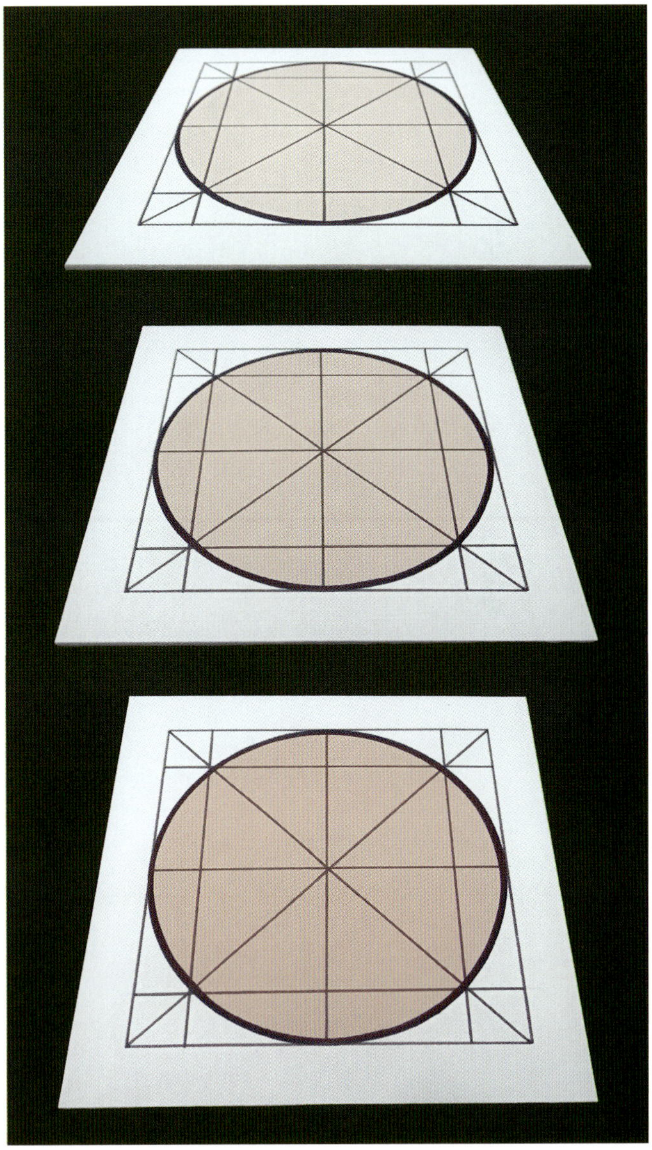

How to use the circle guide: position the card at the eye level required, then gradually tilt the card away from you. The circle will gradually become an ellipse. The steeper you tilt the angle of the card, the greater the angle of the ellipse. The pre-drawn lines on your template form useful construction aids when drawing an ellipse.

Project: Ellipses

Aim: To develop your skill in drawing ellipses.

Art materials required:

- A circle template drawn onto a piece of card
- HB pencil
- Cartridge paper 150gms
- A small round cup such as a clinical wash bath

Project: First, create your own circle template on a square piece of white or cream card. Draw a circle within a square, bisected by diagonal grid lines as shown in the previous image. You may find shading the inside of the circle, here shaded light red, makes it easier to see the circle when you tilt the card. A clear plastic case is perfect for keeping the circle card template clean and stored safely.

After you have completed the template, initially hold the card flat, then gradually tilt the card with the furthest edge moving down and away from your eye-line. You will see how the shape of the circle becomes an ellipse, and the greater the tilt away from you, the narrower the ellipse becomes. Once you have practised drawing ellipses using the template as a guide, try drawing a round 3D object, such as a clinical cup.

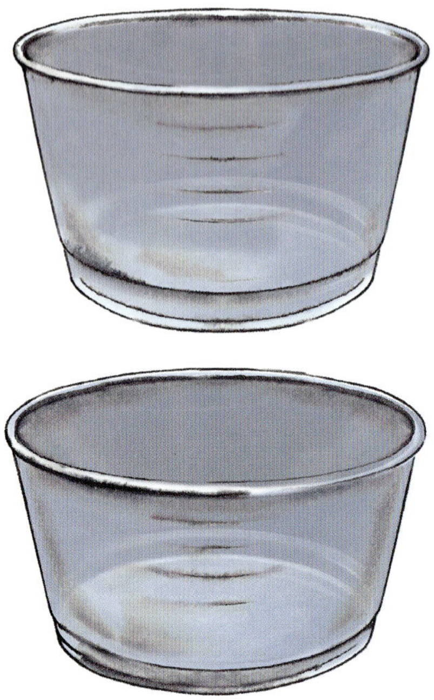

Select one or more cups and practise drawing the structure of the cup with the ellipses in perspective, remembering to curve the outer curves 'around'. The measurement lines on the cup will help you see and form gradated ellipses increasing in size from top to bottom.

SCALPELS

In medical art, we are often called upon to prepare artworks for anatomy and surgical sequences, with each image drawn in perspective – for example, a nurse or surgeon holding a scalpel correctly positioned.

The scalpel, a small sharp-bladed knife, is the surgical instrument a medical artist is most frequently requested to draw. Scalpels today are made from a variety of materials such as stainless steel, carbon or titanium. Medical artists need to become familiar with drawing this small yet important surgical tool, illustrating both the hand and scalpel in perspective.

There are many styles of scalpel blades and handles available. Each will have been designed for their own specific surgical discipline, and individual surgeons will also have personal preferences for specific styles, shapes and brands. Blades may be straight or curved. Handles may be of the standard style and length as pictured here or come with a longer handle, giving the surgeon additional depth. Other handle designs may be wider for strength, or fine and narrow for delicate procedures where precision is required.

Grip

The two most common positions an artist will draw a scalpel being held in by a clinician are the commonly known 'pencil' grip and 'palmar' grip; the latter is also known as the 'dinner knife' grip. In the pencil grip, the scalpel is held between the tips of the thumb and the

GLOSSARY

Eye-level The horizontal view in line with the level of your eye

Horizon line The level of the horizon, often the same as your eye-level

One-point perspective Often referred to as a flat plan – that is, not viewed from above or below

Two-point perspective The vertical lines remain vertical, and the horizon line/eye-level remain horizontal, with all other lines of the object/s or view converging upon the two vanishing points

Three-point perspective The vanishing point is not on the same level as the horizon line/eye-level, so you are either looking up or down at an object, thereby giving the view a third vanishing point

Ellipse A circle seen in perspective. The vertical and horizontal lines remain constant

Recession The illusion that an object recedes into the distance

first and second fingers, with the handle resting and supported against the arch of the hand. For the palmar grip, the handle is first placed firmly in the centre of the palm of the hand, then held between the thumb and second, third and fourth fingers, as when holding a knife.

Hands within a clinical setting will always be drawn and represented wearing surgical or protective gloves unless specified otherwise. When preparing your drawings, always remember therefore, that you will not be able to see their fingernails in any detail – these will just be seen as an indent or an impression through the glove.

Once the hands are inside opaque gloves, they often cause problems for the artist trying to represent anatomically correct hands when only an overall hand impression can be seen.

In the following examples (see pages 74&75), the gloved hand is shown both in full colour and then tonally as a black-and-white image for comparison. When translating a colour photo into a black-and-white drawing, converting the image into a black and white tonal image first will give you a useful reference image for light and depth when planning your artwork. An illustrated version of the gloved hand was then drawn using an ink dip pen. The final image of an ungloved hand illustrates the anatomical position of the hand, but remember it should invariably be gloved in your final artwork.

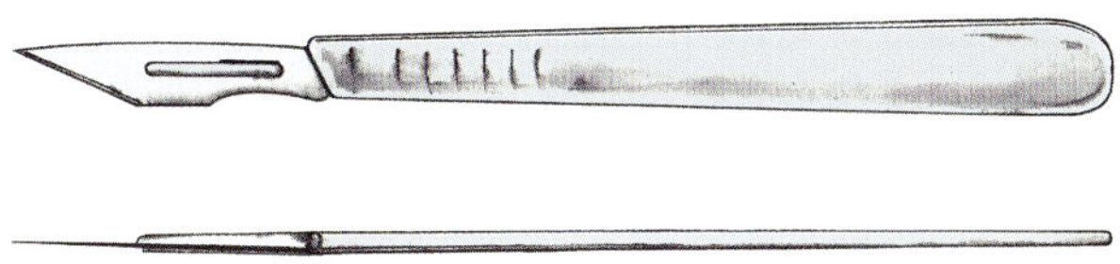

A traditional surgical scalpel has a reusable flat handle, here viewed from the side and the edge. There are many blade and handle designs, each intended for a different purpose. The handle shown here has an attached straight-edged blade, a style also commonly used within the studio, for cutting paper or card for example.

Project: Hand Studies

Aim: To draw one or more hands in a variety of positions.

Art materials:

- HB pencil
- Cartridge paper 150gms
- Disposable gloves

Project: Practise drawing your own hands or those of someone else, observing the shape, structure, and position of the fingers. Set the hand position holding a pen, pencil or instrument and draw the hand from a variety of viewpoints, with and without gloves. Each view will give the hand a very different appearance in perspective. Disposable medical-grade gloves may either be latex, which is made from natural rubber, or nitrile, which are made from synthetic rubber. If you think you may have an allergy to any of the glove's materials, always check first with the supplier or manufacturer.

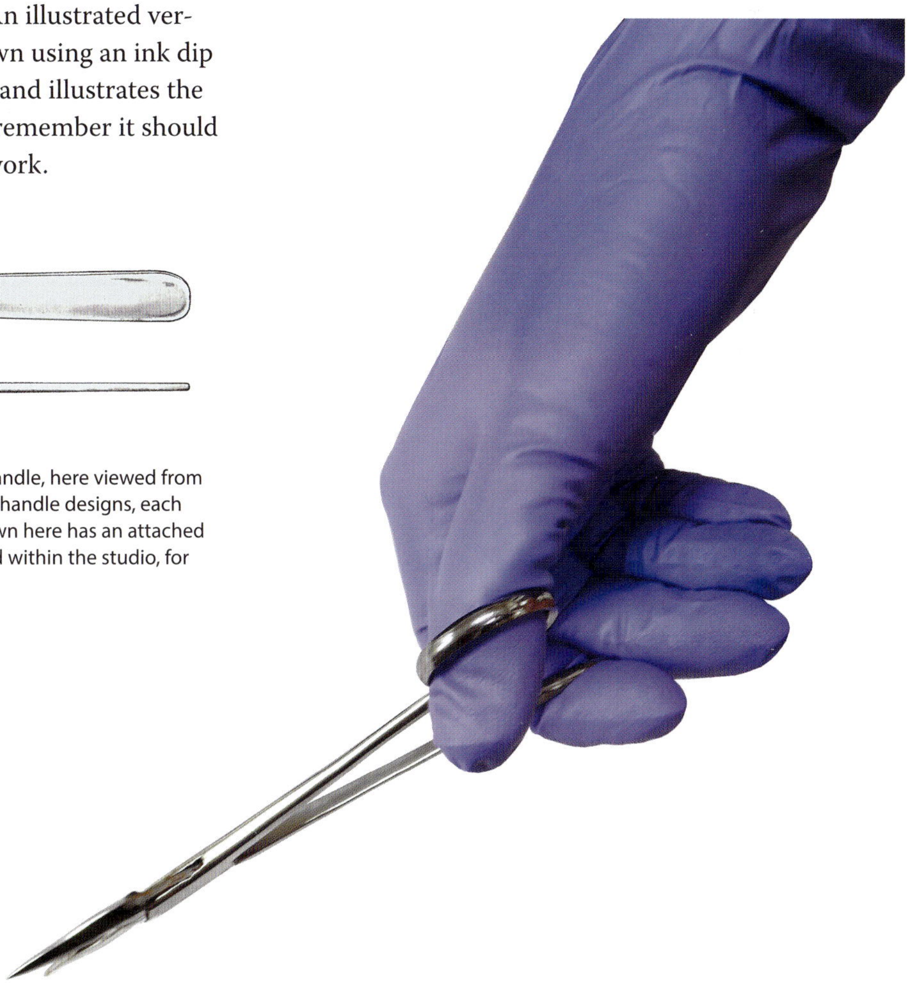

Hand positions

Compare the hand images: between an ungloved hand to a gloved hand, to a tonal image and an ink-line artwork.

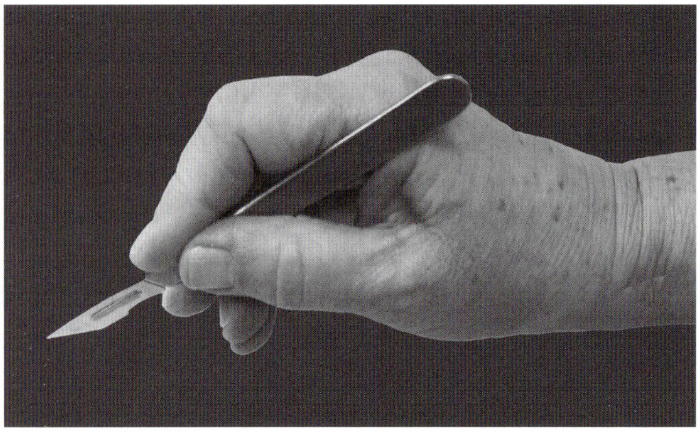

1. The hand holding a scalpel using the pencil grip positiion, without wearing a glove to show the anatomical position of the hand.

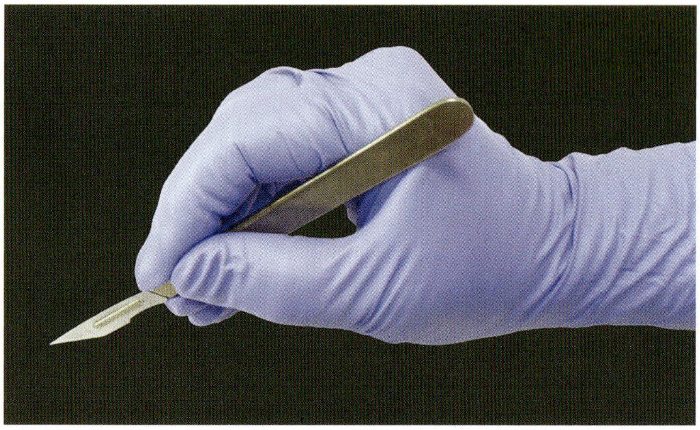

2. The hand wearing a blue clinical grade disposable gloved, resulting in the anatomical features of the hand becoming less distinct.

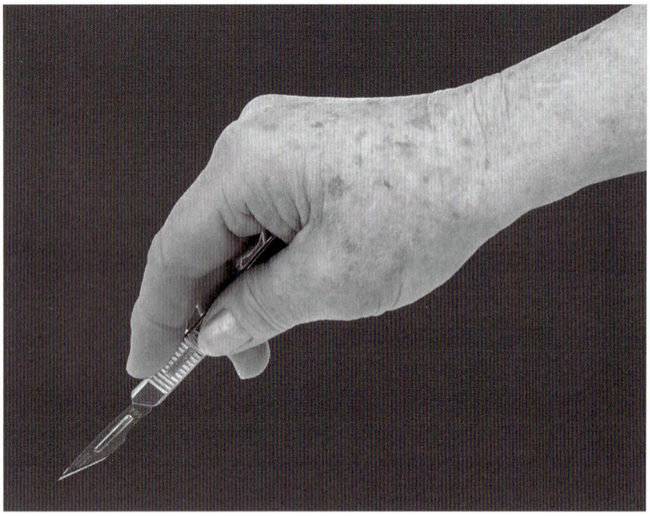

1. The hand holding a scalpel in the palmar grip position, without wearing the glove to show the anatomical position of the hand.

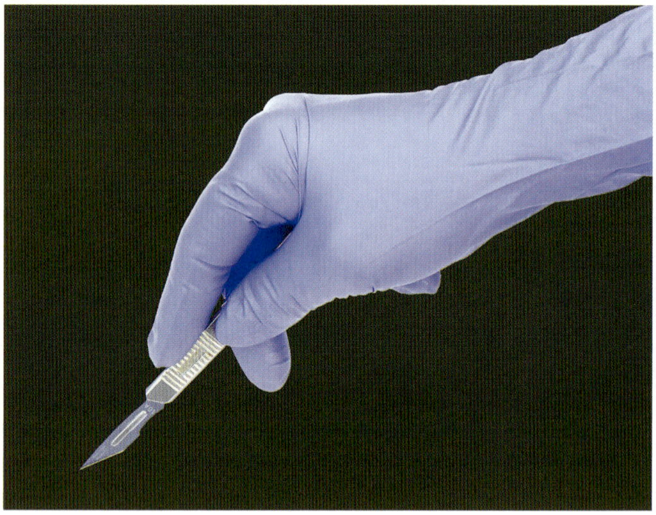

2. A gloved hand for comparison.

A cream latex glove gives a different and smoother visual interpretation of the hand within the glove.

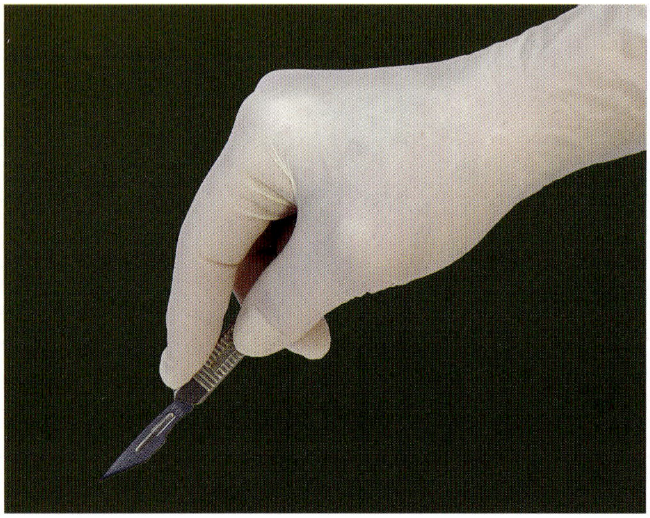

1. The hand wearing a cream latex glove, for comparison with the blue clinical grade disposable glove featured above.

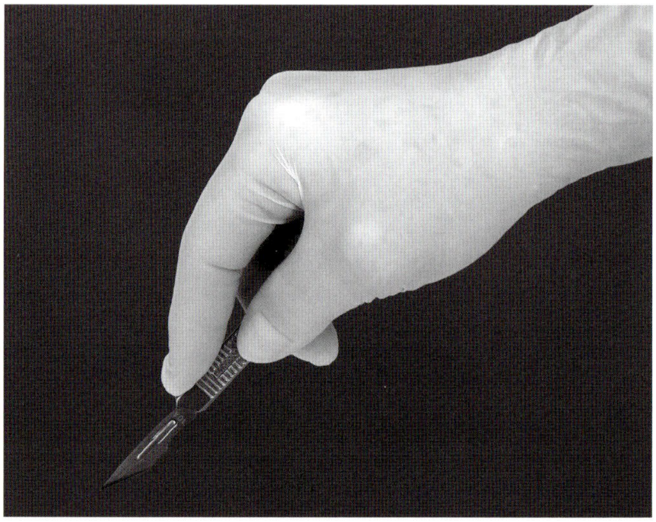

2. The latex gloved hand shown tonally in black and white.

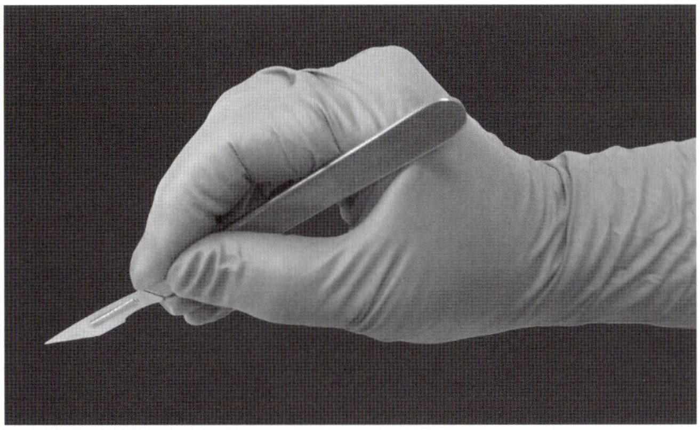

3. The gloved hand shown tonally in black and white. A useful conversion technique for interpretaing light and shade within an image.

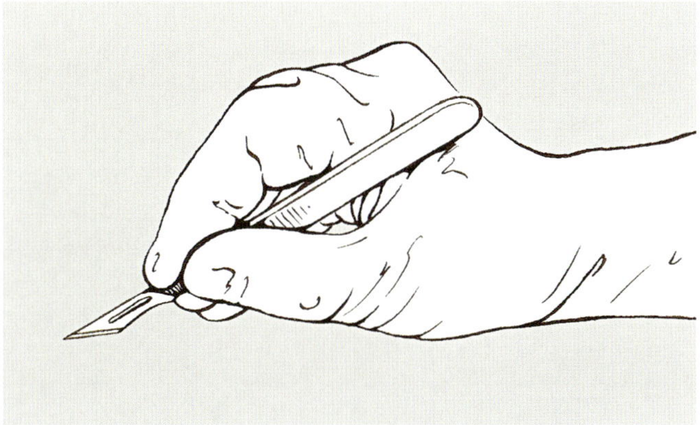

4. The image translated into an ink-line drawing using a dip pen.

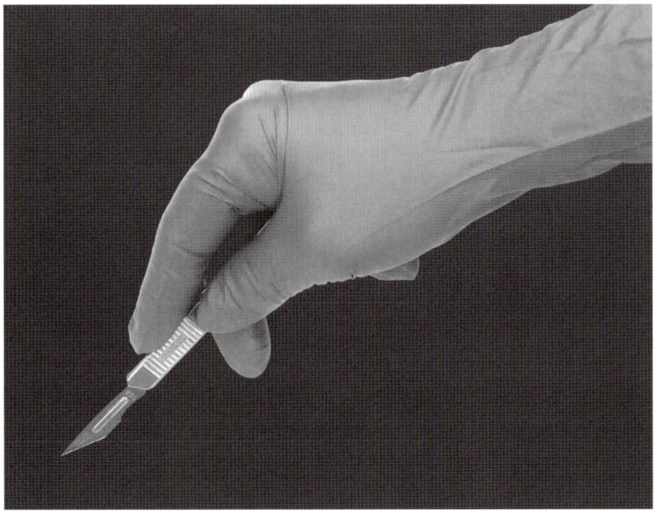

3. The gloved hand shown tonally in black and white for comparison.

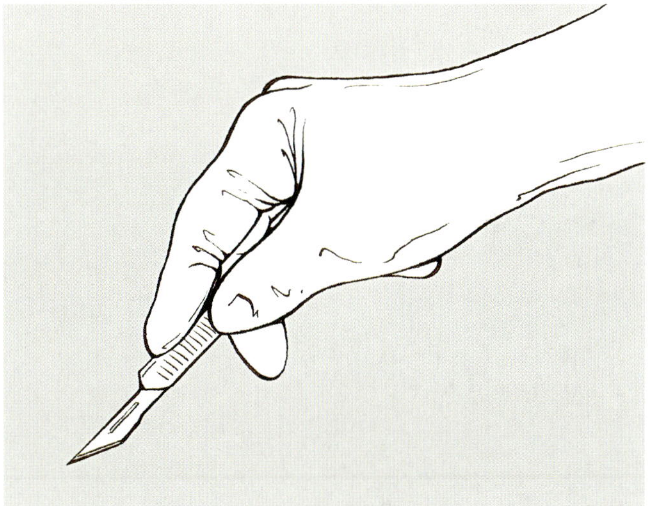

4. The image translated into an ink-line drawing using a dip pen.

A hand holding a pair of tweezers wearing a cream latex glove.

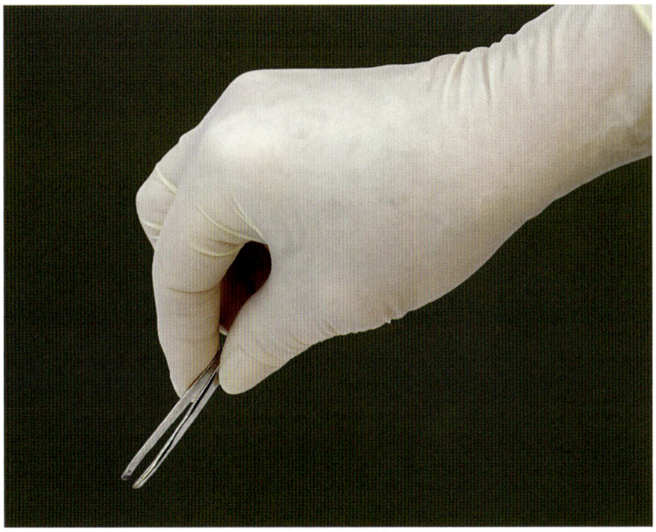

1. The hand holding a pair of tweezers and wearing a cream latex glove.

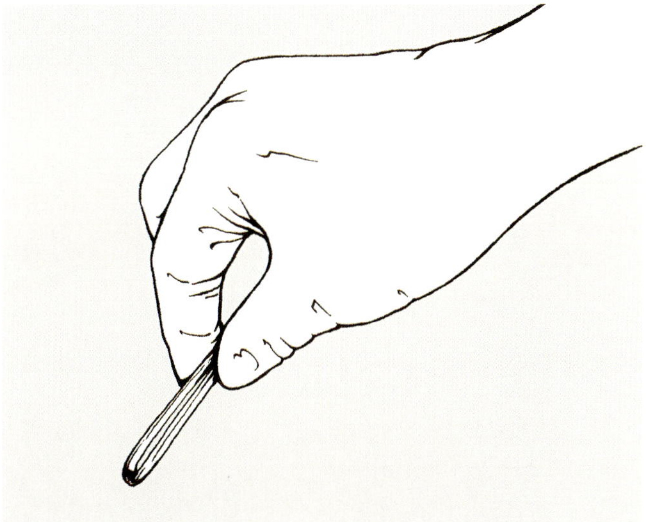

2. The image translated into an ink-line drawing using a dip pen.

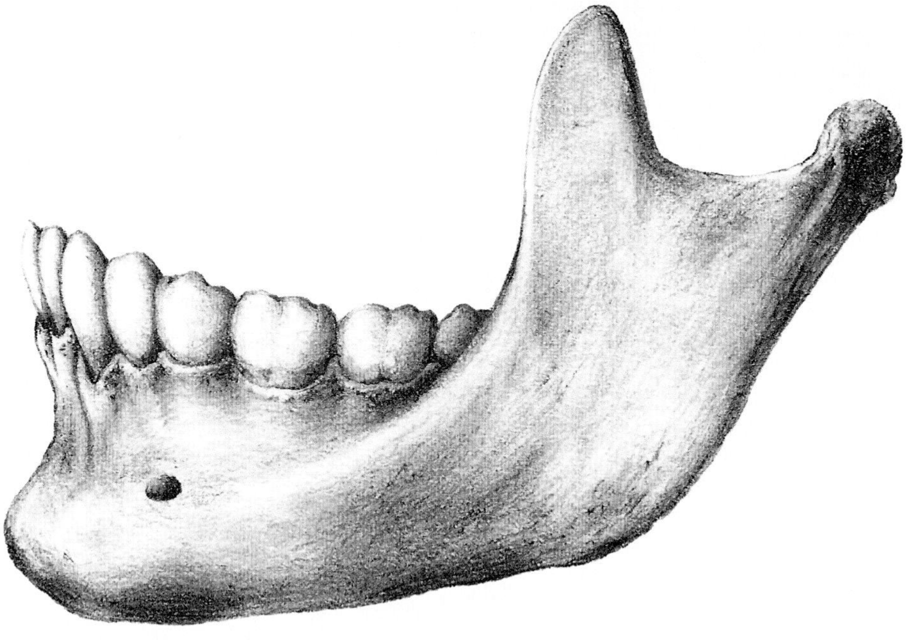

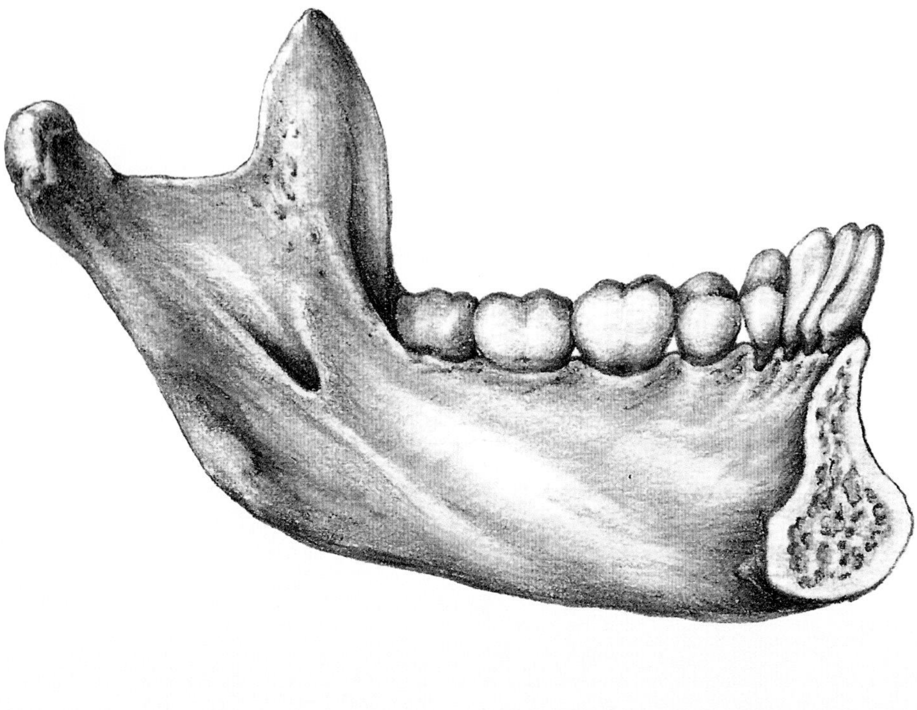

CHAPTER 8

OBSERVATIONAL DRAWING

Eyes are your vessel of observation
The subject being the human form
We bring reality and rationalisation
On any media our work adorns
The lines and colours display the truth
From nowhere is revealed
Your living proof

John Rutherford 2024

Drawing with graphite or pencils is by far the most commonly used and reliable medium to record information, whether creating artworks for pleasure or for work, for sketching or producing detailed graphite line and tonal illustrations for publication. Artwork is increasingly required to be supplied in a digital format; however, whether you begin by drawing with a pencil or on a digital tablet, drawing is the key. Drawing by hand has a more fluid and expressive result, compared to digital illustrations. Primarily we observe and learn visually, meaning we need to be able to see, learn and interpret through direct observation in conjunction with verbal and written communication. This section will look at graphite pencil line drawing and shading tonal values.

DIRECT OBSERVATION

Every artist begins by observing, drawing and creating observational sketches and artworks. Medical art is often described as functional, in that the resulting illustration has had all unnecessary and superfluous visual elements carefully selected, edited or removed, essentially whittling down the information to concentrate and focus on the most important elements. Whether the initial sketches ultimately become a final hand-drawn artwork or are converted into a digital format, good observational and drawing skills underpin a successful result.

Before placing pencil on paper, take time to study your subject or specimen. Spending time really looking in detail is that first important step in understanding what it is that is in front of you. In addition to looking, also feel the object if possible. If, for example, you pick up an apple, first study the subject from every angle, beginning with what shape is it? An apple is never quite round. What does the surface texture look and feel like – is it rough, shiny, textured or smooth? An apple feels surprisingly cold if you close your eyes. Does it feel soft, hard or malleable to the touch? All these observations will enable you to make a more accurate representations in your drawing.

It is very difficult to convey information precisely through your drawing without first understanding the subject thoroughly and knowing exactly what you are looking at, which in medical art is especially relevant. Practise by taking a very familiar object and really studying every aspect. You may find you see many facets that you had either forgotten or simply taken for granted, and features you thought it had that are not actually there at all!

Tonal drawing of a mandible (top: left medial view, bottom: right lateral view).
Graphite pencil tonal work, with shading accomplished using pencil grades between H and B.

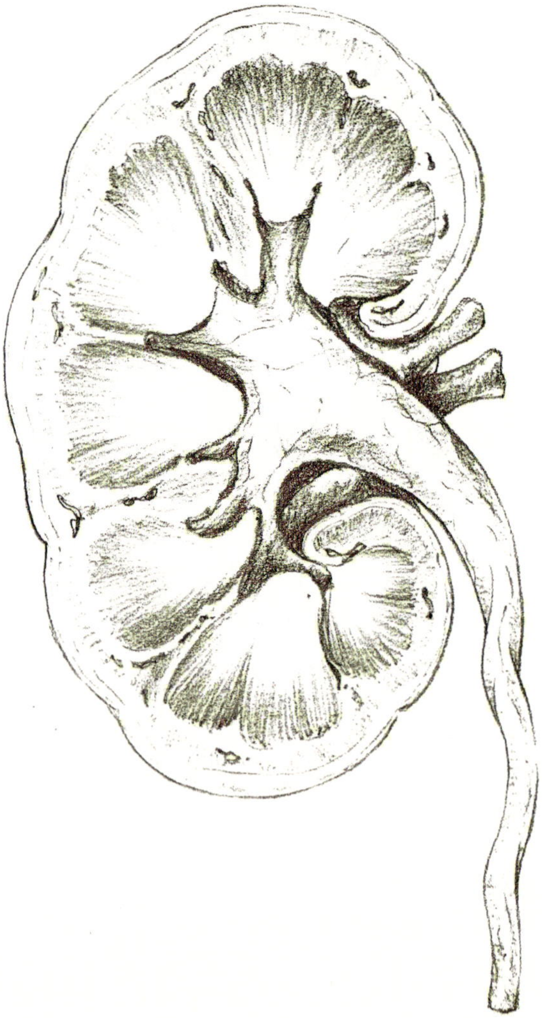

Kidney cross-section. Graphite pencil sketch.

DRAWING IN PENCIL

Pencils are the most frequently used tool of any artist and are indispensable in the studio or portable art case. Graphite pencils (as opposed to coloured pencils) come in different grades, ranging from the harder H (hard) grades through to the softer B (black) grades. By using different pencil grades, this will give you line and tonal flexibility throughout your drawings.

Graphite pencils as we know them today are a fairly recent invention, only coming into significant use from the sixteenth century onwards. Before this time, lead was commonly used, but is not recommended today. Graphite is a crystallised form of carbon, which makes this a very versatile drawing medium. Today pencils have an outer wooden covering, making this format exceptionally easy and comfortable to use.

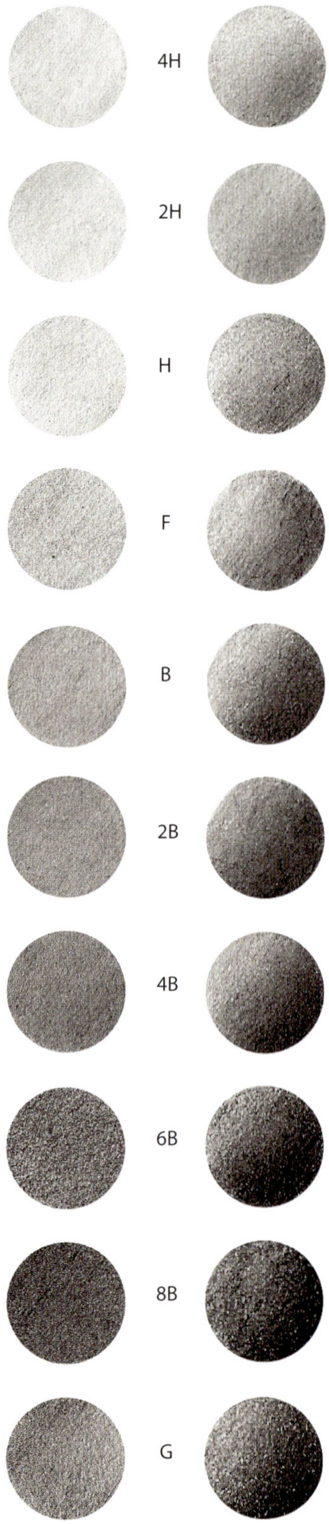

1. The sequence of circles on the left demonstrate pencil grades as evenly shaded tones from 4H down to 6B and a graphite only pencil (G) for comparison. Examples were drawn on heavy weight cartridge paper.

2. The sequence of circles on the right shows the same pencil grades, shaded with added pressure to create a graded tone from left to right. Note that different papers will create different tones and effects.

Graphite Pencils

Observation and drawing with pencils will build your skill by training your hand and eye together to interpret light, tone, shape and texture into a 3D form on paper. Graphite pencils can be purchased singularly or as a box set containing a range of grades between the hardest H grades and the very soft B grades.

H grade pencils contain less graphite and create a paler tone. The hardest grade available is 9H, followed by 8H, 7H, 6H, 5H, 4H, 3H, 2H and then H (the least hard of the H range). The B grades produce increasingly darker tones due to the softer grade of mix with carbon. B grades range though HB, B, 2B, 3B, 4B, 5B, 6B, 7B, 8B, 9B to 9xxB. Between H and B grades, you will frequently find an F (fine) grade pencil. Most boxed pencil sets on the market will contain a reduced range of these grades, often every other number, for example, 6H, 4H, 2H and so on. Every artist develops a preference for a few favourite pencil grades. Choose high-quality artist's grade pencils, which will be more refined and therefore feel less gritty and will give you a smoother result when drawing.

The circles shown in these tonal shaded examples (see left) demonstrate the pencil tonal ranges from 4H to 6B, these being the most common grades found in a pencil set. The second set of circles shows the range in the tonal effect possible with each pencil. An ungraded graphite (G) pencil has been included for comparison.

Project: Pencil Grades

Aim: To create your own pencil tonal charts reflecting the pencils you use.
Art materials required: A set of graphite pencils.
Project: This is a good way to get to know how your pencils work, how they feel and what tone they produce, becoming a useful reference guide for the future. Begin by drawing two sets of circles or squares, allowing one circle or square for each grade of pencil for each set.

Tonal set 1: Shade each circle evenly, working in order from the lightest H grade to the darkest B grade pencil. Label each circle with the pencil grade used.

Graded tonal set 2: Shade these circles in the same order from H through to B, but this time shade lightly on one side and gradually deepen the tonal shade across the circle to very dark, creating a graded tone. Label each circle with the pencil grade you have used.

Expressive Graphite Pencil Lines

When drawing, consider the amount of pressure you are applying to create your line. By using more or less pressure will create darker or lighter lines, or a gradation of line weight. This will in turn support the shape and form you are creating without needing additional tonal shading for just the outline. The change in pressure will create a different interpretation, upgrading a 'flat' drawing to one with three dimensions. Being clear about

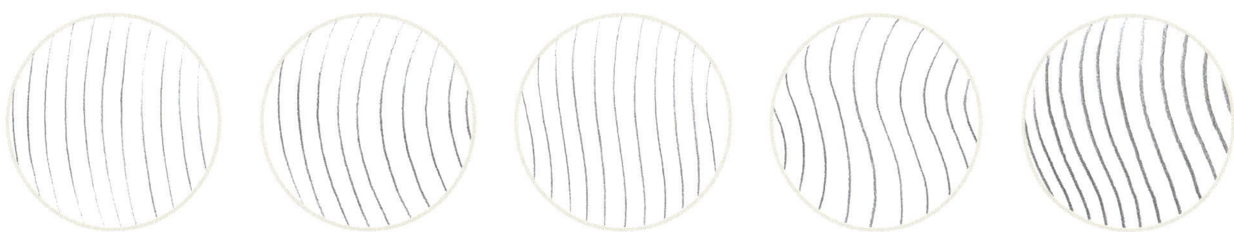

H B 2B 4B 6B

Pencil lines drawn with varying applied pressure to create expressive lines. Pencil grades from left to right: H, B, 2B, 4B and 6B.

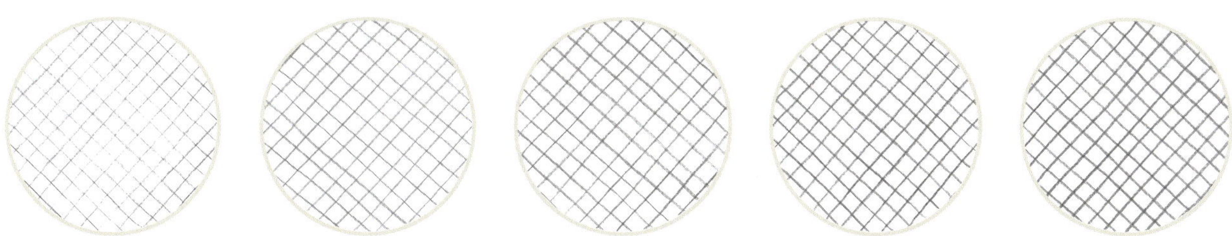

H B 2B 4B 6B

Cross-hatched pencil lines creates additional texture and depth.

what it is you are trying to convey in terms of shape, light and shade will develop with practice. Mastering pencil pressure and tone will carry you though into ink line work and many other media.

Tonal Value for Creating Form and Depth

First look to see where the main direct light source falls onto your object, to find where the highlights, and correspondingly shadows will fall. Identifying which areas are affected tonally by these changes in light is important. Lighting is covered in Chapter 6. In developing your drawing, think of each area you are incorporating, similar to if you are creating a landscape drawing. In general those objects closest to you will have a stronger or darker tonal depth, and those areas further away will have an increasingly softer and lighter tone as they recede into the distance. We naturally perceive darker areas as being closer and lighter areas as further away from us. If you observe a dark-coloured object at a distance, it will be tonally aligned with similar objects at that same distance and will be illustrated tonally equivalent to those surrounding it. Visually this may seem counterintuitive, but creating recession through tonal interpretation will enhance the illusion of three-dimensional depth within your artwork.

When creating pencil tonal drawings, relate the pencil grade to the area you are working on – i.e. use a harder pencil for a lighter area. Then if you find you are beginning to press harder into the paper trying to achieve a darker line, then it's time change the grade of pencil. This will help keep a soft surface appearance to your work and prevent pencil line indents caused by applying too much pressure onto the paper.

Project: Graphite Tonal Studies

Aim: To develop your observational drawing and tonal skills.

Art materials required:

- Pencils ranging from 4H to 4B
- Cartridge paper 220gms
- Putty rubber

Project: Select one or more objects with which to practise observational pencil tonal work in your sketchbook. This may be a bone, a natural history object such as a leaf, acorn or a flower, or any readily available familiar object such as an egg, fruit or vegetable.

Creating Depth

Understanding tone will enhance the illusion of a three-dimensional depth within your work. Begin by choosing the pencil grade you will need according to the tonal value or shade of grey you are trying to achieve. Tone and depth are easier to differentiate when viewed without colour. This is why many examples throughout this text are shown tonally as black-and-white images alongside the colour version for their comparison.

Light and Shade

The light that falls onto an object will determine how you draw, translate and tonally shade your artwork to create your three-dimensional image. Once you have identified where the light source is coming from, there are further considerations to be taken into account:

- Is the light coming from the sun or from a lamp?
- Is there more than one light source – for example, daylight and a desk lamp?
- Is the light source creating a strong and bright light or a soft, diffuse light?
- Is the object in the light, or partially in the shade of another object?
- What material is the object made of? Does it have a shiny or matt surface?
- Is the object a light or dark colour? A very dark object will absorb the light and may not display strong highlights or shadows.

GLOSSARY

Graphite The tonal medium used to create a pencil drawing
Highlight The lightest area indicating where the main light source shines onto your subject
Lead The graphite in the pencil, which is the part that makes the marks (formerly lead was used)
Tone The quality of light/dark
Tonal value The range of tone
Putty rubber A soft, flexible, kneadable rubber
Light source Where the light comes from that is shining on your subject
Shadow or shade The opposite side of the object from where the direct light falls
Reflected light Light that is reflected and/or bounced back onto an object from either the surface it is sitting on or a nearby object. An object may have more than one reflected light source

Tonal Values

The following examples, using a small ball, show the effect of the light source and how this creates the highlights and shadows. The pale ball has a soft surface texture, forming a soft diffuse, shadow with no sharp edges.

Each ball has a highlighted area and a complementary darker shadowed area on the opposite side. In addition, there is also what is termed a reflective light – here this is where you can see the surface of the paper reflecting light back onto the underside of the ball.

The reflected light is not usually brighter than the highlight because it has been bounced back from another surface, thereby reducing its intensity. Every object will be subject to its own reflected light, whether this is from the surface they are resting on or from other items nearby. Reflected light is how we interpret objects in three-dimensional form and is an important element within any drawing. In the examples shown here, each image has also been produced in greyscale – i.e. using only black and white tones – for comparison with the colour image to make it easier to observe the

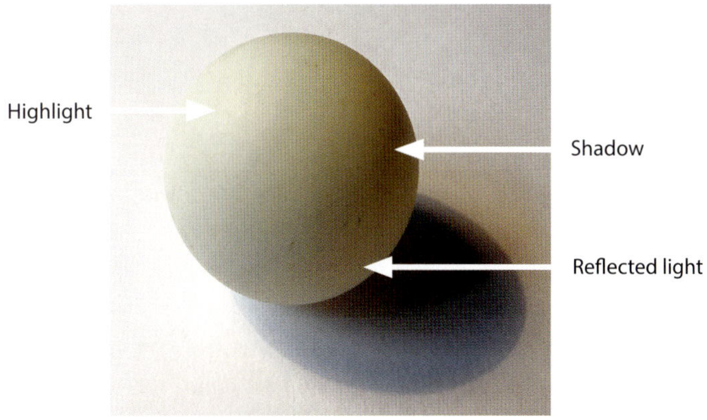

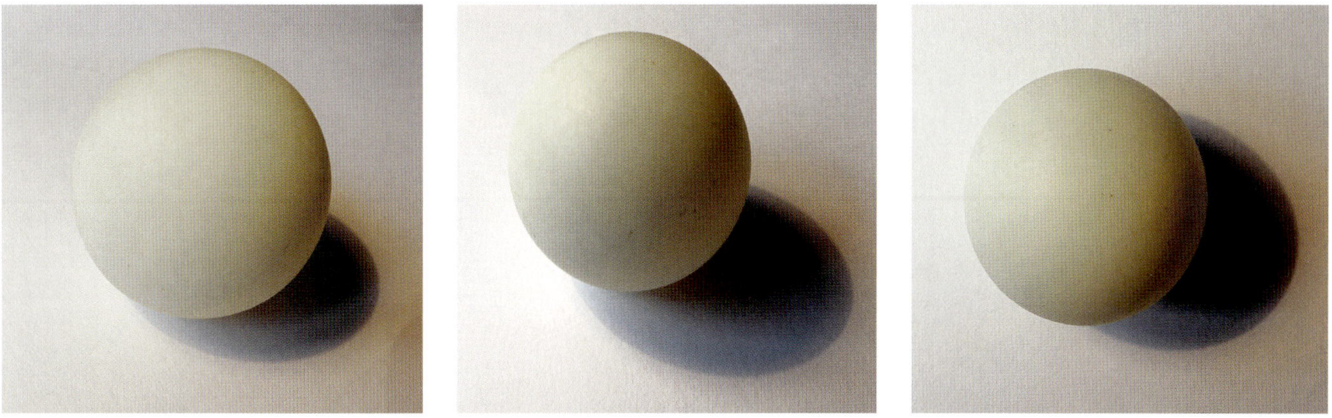

Each individual ball will be influenced by the direcion of the light source as well as reflected light from the surface the ball is placed on. Here you can see how different angles of light and the different viewpoints, affect how and where the highlight, shadows and reflective light fall on each ball.

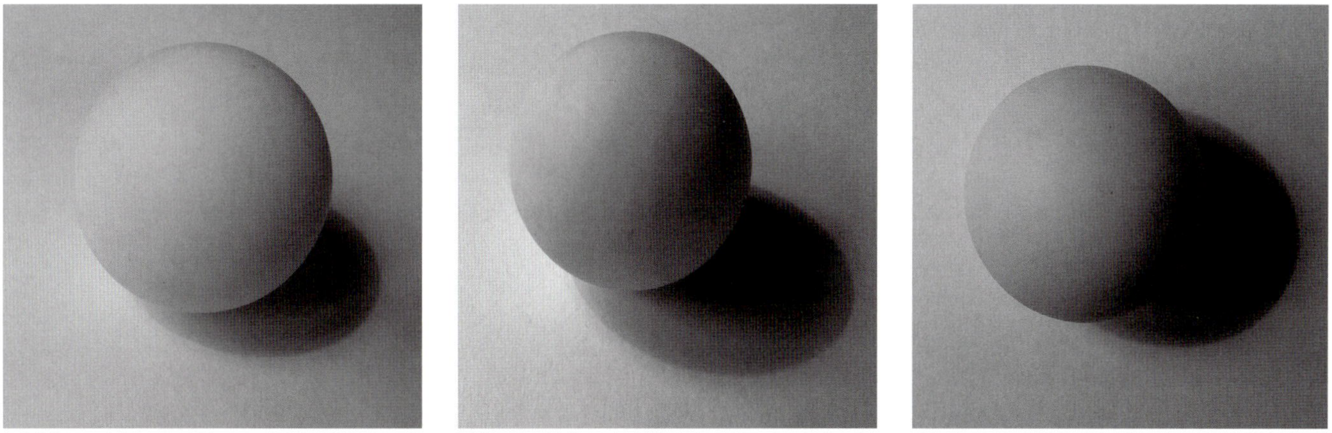

The same balls showing the corresponding highlight, shadows and reflected light as black and white tonal images for comparison.

subtle changes in light and shade. Note that darker colours may be misinterpreted as a shadow.

Note the significant reflected light appearing on each egg being reflected sideways onto the other and how this affects the tonal shading on these neighbouring areas. You can see where the cream egg is reflecting light back both onto the light-coloured egg and onto the darkest egg, which in turn throws a cast shadow over a portion of the cream egg.

Whether you are drawing a ball, an egg or the human form, being aware of how light is directed onto and between structures is essential. Observation of the direction of the primary light source and the areas of reflected light between nearby structures or objects will influence your light and shadow interpretation, whether this is within your pencil, line, tonal or colour artwork.

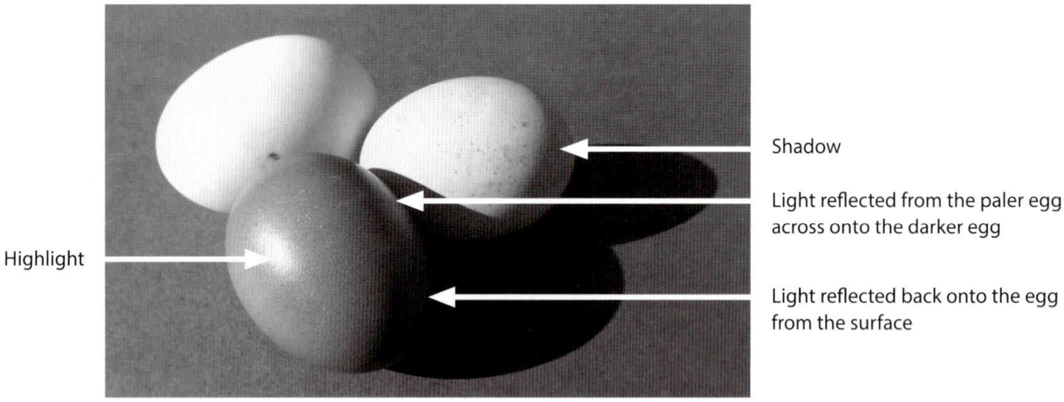

Lighting: areas showing where light creates a highlight, a corresponding shadow and reflected light. Reflected light occurs from both the surface below and from the neighbouring eggs onto each other.

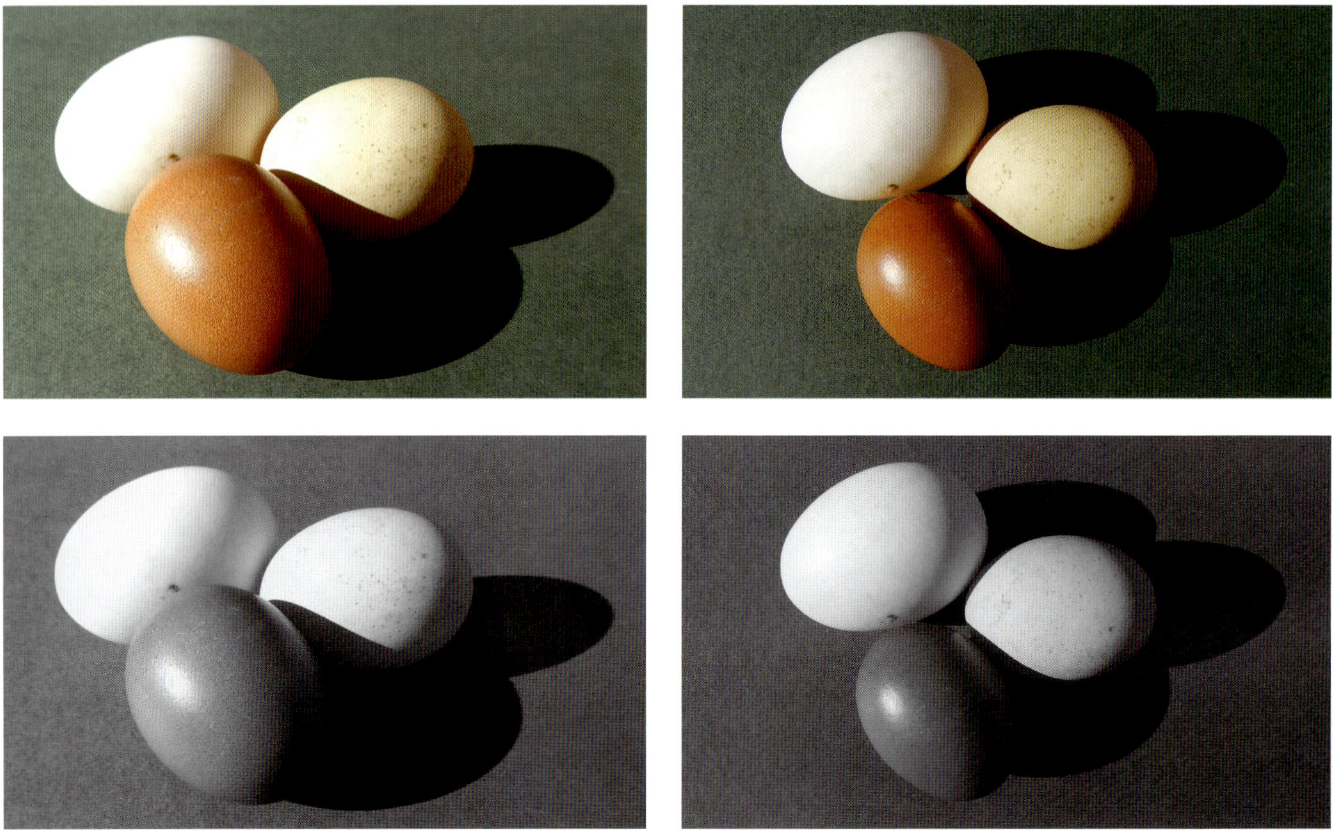

Note the three differing colours or tones of these eggs. The lightest-coloured egg shows the least amount of focused highlight – this is diffused because the light surface of the egg reflects the light back away from itself. The cream-coloured egg also has a diffused surface highlight, whereas the dark brown egg has a more clearly defined highlight with a slightly shinier shell surface.

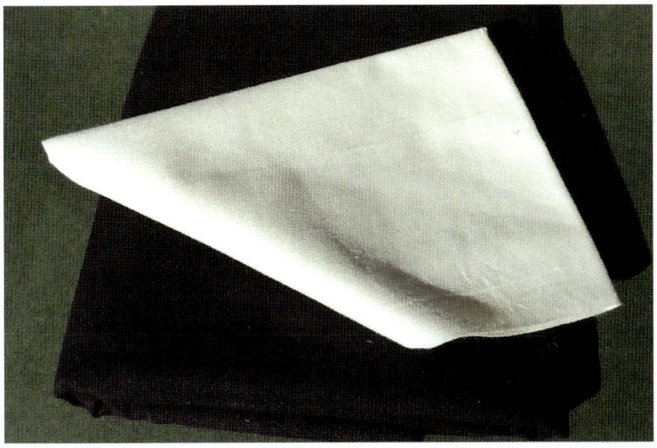

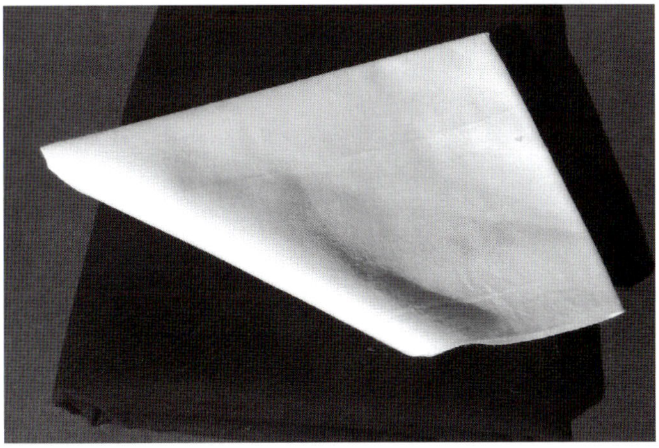

In these cloth images, you will see the darker material absorbs light, leaving only a limited amount of light being reflected back onto the pale cloth above. The black folded cloth beneath the white cloth therefore appears to have little definition in terms of highlights and shadows.

KEEPING A SKETCHBOOK

Keeping a sketchbook for drawing, observation and notes is a frequently underestimated yet important reference tool for any artist. Sketchbooks come in many sizes, but the most portable options, such as A6, A5 or A4, are the most practical. Ideally, your sketchbook will be hardback, to provide a firm supporting surface on which to work, and spiral-bound, so the pages are held securely, can be turned easily and stay open at the desired place. Loose-leaf sketchbooks – those glued along the spine – have the disadvantage that pages may become detached.

Select a good-quality cartridge paper sketchbook for recording your observations and notes. These sketchbooks create records for future work, each note or sketch reminding you of your observations from the day, and will become an essential reference for your final artworks.

Sketchbooks for Medical Artists

Sketchbooks become important reference material for working medical artists, who need to record every detail from first impressions, to where the light source is, to shade, tone and colour indications, size, relative proportions and perspective. All these recorded details will ultimately contribute to creating accurate medical illustrations.

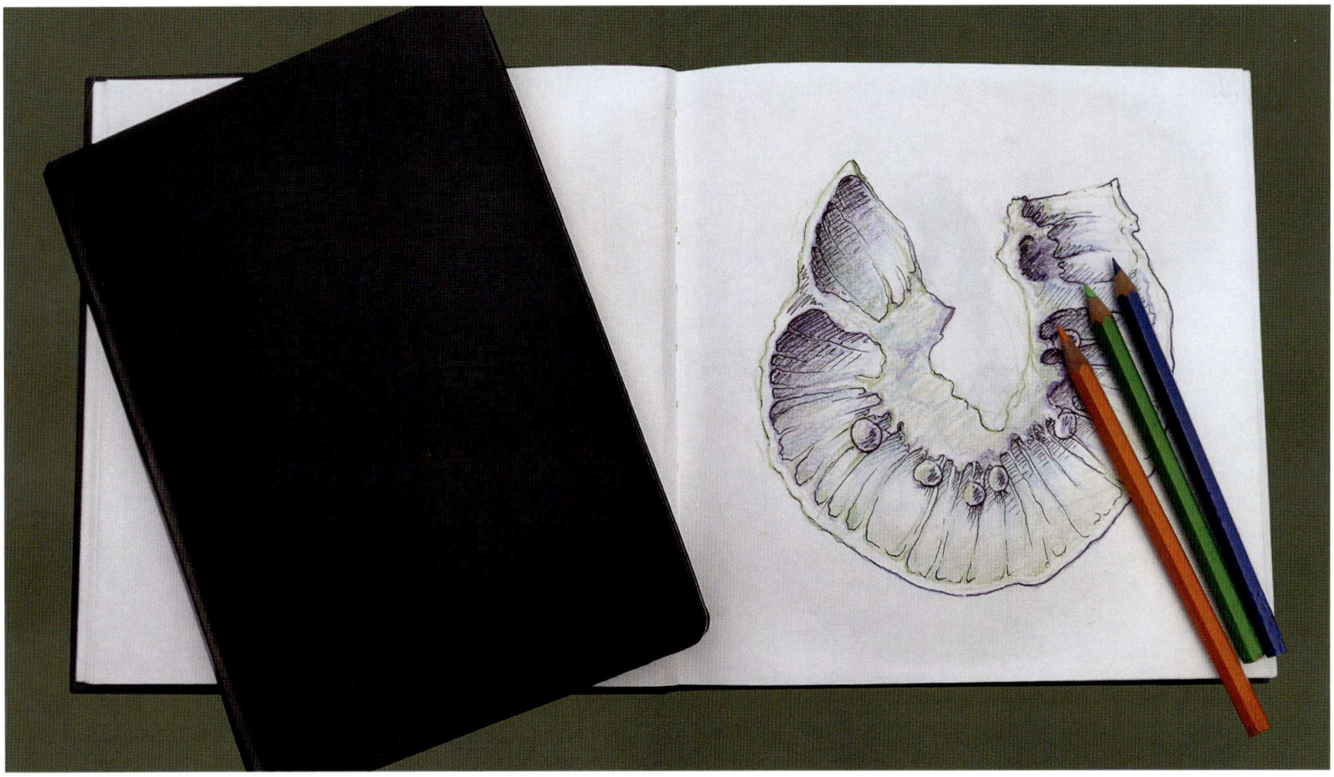

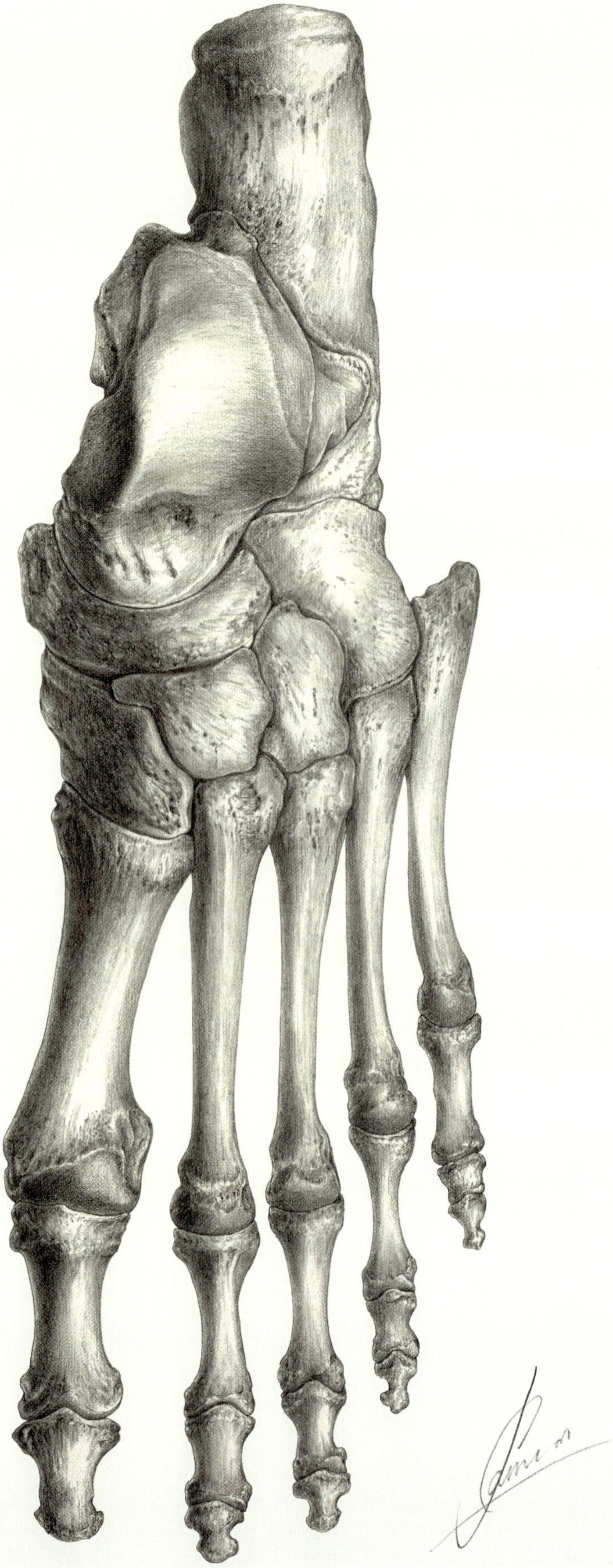

CHAPTER 9

DRAWING BONES

This section looks at how to observe and draw a bone specimen, combining pencil outlines and graphite tonal work and concludes with a step-by-step illustrated bone example to follow.

Working with graphite pencils will give you accuracy and versatility, working from initial sketches through to your completed artwork. Pencils allow you to develop your drawings and artwork tonally. Note-taking and gathering preparatory observations in a sketchbook have been covered in Chapter 8. For bone or any other specimen, it is important to record all the details regarding size, shape, proportions, form, tone and colour precisely.

Today, many bones and specimens are available as a public resource either through visiting a museum or collection in person (*see* Chapter 4) or viewing online databases for reference.

Note, however, that online resources are presented in photographic form, which, of course, is very useful for research, but doesn't compare with working from your own direct observations when it comes to producing accurate drawings. To be able to draw a specimen without having seen the original requires a detailed drawing knowledge acquired through practice and observation. Here we will stay with the basics and practise drawing directly from the specimen and not from a photograph or an online image.

Accurate drawing will develop with practice, and building on your drawing skills by direct observation will stand you in good stead. 'Direct observation' in this context means observation directly by eye, followed by your eyes and hand working together in coordinaton to translate what you see into artworks.

EQUIPMENT

Pencils

Select artist quality pencils whenever possible, as these will invariably have a finer graphite lead and therefore, be smoother to work with. Pencils and their grades are covered in Chapter 8.

Paper

Pencils may be used on a variety of surfaces. For medical art and illustrations, a high-quality heavyweight cartridge paper in the region of 200gms-plus with a smooth surface is recommended.

Rubbers

There are a plethora of options available, and it is a good idea to try as many as you can to determine the materials you prefer to work with. Note that while one rubber might be perfect in a studio setting, another may be more appropriate for taking out and about. Keeping your rubbers or putty rubber in their own small case or tub will keep them clean and dust-free.

Bones of the left foot. Graphite pencil tonal drawing.

SETTING UP

First, before you begin drawing your bone, there are two key elements to consider: the lighting or light source and how you subsequently position the specimen ready for drawing.

Light Source

Before you begin drawing, always consider where your light is coming from because it will have an impact on your work. Is the light source coming at the top left, top right or directly above you? Consider whether you are in the best position. Do you have clear light onto the specimen and a well-lit area in which to work, or will you be potentially drawing in the shadow of your own hand? For right-handers, it is best to have the light coming from top left, and for left-handers, from top right.

The position of your light source with regard to your subject is very important when considering how to interpret the form and structure, and how to create this on paper. In essence, you are converting the 3D object in front of you into an image on a 2D paper surface, interpreting it through your pencil lines and tonal work back into a visually understandable 3D object! Planning a well-positioned light source will significantly help you to achieve a more realistic drawing.

A drawing may take many hours, so it is important to have considered all these elements before you start.

Number of Sessions

Whether or not you can complete your preliminary drawings in one session is an important consideration for any sizeable project because of the need to ensure consistent lighting. If you are drawing in a museum, for example, and need to make more than one visit, are you able to come at the same time of day on each occasion, which would be advisable to give you the best chance of consistent lighting. Morning light is very different from afternoon light. Even if you plan to rely solely upon artificial lighting, this may still be affected by daylight creeping in. For larger projects, an initial pre-drawing visit to the venue is advisable to select the best time for drawing.

MAPPING THE BONE SPECIMEN

Your eye position in relation to your bone specimen is important. Whatever the size, it is essential to be able to examine the whole length of the bone at eye level, a process called mapping. If the bone is held vertically within a clamp, or attached by a wire to a supporting backboard, you may then slide the bone up or down the clamp or wire support by small increments so that a different part

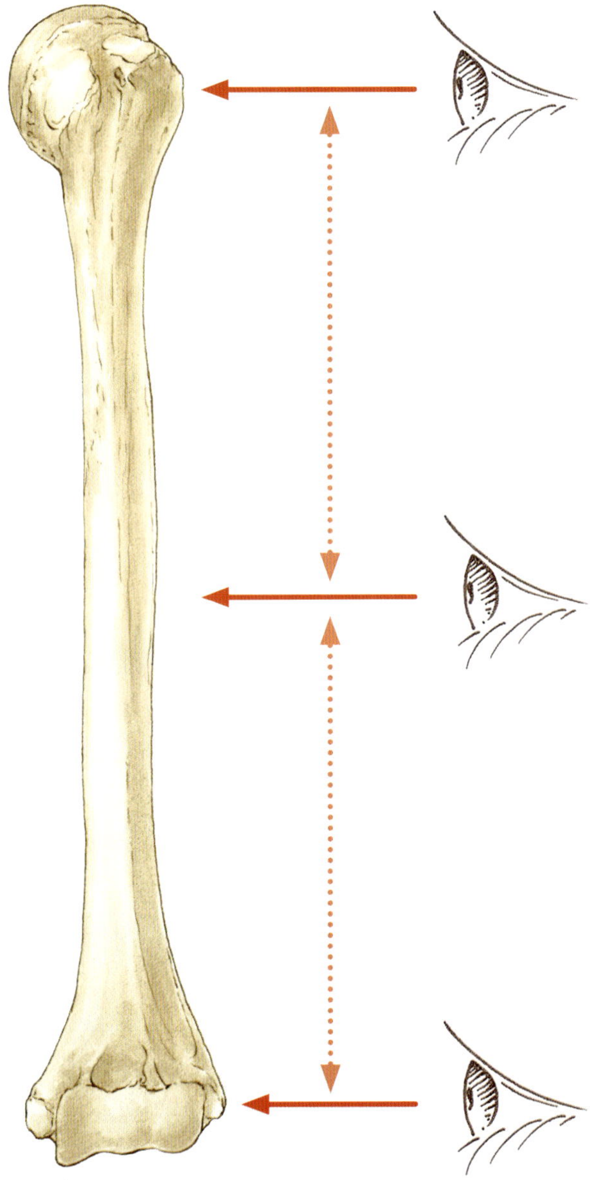

Mapping a bone
It is essential to be able to view the whole bone from end to end progressively from top to bottom and not from just a single viewpoint. A single viewpoint will give you a distorted and limited view of all the elements. To achieve a full 'mapping' of the bone, move either the bone or your eye view (see right) until you have observed the whole length of the bone straight on from end to end.

of the bone is at eye level each time. Continue moving the specimen until you have studied and recorded the whole length of the bone.

BONE FEATURES

Every bone in the human body has developed its own specific shape, with each feature having a particular purpose. For every lump, bump or indent, ask yourself, 'what it is for?'. What is the purpose of each smooth, rough or textured area or prominence, is it developed by use or evolution? Considerations could include questions such as, does a muscle or ligament attach or insert here? Does a smoother area indicate a joint or articular surface with another bone? Specific foramina may indicate nerves or vessels arising within or circling around the bone. Alternatively, could the feature be the result of an accident, such as a fracture? Studying your bone in conjunction with an illustrated anatomical textbook is recommended.

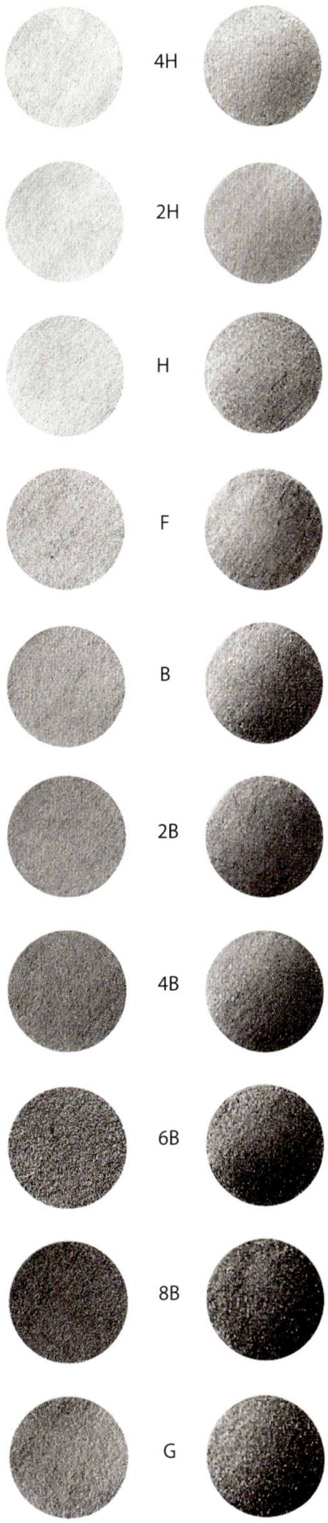

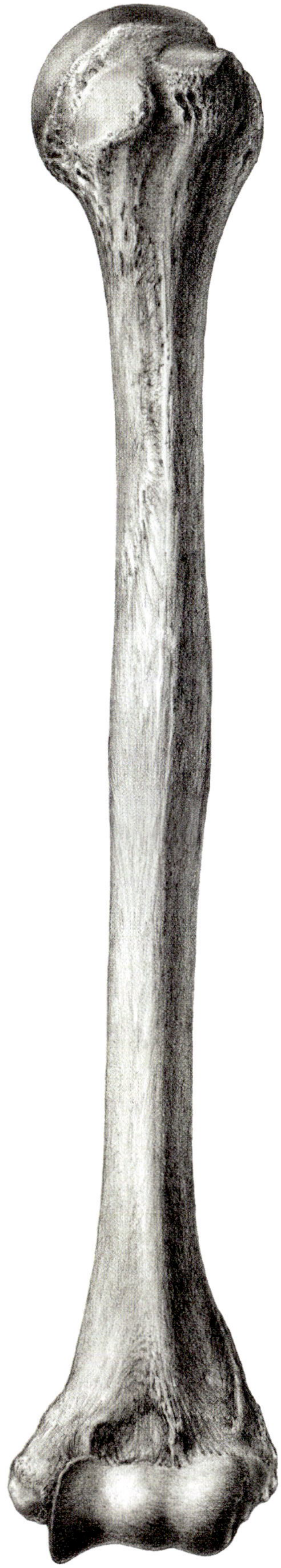

Anterior view of the left humerus.
Tonal graphite pencil drawing.

The humerus links anatomically to the clavicle and scapula superiorly, and at the elbow joint which includes the ulnar and radius bones of the forearm.

Tonal ranges of pencil weights, progressing from the lighter H grades to darker and softer B grades have been included here for comparative information (also refer to page 78).

The Humerus

As a good example, this section will look at the humerus (the upper arm bone), selecting a few surface details and structures that can be clearly distinguished.

The smooth areas at either end of the humerus are the respective joints' (elbow and shoulder) articular surfaces. These surfaces are smooth compared to the rest of the bone, allowing the joints to move freely during movement. These joints have their own capsule, circumnavigating the whole joint as a slightly irregular raised line and sited just below the smooth articular surface.

The medial humeral head has a deep groove through which one of the two tendons of the biceps muscle pass ('bi' meaning two). This tendon arises from the coracoid of the clavicle, passing over the top of the shoulder joint and down through this groove. The biceps muscle then attaches to a broad area lower down the humerus. This can be clearly seen on the anterior medial surface near the humeral head.

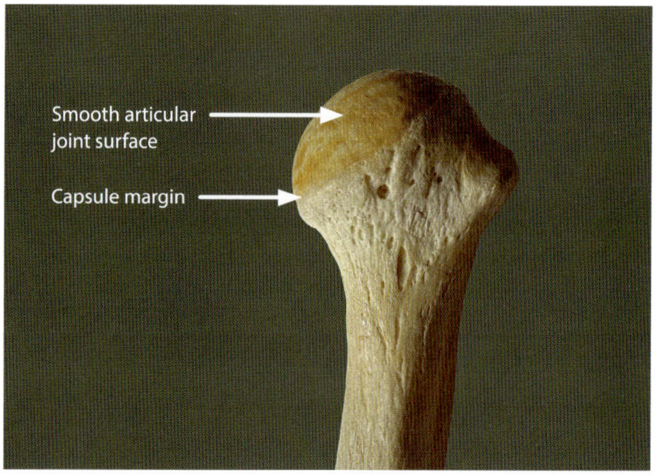

The smooth articular surface of the humeral head is distinct from the rest of the bone surface, separated by the capsule margin.

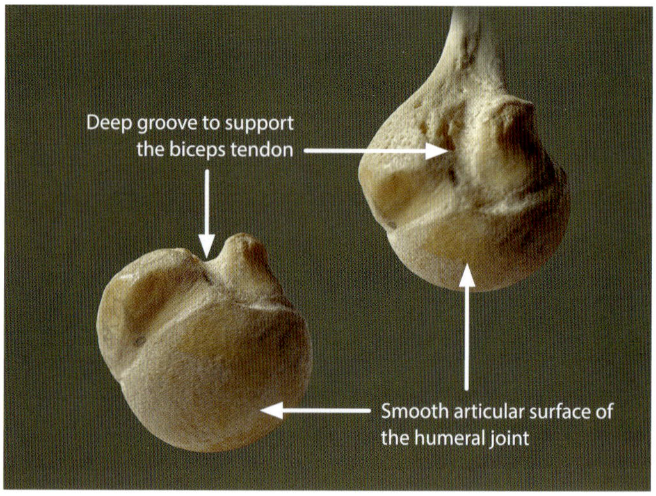

The humeral head viewed from above – superiorly, showing the deep groove which supports the strong biceps tendon.

Project: Bone Studies

Aim: Mapping a humerus bone and developing a graphite tonal pencil drawing.

Art materials required:

- Pencil grades 4H to 6B (for a more subtle result, limit range to 2H–2B)
- A3 cartridge paper 220gms
- Pencil sharpener
- Putty rubber
- Callipers or measuring device

Project: To observe, map, accurately measure and record an anatomical humerus bone specimen.

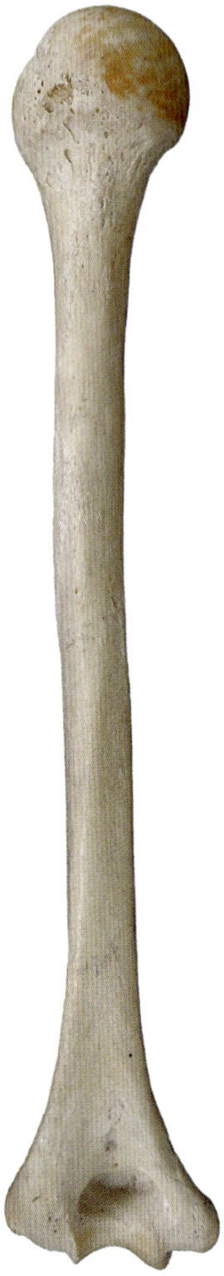
Humerus: posterior view.
Note the areas of surface damage around the lateral distal end.

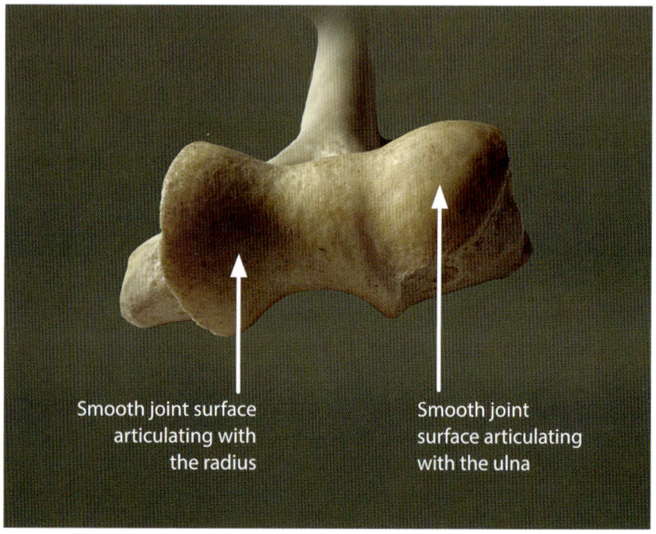

The distal end of the humerus at the elbow joint has a set of distinctive irregular ridges forming a smooth joint surface, articulating with the radius and ulnar bones of the forearm.

ARTICULATED SPECIMENS

Bone specimens are prepared and stored either as individual bones or as collections (*see* Chapter 4). The human body has around 350 separate joints. Joint articulation refers to where two or more bones align together; these joints may or may not move. The images here show the bones of the foot articulated with a clear wire line. This is a specialised skill where the bones of the body have been placed in the correct anatomical position and joint alignment and joined together, representing how the bones would be inside the body.

The foot example below shows several bones articulated to more than one other neighbouring bone. Holes have been drilled through each bone and threaded with wire, leaving a flexible space between each bone. This has been done for educational teaching purposes, enabling the joint to be viewed from all aspects. When the wires are pulled tight, the bones fit back together in the correct anatomical position. Note, however, that the metatarsal and phalangeal bones may twist around the supporting wires. They will need to be turned manually to place them in the correct anatomical position before beginning your drawing.

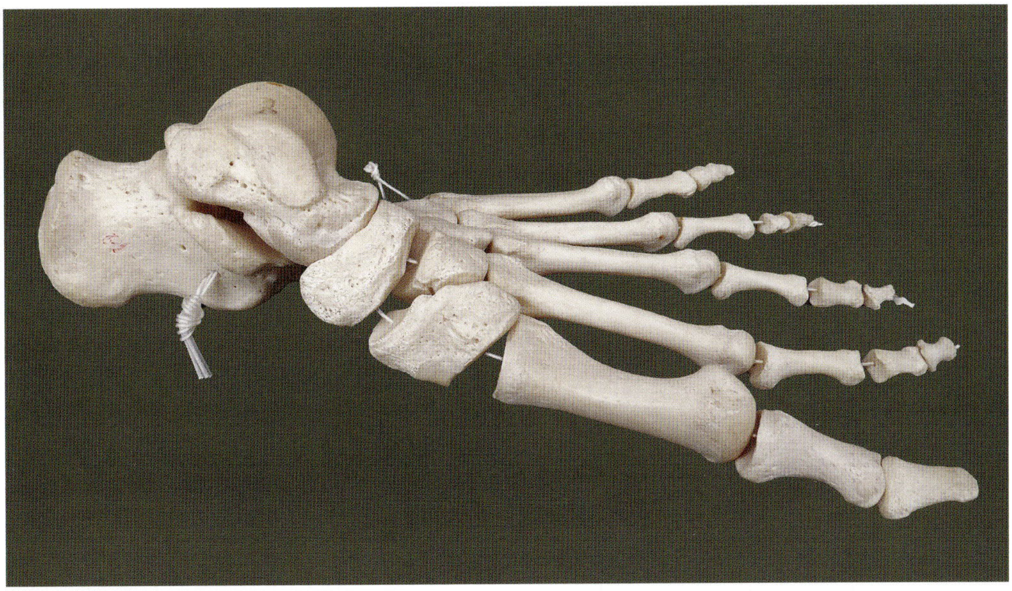

Medial view of the left foot. The bones have been articulated together with wires. Several bones articulate to more than one other neighbouring bone.

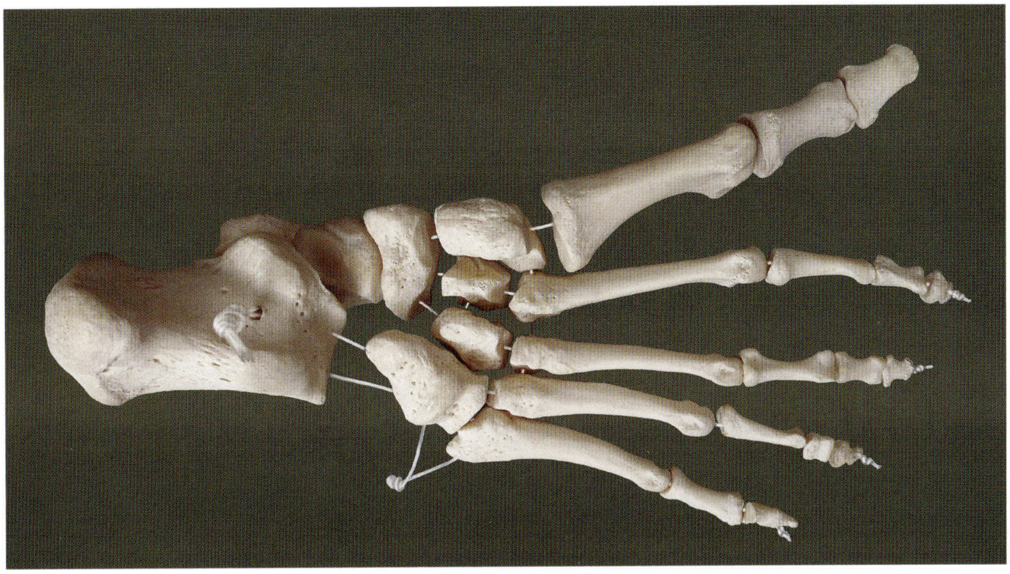

Plantar view of the left foot. Many bones have interconnecting wires across the arch of the foot, i.e. they are wired in more than one direction. You will also see this with articulated bone specimens of the hand for example.

Steps

1. Select your bone specimens and follow the information for observing and measuring your specimens. Measure the three bones of the toe forming an initial accurate outline.

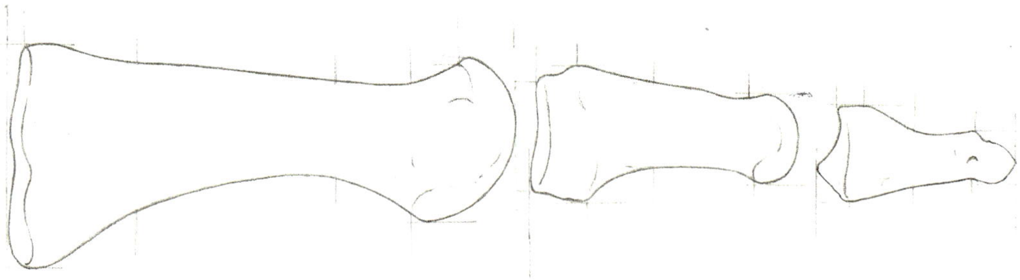

2. Begin building the shape and tone of the three bones.

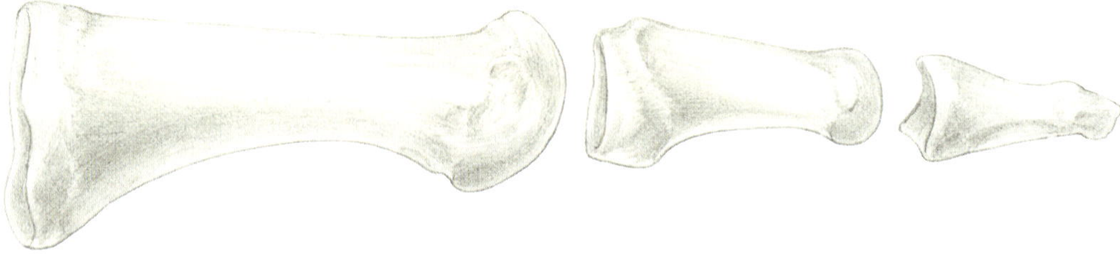

3. Continue building the form 'as a whole'.

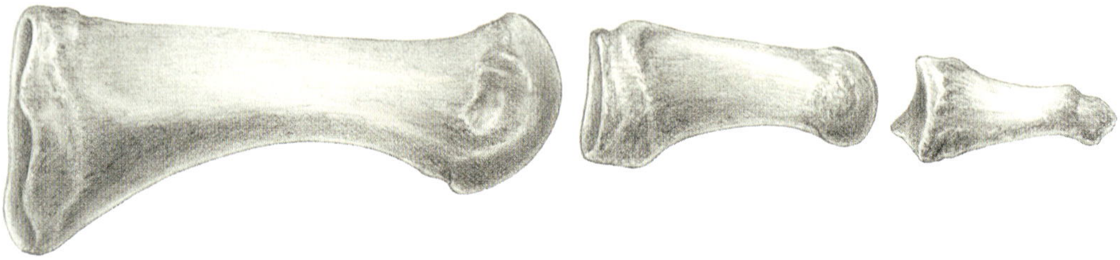

4. Complete the artwork by including all the surface details.

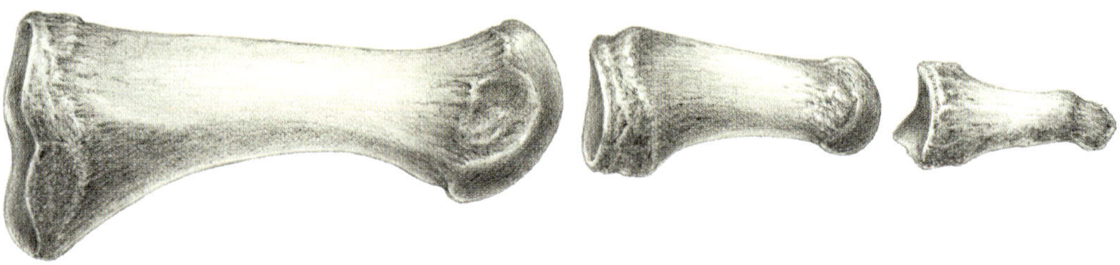

Step by step: Measuring and recording to create a pencil outline, developing into a series of final detailed artworks of the big toe.

Step by Step: Recording a Bone Specimen

Aim: To observe, map, measure and accurately record an anatomical bone specimen. This example demonstrates drawing the bones of the great toe, more commonly known as the big toe. The bones of the big toe include the first metatarsal and the proximal and distal phalanx.

This step-by-step project begins by taking precision measurements in preparation for a pencil outline, before the artwork is completed tonally in pencil, shown here developed through four drawing stages (left).

Steps:

1. Place the bones on a white background, such as a blank sheet of paper. Check your lighting to ensure the bones are lit evenly. Measure the overall length of the bones and mark the measurements lightly on the paper, noting the maximum width and height to enable the positioning of the specimen centrally on your paper. Measure each bone individually, noting any specific points of reference. Collate your measurements and lightly mark points and/or lines on the paper. Keep these lines very light so they can be easily removed by a rubber once the artwork is complete. Once you have placed your measurement points, carefully create a light outline with an H or 2H pencil. It is worth taking great care at this stage in measuring and noting the proportions because it is harder to make changes to the shape and form later.
2. When you have completed your measured outline, start adding light tonal pencil shading, beginning with the more shaded areas. It is best to build the drawing up as a whole, working on each part equally; avoid falling into the trap of completing one area in detail, only to find this may later need to be changed either lighter or darker. Working on the image 'as a whole', ensures an even and consistent approach across the artwork.
3. Continue to build up the tonal range across the whole artwork, including the lighter areas and to begin to work on specific surface details.
4. To complete the drawing, continue working across the artwork as a whole. Gradually increase the tone in all areas and concentrate on the overall form. Add detailed features such as the foramina, show the smooth joint surfaces and the articular ridge, and identify areas where muscle, tendon or ligaments attach.

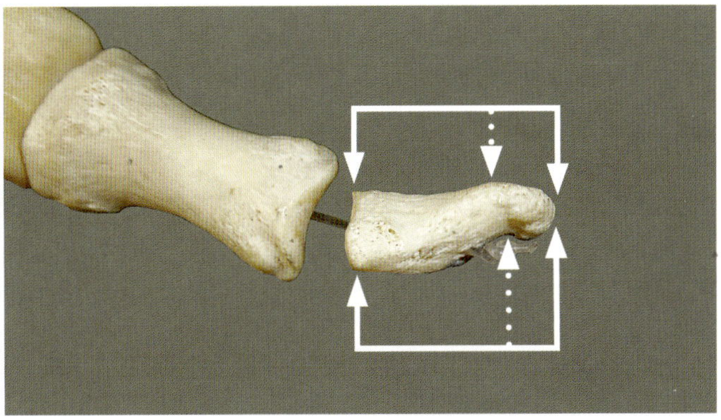

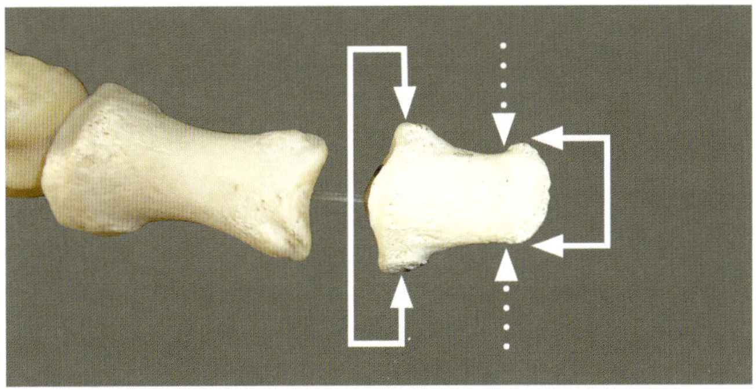

Measure each bone from both the lateral and superior views, together with any additional features.

Project: Bone Studies in Graphite Pencil

Aim: To develop skills in recording bone specimens.

Art materials:

- Pencil grades 4H to 6B
- A4 or A3 sketchbook or cartridge paper 220gms
- Pencil sharpener
- Putty rubber
- Callipers or measuring device

Project: Select a bone specimen, either a human or animal, such as the fox skull below, taking care to choose bones of a manageable size. Begin by observing, then map, measure and accurately record the bone specimen. Keep a sketchbook of your reference studies.

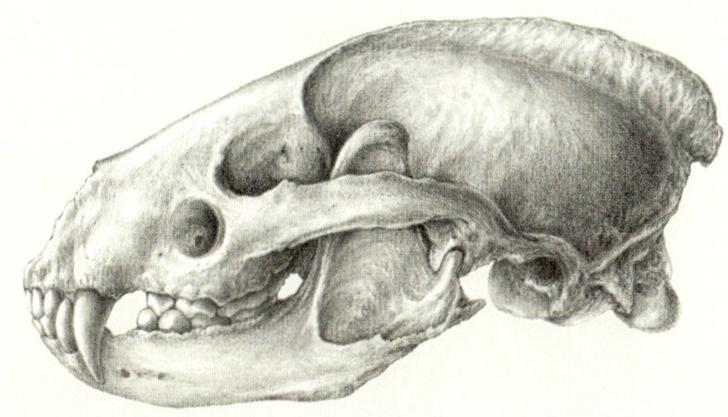

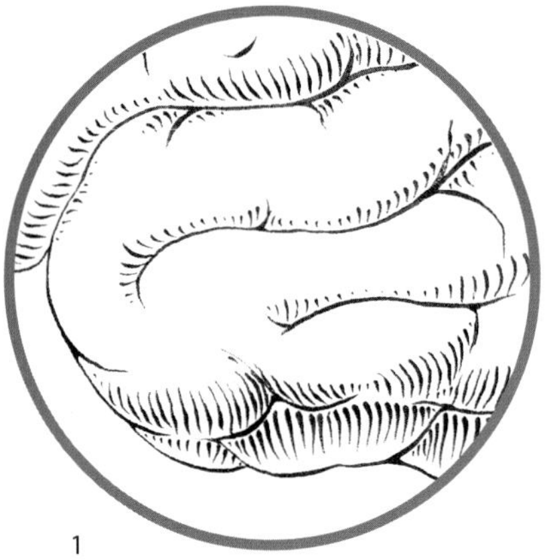

1

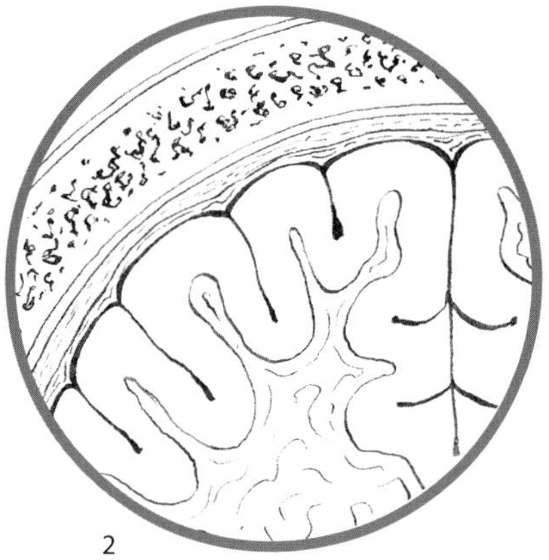

2

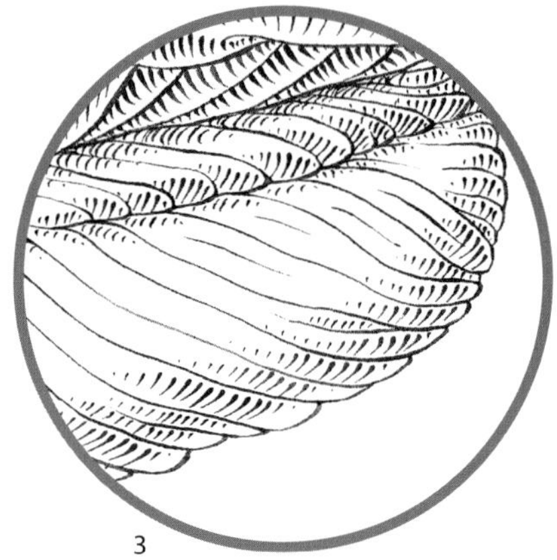

3

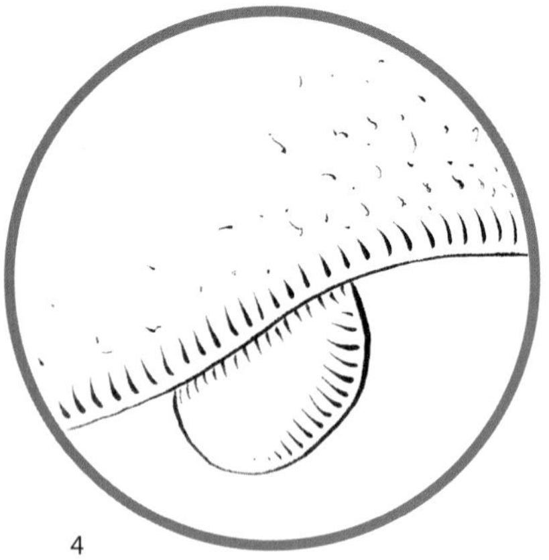

4

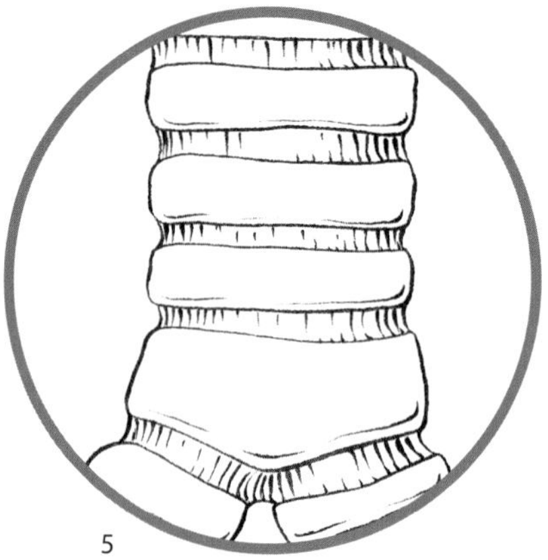

5

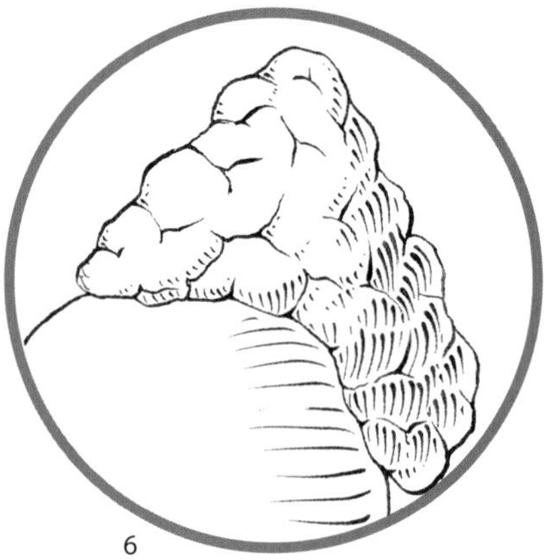

6

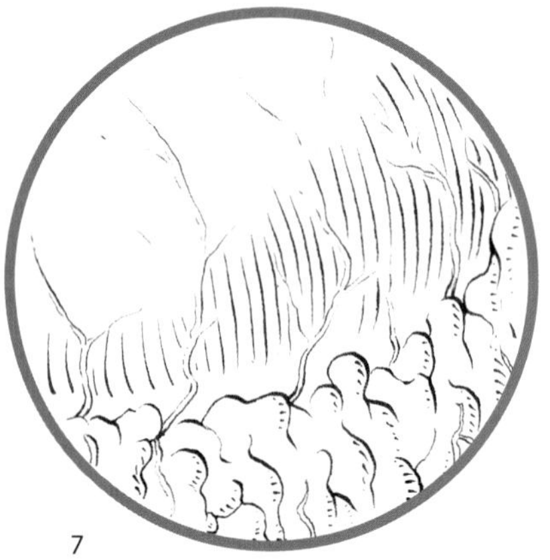

7

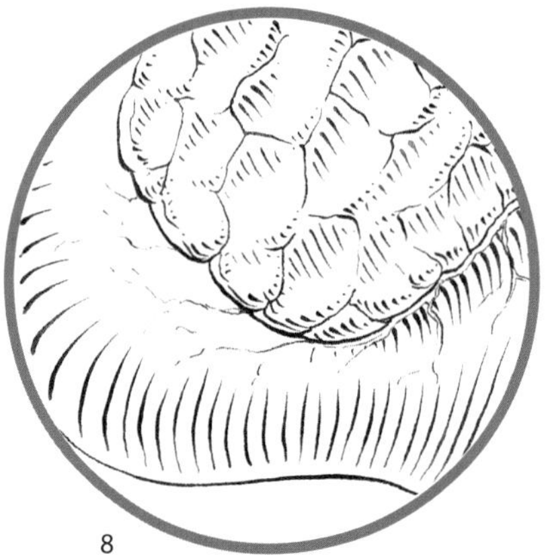

8

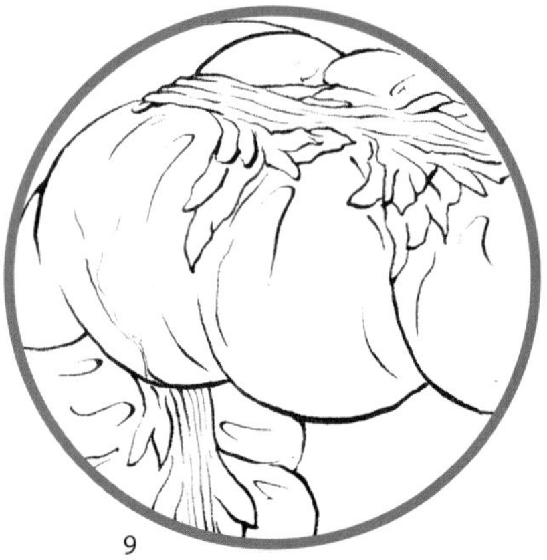

9

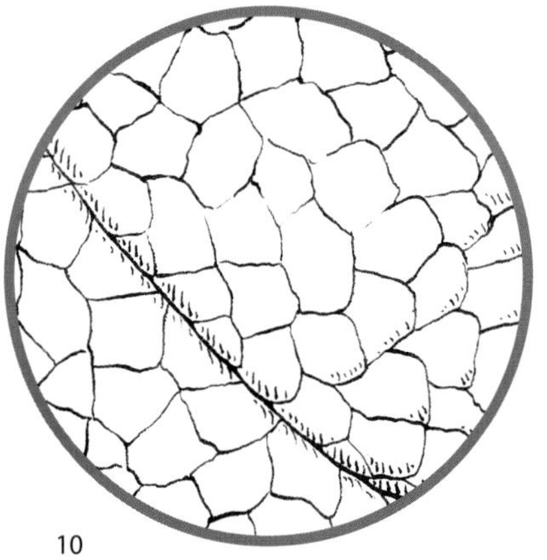

10

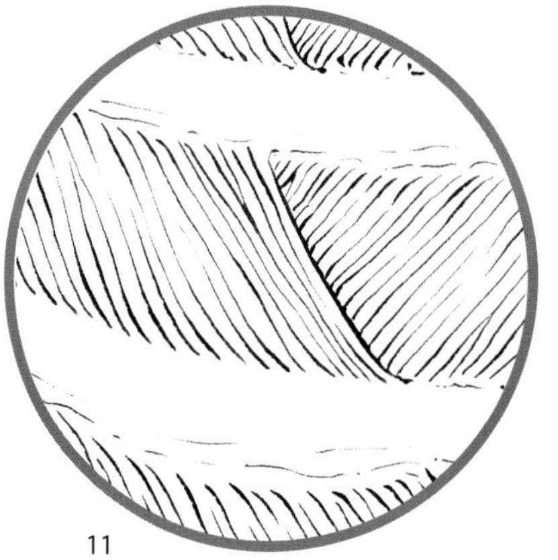

11

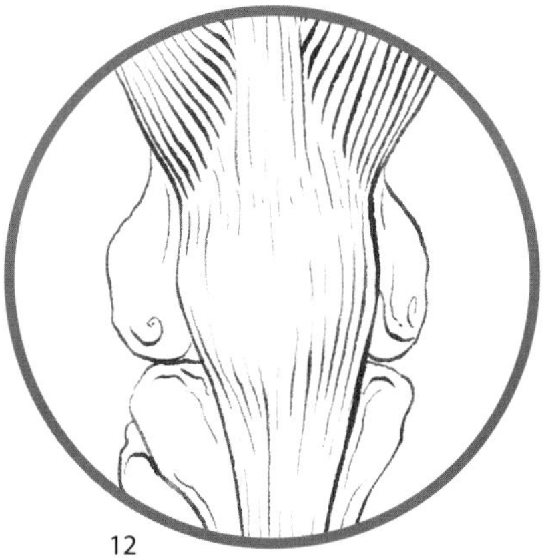

12

CHAPTER 10

DRAWING WITH INK

Producing illustrations and diagrams in pen and ink has been and continues to be a staple medium for medical artists to create clear anatomical illustrations, defining surgical procedures, patient information and diagrams. Black ink on a white paper background is popular for its ease of reproduction and publication qualities. Nowadays, digital illustration has largely replaced hand-created artwork for many areas; however, the expressive nature of dip pen illustration and other forms of ink work means it has endured. This section covers a variety of pen and ink options, concentrating primarily on the dip pen, with anatomical examples to develop your own technique.

PENS

There are only a few materials needed for creating ink work – primarily a variety of pens and nibs, inks and paper. Working in pen and ink creates instinctive and expressive artworks, which digital mediums often lack. Ink artworks are formed primarily with linear strokes, which may be applied evenly, or with gradated pressure forming a changing flowing line, or cross-hatched for form, effect and contrast. Working with ink can be rather addictive once you begin! You may find yourself collecting a range of different pens, nibs, inks and paper and even experimenting to make your own inks.

There are many pen options to choose from, beginning with the traditional feather.

Quill Pen

Feathers were traditionally used for writing and drawing. A large, sturdy feather such as a swan or seagull feather can be used as a pen. These can be collected, cleaned and the ends carefully cut to produce a nib. A feather in the studio is also very useful for brushing rubbings or dust gently away from the surface of your artwork.

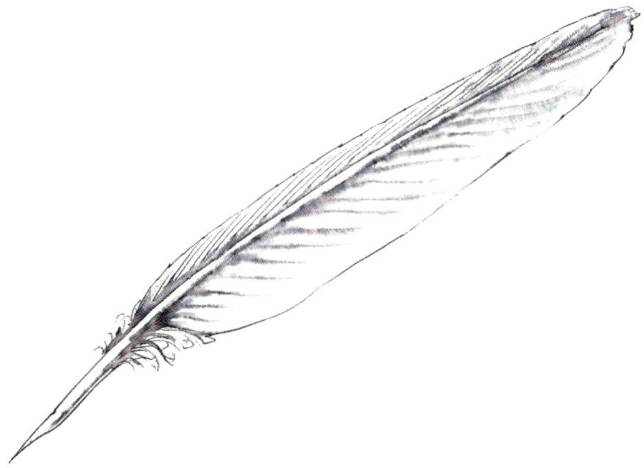

Twelve anatomical representational ink line illustrations.
1 A portion of the left cerebral surface of the brain, lateral view. 2 Frontal cross-section through the cranium (skull), revealing lobes and fissures of the brain. 3 Lateral view of the exterior surface of the cerebellum. The cerebellum lies in the posterior fossa. 4 The inferior margin of the right lobe of the liver, with the gall bladder (in green) below. 5 Bifurcation of the trachea (windpipe), showing the annular ligaments between the tracheal cartilages.
6 Adrenal (suprarenal) gland above the right kidney. 7 Lower portion of the stomach, showing the edge of the greater omentum and its attachment along the edge of the stomach. The omentum is a fold or peritoneal flap covering and connecting the stomach to the other abdominal organs. 8 The duodenum (small intestine) and head of the pancreas. The duodenum is the first section of the small intestine from the stomach. The pancreas is important for digestion, creating enzymes that help break down food. 9 The colic flexure and transverse section of the colon (large intestine). The large intestine often has many small fatty appendices called epiploicae. 10 A fissure separating lobes of the right lung. 11 External and internal intercostal muscles, giving flexibility between the ribs. 12 Ligaments of the patella. The medial and lateral rectus muscles sit above the knee, and the tendon of the rectus femoris muscle runs centrally between these muscles to the patella. The patella ligament is attached inferiorly to the tibia.
The corresponding watercolour images can be found on Page 128.

Dip Pens and Nibs

Here we will focus on the dip pen style nib known as the pointed or quill-style nib, used with a traditional or classic straight pen handle. Working with a dip pen creates natural feel and expressive line by changing the weight, pressure and emphasis down through your hand to the pen. The human body is a natural subject and the expressive lines that can be created with a dip pen suit this and other scientific subjects.

Pen nibs come in a large variety of styles, shapes and sizes, depending on their intended purpose. Those with fine and flexible tips create flowing lines, varying from the most delicate to extra thick bold lines.

Nibs can be bought singularly or as a set and are easy to use and clean. When purchasing pen nibs, always check each one carefully. Make sure that the nib body or shank is straight or slightly curved depending on the design – that is, not bent or out of shape. The nib should taper evenly from the shoulder down through the two tines (the two split nib sections) to the very tip. Check from the breather hole to the tip end, looking to see that both sides of the tines are even and straight – that is, one

ANATOMY OF A DIP PEN

Tip or point May be made of either the same or a different material
Tines The nib is divided into two tines, with a slit between them; when pressure is applied they will spread apart to create a wider line.
Vent or breather hole This area acts as an ink reservoir from which the ink flows down to the tines. Pens may sometimes have an integral reservoir built into the handle.
Shoulders The widest part of the nib supports the two main tines. Some nibs may also have further slits either side of the vent hole for flexibility.
Body or shank The main part of the nib, which is inserted into the pen holder
Tail or heel The rounded end of the nib
Imprint The make and style of the pen usually printed along the shank
Ferrule A ring, often made of metal, which holds the nib securely in place
Holder or handle The body of the pen, which holds the nib

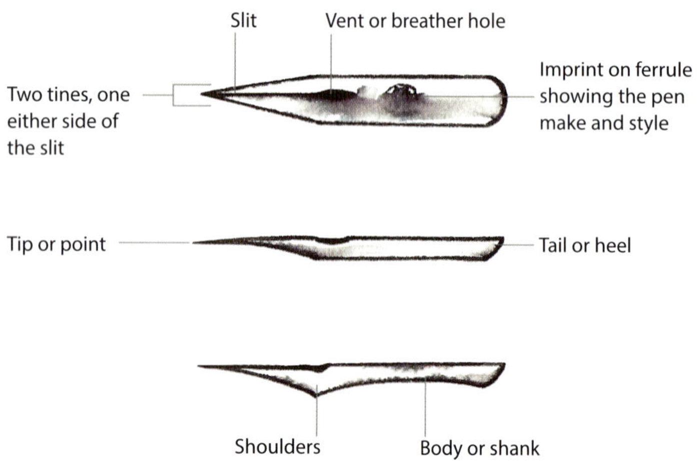

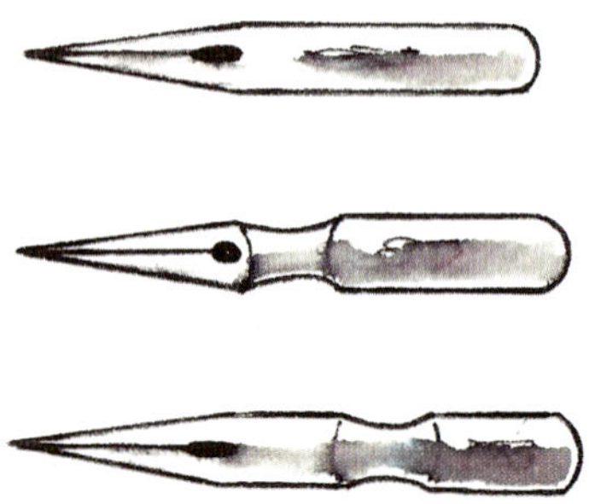
Ink nibs come in many different styles

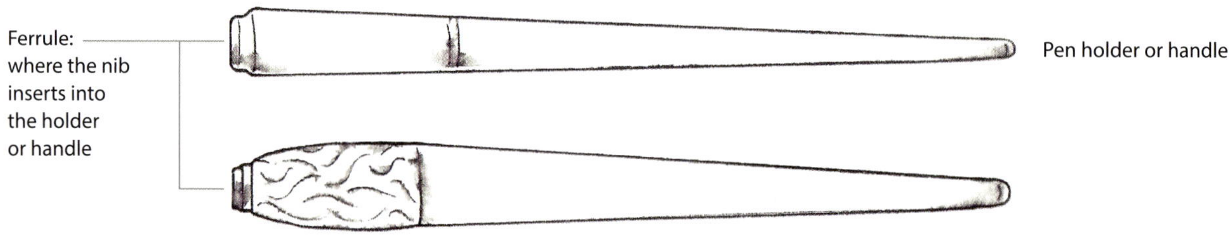
Ferrule: where the nib inserts into the holder or handle
Pen holder or handle

side should not be larger or longer than the other; this rarely occurs, but if the tines are uneven in either width or length, the ink will not flow smoothly and the nib may snag on the paper.

Drawing with a dip pen gives you the greatest versatility and expressiveness of line. Classic-style dip pens have the advantage of being equally suitable for right- and left-handers. Varying line widths are achieved by changing the amount of pressure you apply with your hand; increasing the pressure pushes the tines of the nib slightly further apart, gradually creating a thicker line by allowing more ink to flow onto the paper. If you are unsure about a style of nib, always ask the sales assistant; they may allow you to try a sample nib before purchasing. Nibs are inexpensive, so it is advisable to purchase a selection, acquiring a few as spares and for replacements, while working there will be the inevitable breakage over time.

Dip pens also have the advantage that you can switch quickly and easily between pen nibs, sizes and styles to suit the work required. After use, always remove the nibs from the holder to clean, dry and store them ready for next time. Follow the maker's instructions for cleaning before you use a nib for the first time, as some have an initial protective coating. For most nibs, cleaning with water and a paper towel will be fine; however, stronger cleaning fluids such as alcohol may be needed for cleaning if the ink has become too dry and caked onto either the nibs or handles.

Pen holders come in different lengths, weights, styles and made of different materials including plastic, wood and metal. Try different handles to see which style suits you best. Select your choice primarily for comfort. A wooden handle for example has a nice natural feel and weight.

Pen holders will have ferrule ends for different sizes of nib. Most nibs fit a standard holder but do check that you have a matching set in size and style for both handle and nib. The nib needs to fit firmly and securely within the holder.

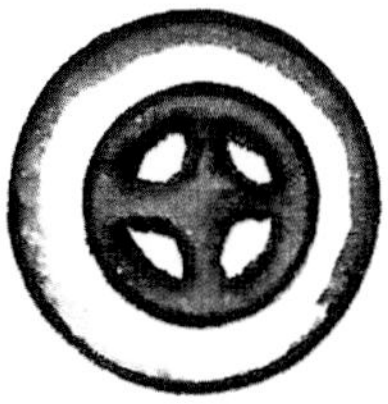

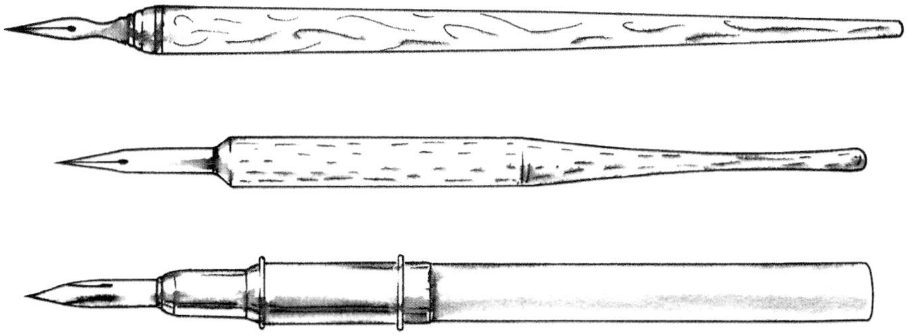

A universal style ferrule (above) is embedded deep within the shoulders of the handle. Pen holders and their ferrules may vary in style, these hold the nib firmly in place between the outer metal or wooden rim and the inner curved flexible grip/s.
Pen handles also vary in style (above right), with wooden handles being the most comfortable to hold.

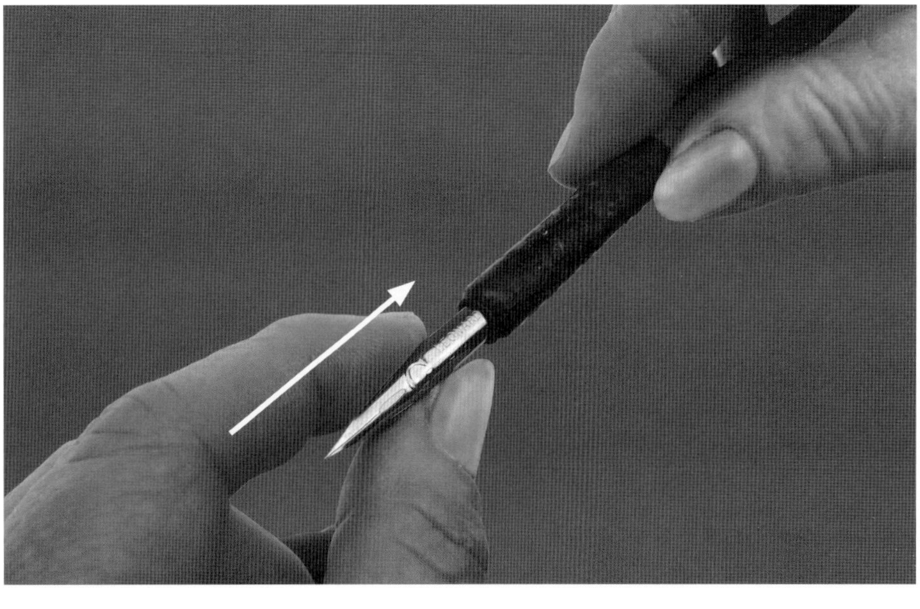

To insert a pen nib into the ferrule, hold the nib very gently along the sides of the shank of the nib, avoiding the delicate tines and tip. Gently slide the tail end of the nib into the pen holder ferrule until it is being supported firmly in place.

Fineliners and Brush Pens

Fineliner pens come in a range of tip sizes and are designed for very detailed work. The line produced has a consistent thickness. These pens have the advantage of being more portable than ink dip pens, however, if you choose to use this type, keep a range of pen styles and thicknesses. The nib size will be indicated as a point size, so that you can create a variety of line techniques.

Brush pens are very useful for creating flowing and expressive lines similar to those of a dip pen, i.e. where you can vary the line thickness according to the pressure applied. They have the advantage of often being water soluble, working in conjunction with a water brush pen.

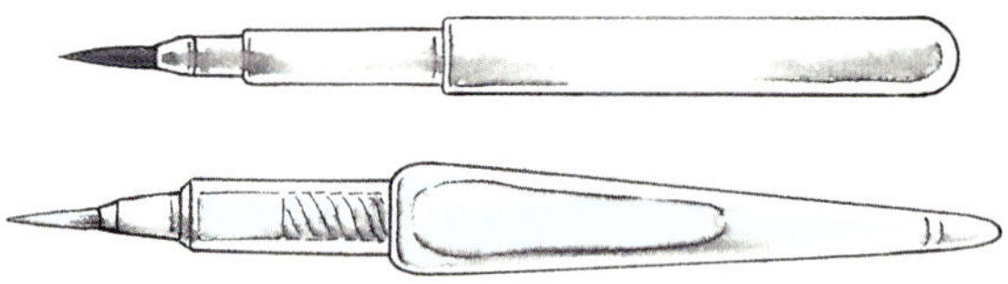

Ink brush pen (above) and water brush (below).

Technical Drawing Pens

These are designed to create consistent lines every time. The traditional high-quality metal-tipped technical drawing pen is designed to last. It can be used with either a changeable ink cartridge or a refillable ink chamber. It is essential to remove the nib section for cleaning after every use, either rinsing with water or placing it into the manufacturer's recommended cleaning fluid. The fine nibs create very even, fine and consistent lines, but be aware the very fine nibs can clog or be easily damaged without regular care and attention.

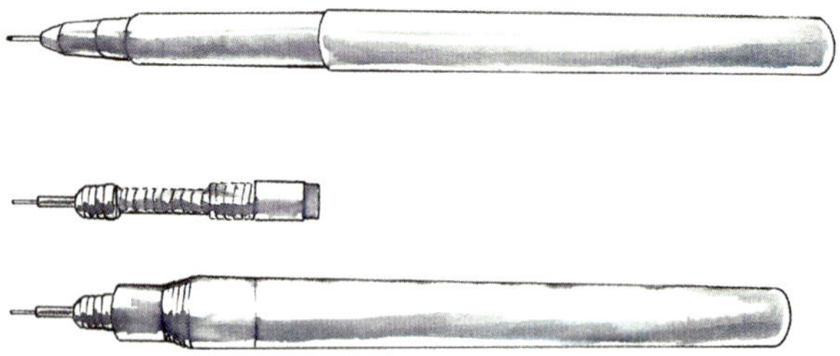

A fibre-tipped (above) and a technical pen shown with replacement nib option (below), both designed for detailed illustration or drawing.

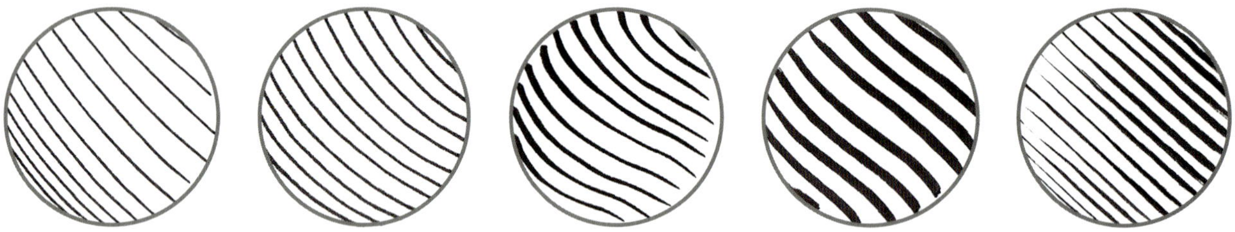

Brush pen strokes give a softer result, closer in style to using a paintbrush.

Paper for Ink

Select an extra-smooth paper that has been specifically designed for ink work. With rougher paper surfaces, there is a risk of the nib snagging in the texture, leaving jagged lines or blobs of ink and damaging your pen nib. Your paper choice may be dictated by whether you wish to add colour to your artwork. Some very smooth surfaces may not carry or hold watercolour paints.

Stippling Technique

Stippling is creating artwork by placing successive dots of ink, building up detail, tone and depth. Small dots are evenly spaced apart create a lighter tone, and larger dots closer together create a darker tone. Fine liner style pens are a good choice for this technique. Changing pen point sizes changes the dot sizes; gradually moving from small to larger dots creates a gradated tone.

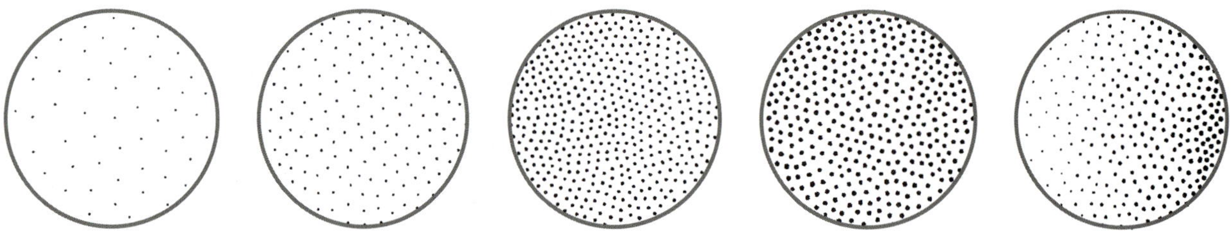

Stippling creates tonal progression by changing the size, density and gradation of the dots, which will in turn create tonal changes and form.

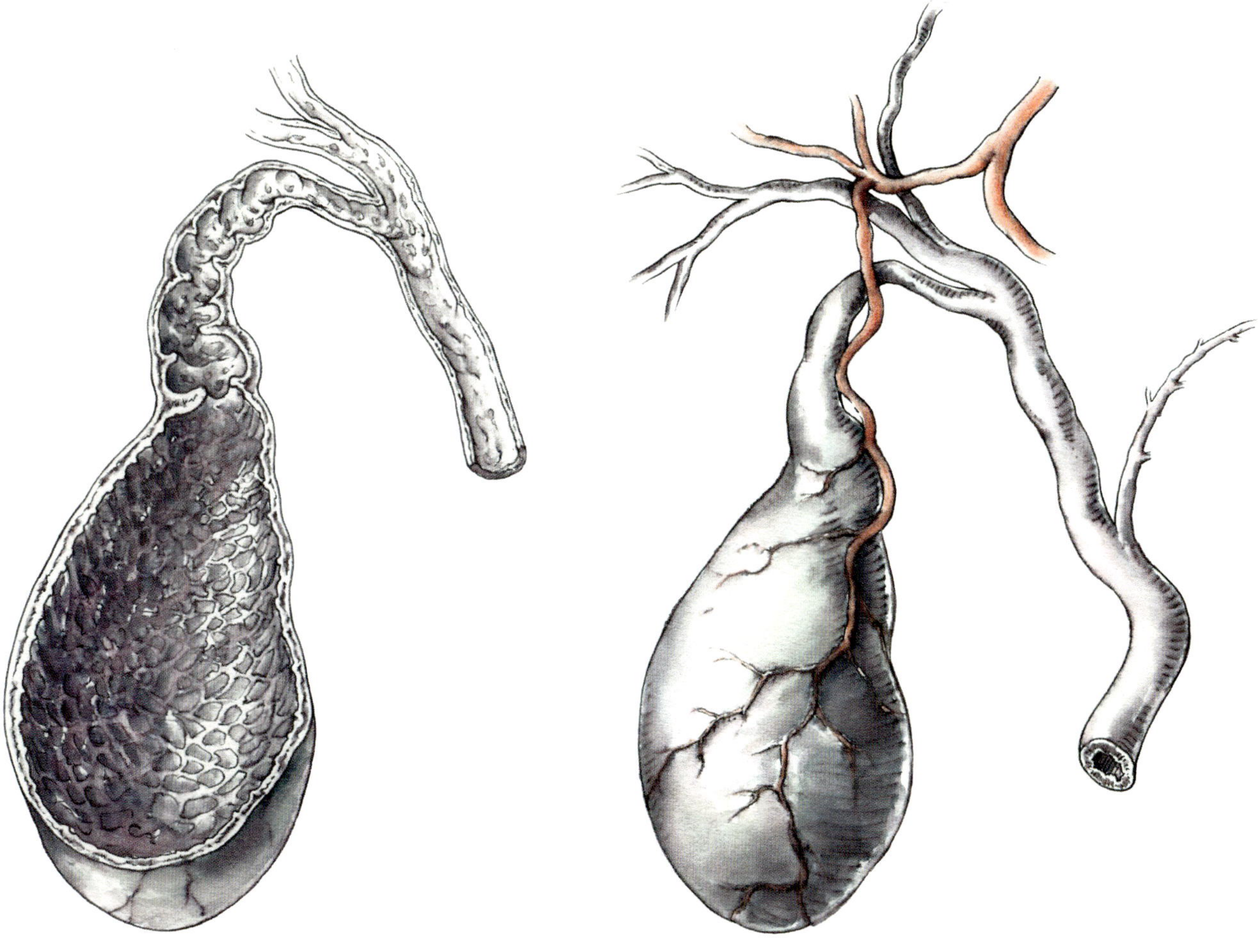

An ink pen line illustration of a gall bladder in section (left) and anterior external view (right).
The artwork has been developed further by applying additional ink colours, added and blended with a water brush pen to create form and tone.

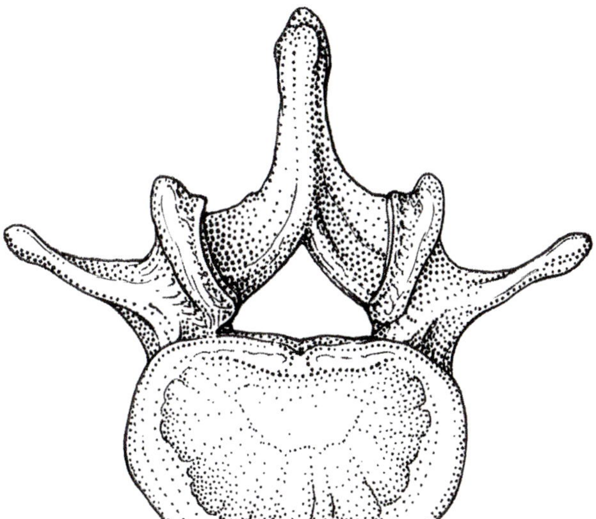

A stippled line illustration of a typical lumbar vertebra (superior view).

INKS

Inks come in a plethora of colours, styles and makes, and there are many elements to consider:

- Is the ink waterproof or soluble?
- Is it light-fast or permanent?
- Does it have a consistent flow?
- How thin or viscous is it?
- Will it dry glossy or matt?
- How long will it take to dry?

Ink will dry at a different rate depending on whether it is matt or glossy. Glossy, thicker ink will take longer to dry as it has a tendency to sit on the surface of the paper. Temperature also has an effect: if it is a hot, dry summer day, drying time will be quicker, whereas a cool or humid day will slow down the drying process. Ink can sometimes take a lot longer to dry than you may expect, so allow for this while working. It may be efficient to work on multiple artworks together, so while the ink is drying on one piece, you can continue working on another.

An ink you choose for brushwork may not be the same ink you would choose for a detailed technical pen and ink drawing. Always read the manufacturer's information about the ink before purchasing. Over time you may find yourself collecting many different bottles of inks, each for a different purpose. Each will have its own character and use. Here, inks have been divided into the following categories:

Black drawing inks These may be light, blue-black or an intense black, and once dried on the paper, may be either matt, semi-matt or gloss. No two black inks are the same, so selecting the right ink for your use is essential. Black inks are the most numerous on the market, and range from deep, intense blacks to more fluid drawing inks. A Chinese style and general drawing inks are both good to begin with. It might be possible to dilute a dark ink, which becomes a thinner or lighter black ink. If you work is going to print, choose a good quality black ink that will reproduce well.
Coloured inks These can also be used for drawing. Three of the colour swatches below include Blue-Black ink, Sepia and Sienna for comparison. Some inks have wonderful names, such as Doomsday and Prouts Brown. A colour that is not as intense as black may be preferable for your subject matter, so always consider a range of colour options.
Homemade inks These are relatively easy to make and fun for artwork and drawing experiments, bringing a softer, natural look to the subject, for example the Oak Gall and Walnut swatches below have both been home-made. If you are considering making your own ink, it's worth investing in an outside camping stove rather than using your clean kitchen hob!

Storing Ink

When storing your inks, if possible, keep them away from bright sunlight, unless you are working with them because some colours may be affected by light over time. Choose sturdy pots in which to store your ink when travelling. If you are making your own ink, consider dark-coloured glass pots to preserve the inks longer.

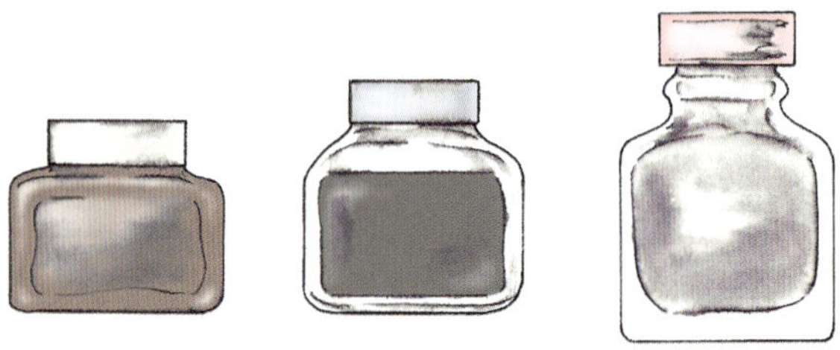

Blue-Black Sepia Oak Gall Sienna Walnut

USING A DIP PEN

Begin by holding the pen between your thumb and forefinger, not overly tightly, then let the pen handle rest gently on the curve of your hand between thumb and finger, an area called the perlicue. Place the tip of the pen on the paper at approximately a 45-degree angle. If the pen is held too vertically, the ink will not flow evenly down through the tines, which may cause the pen tines to split apart and then snag across the paper.

Ink up your pen nib, then pull the pen evenly towards you at a gentle angle and steady speed. Keep applying an even pressure to the tines to create long flowing lines.

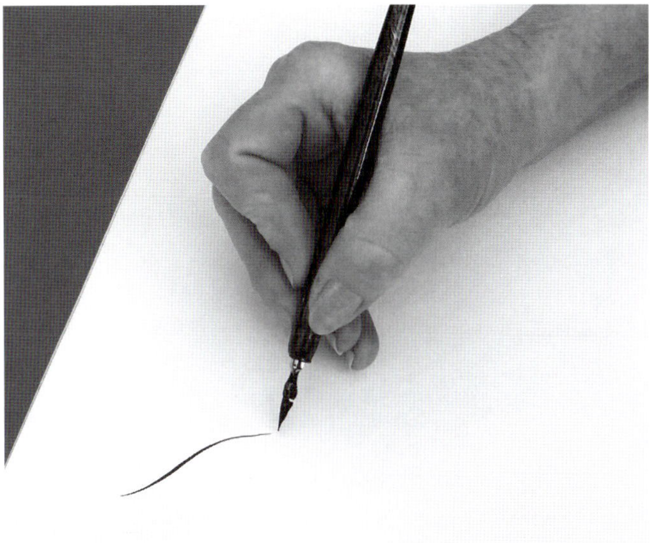

Hold the pen gently yet firmly at an approximate 45-degree angle. Varying the pressure you apply through your hand to the pen nib will change the width of line – greater pressure will result in a thicker line.

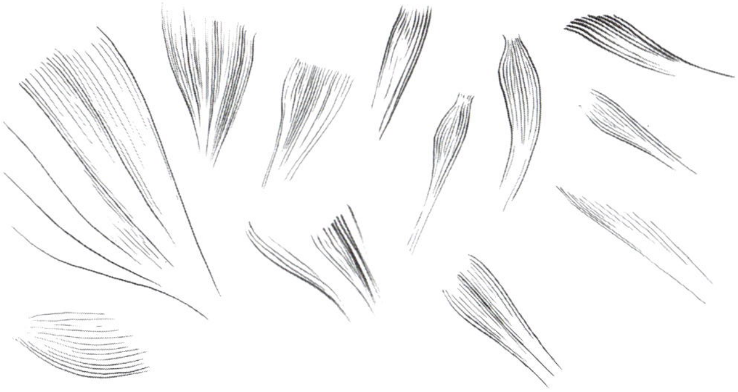

Begin by making simple pen strokes with the dip pen, then begin to form shapes and structures varying the line width to create form.

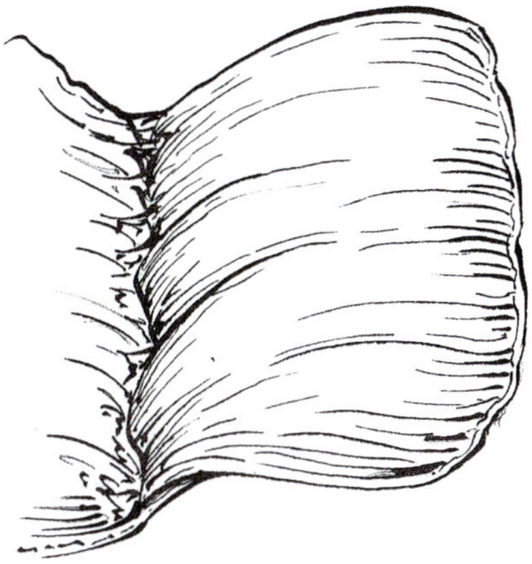

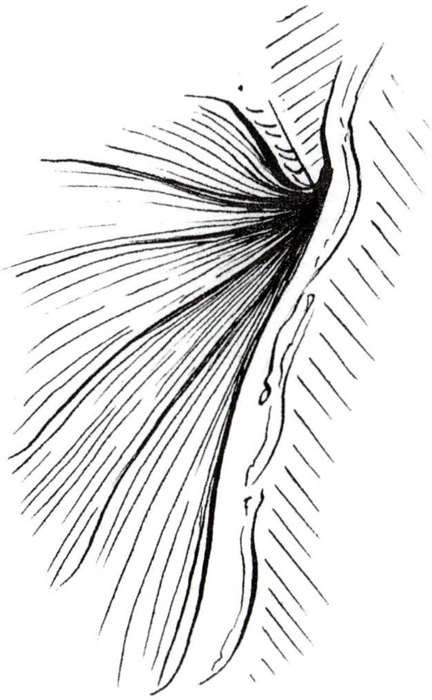

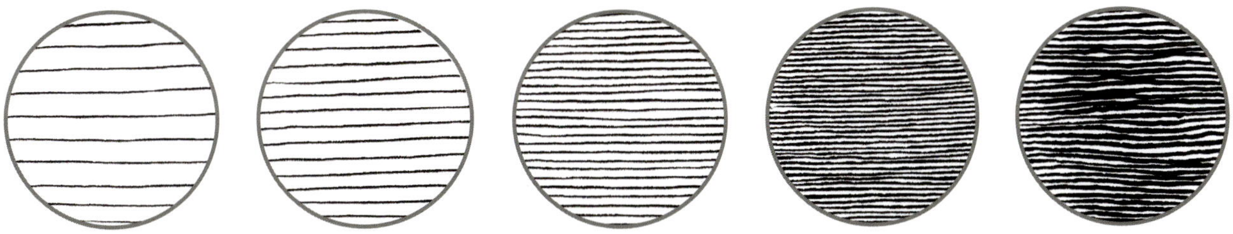

Tonal shading with a dip pen. Here the lines gradually form increasingly darker tones, by either placing the lines closer together or the line thickness has been increased by applying more pressure allowing more ink to flow down through the nib, or by a combination of both methods.

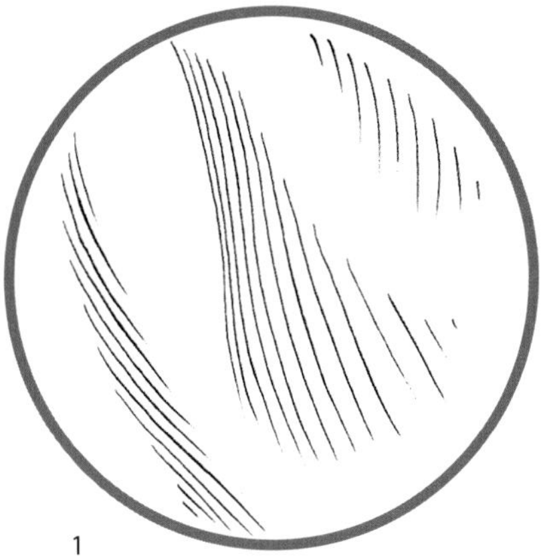

1

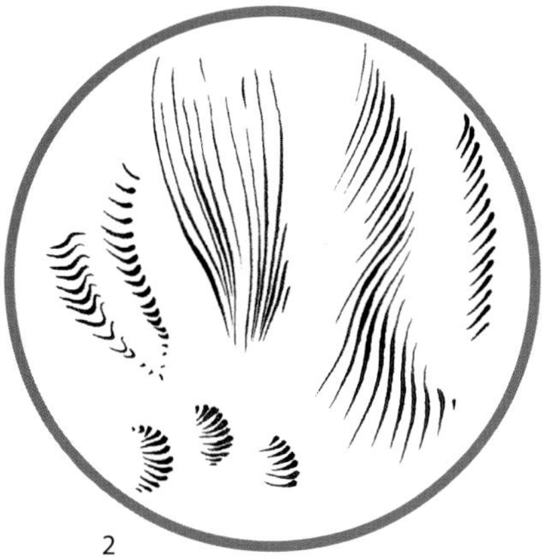

2

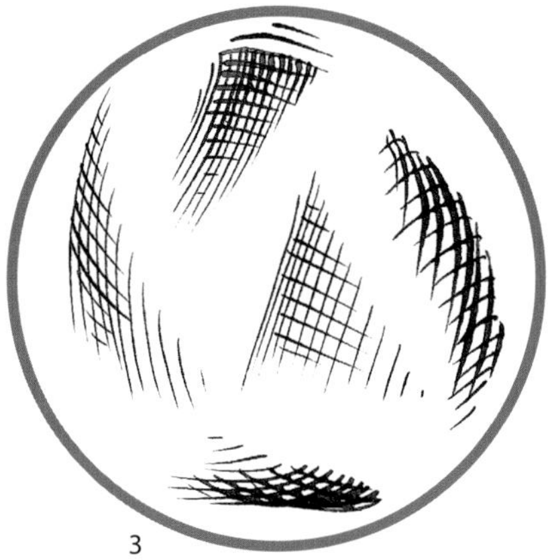

3

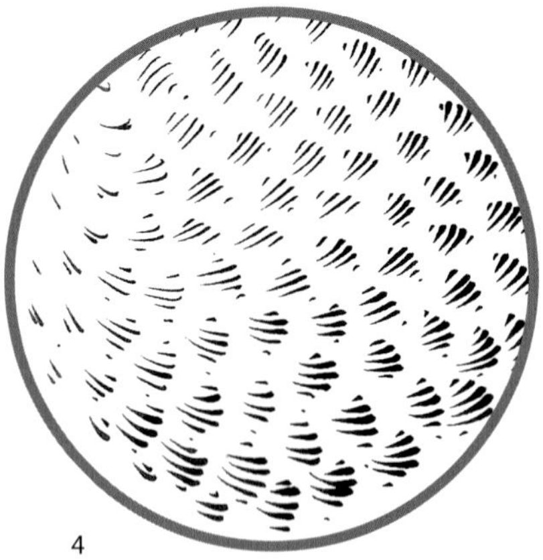

4

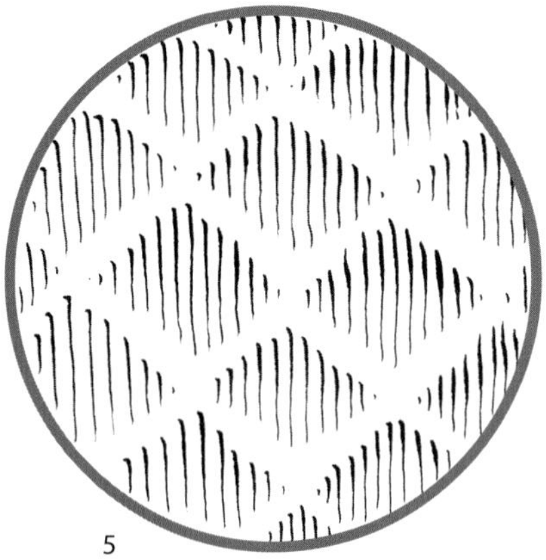

5

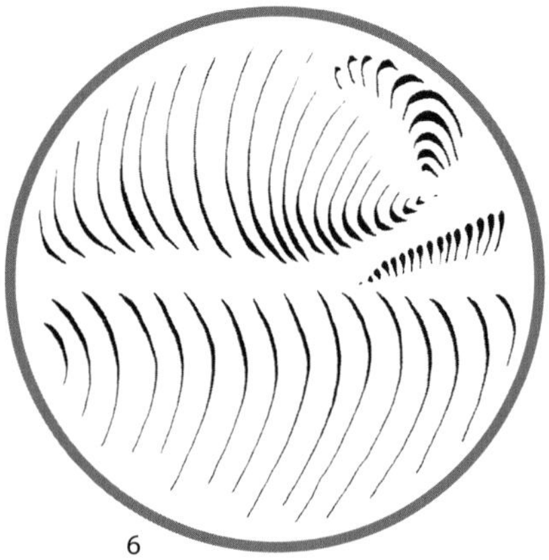

6

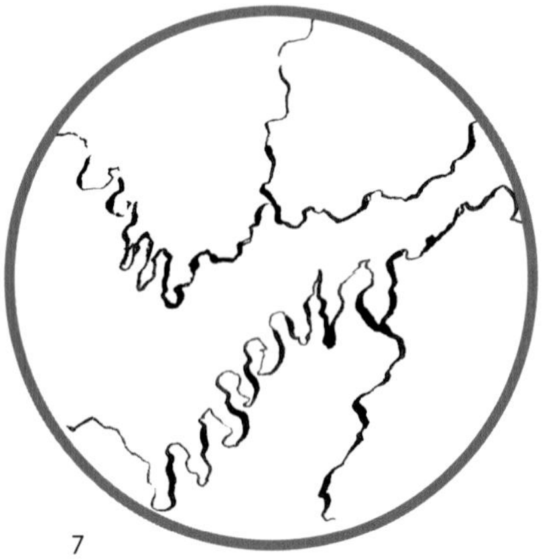

7

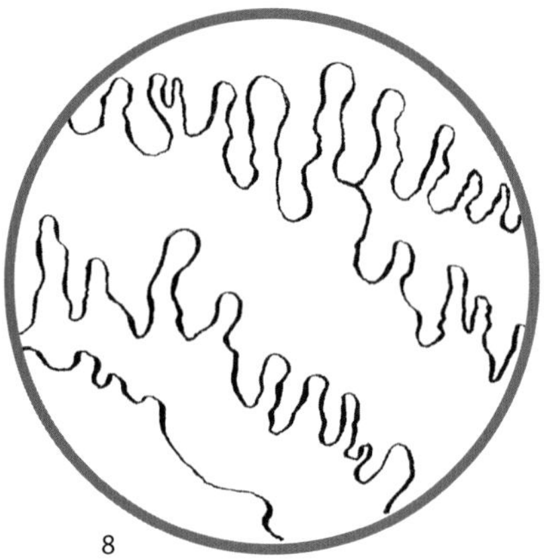

8

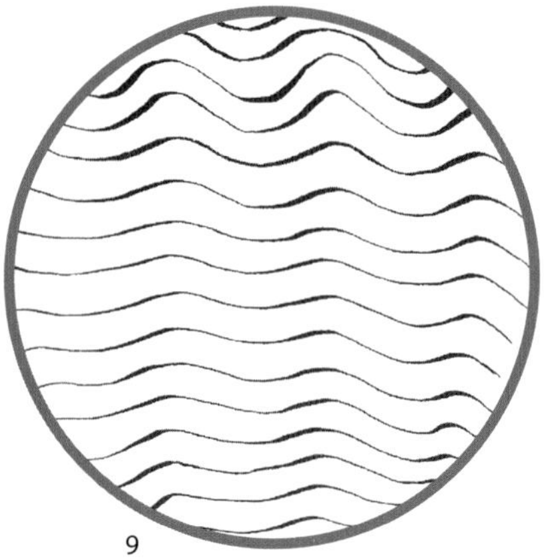

9

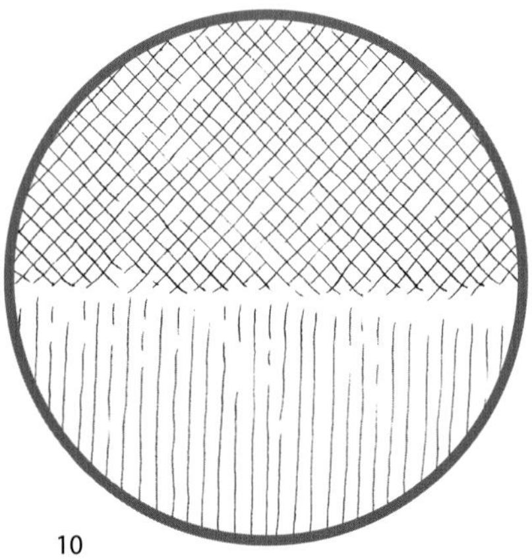

10

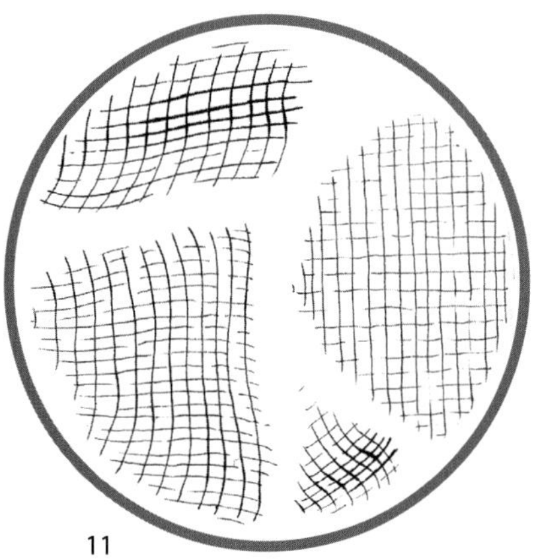

11

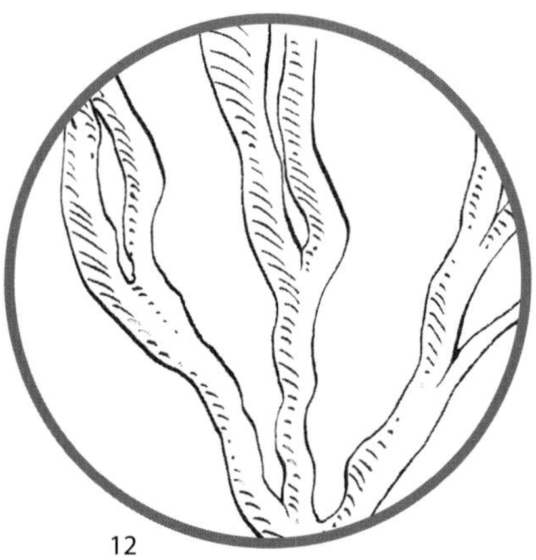

12

Project: Dip Pen Line Work

Aim: To practice drawing lines with an dip pen, from simple straight and curved lines, gradually changing the line pressure to create distinctive forms and shapes.

Art materials:

- Ink
- Dip pen holder and nib
- Choose paper with an ultra-smooth surface, for example Bristol board paper 250gms, A4 or A3 pad

Project: Experiment initially by creating slightly curved lines with your dip pen, occasionally changing the pressure down through your hand to the nib to change the thickness of the line. Your lines will become smoother and more confident with practice until you are creating gradated flowing lines. These eighteen examples, develop from simple curved lines, to cross-hatching, to bone and fat textures, alongside features found within medical illustration.

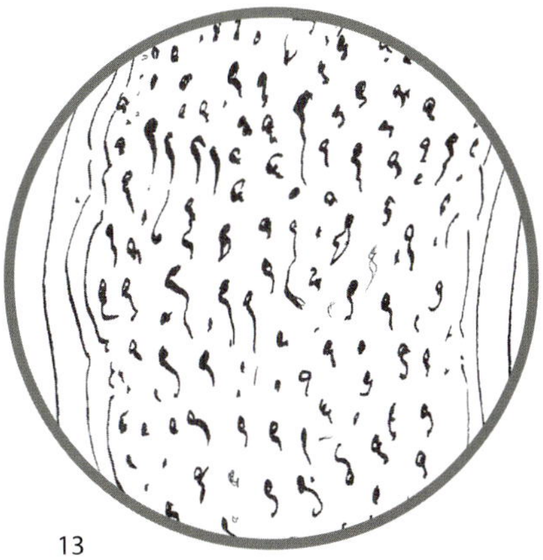

13

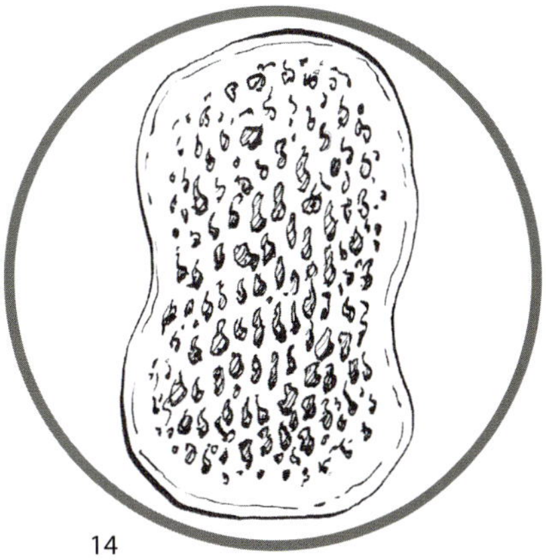

14

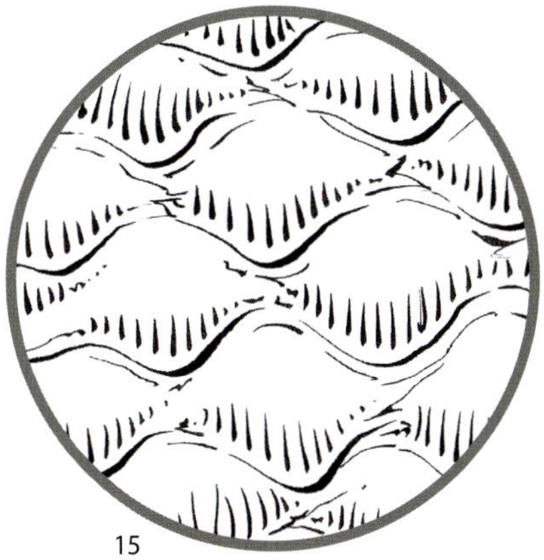

15

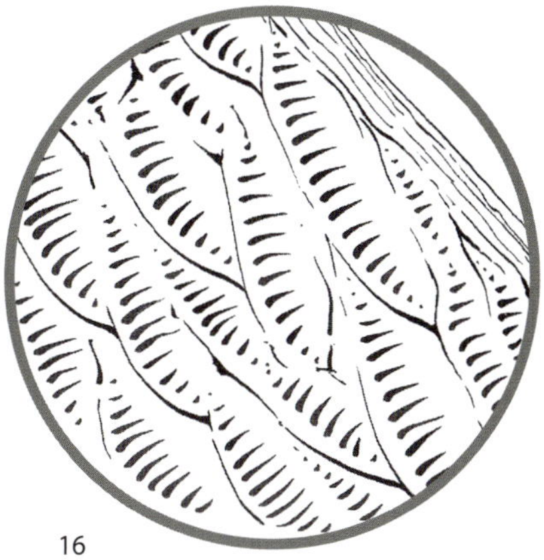

16

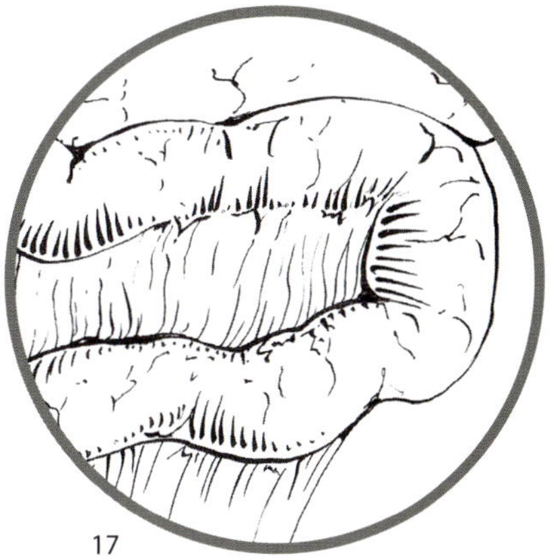

17

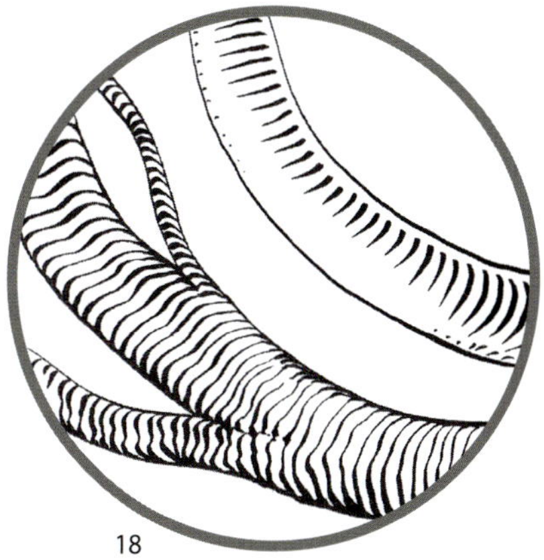

18

1 Gentle flowing lines

2 Gradually increase the pressure through each line

3 Cross-hatching creates form, shadow and depth

4 Short expressive slightly curved lines

5 Longer, straighter textural lines

6 A variety of curved lines formed by gradually increasing pen pressure

7 Bone sutures created with tightly curving lines. Keep those lines travelling in the same direction thinner, than those on the return curve

8 Bone sutures formed withmore widely spaced curving lines

9 Gradating the lines gives the impression of underlying structures forming raised forms and undulating ridges

10 Mesh interpretated with thin straight lines and cross-hatching

11 Cloth gauze texture with gently flowing lines and cross-hatching

12 Dividing structures, with shaded lines following their form

13 Bone structure in cross-section, created by short, curled expressive lines. The darker sweep of the line forming the shadow

14 Bone structure in cross-section, created with short controlled curled lines, reflecting the inner trabeculae network with an outer bone edge

15 Globular effect, combining expressive lines to create form and shadow

16 The soft, curving globular nature of fat, is perfectly suited to being interpreted with a dip pen

17 Section of the small intestine, a curving tubular structure, with an outer line and added tonal shading to create the shape and form

18 Blood vessels can be distinguished by changing the line effect. Arteries, being rounder and more tubular in shape and veins, with thinner structural walls, have a flatter, darker and more irregular appearance

Project: Anatomical Studies

Aim: To develop your dip pen skills through a series of six anatomical studies.

Art materials:

- Black or sepia drawing ink
- Dip pen nib and handle
- A4 or A3 Bristol board paper pad 250gms

Project: For each of following studies, there are two or three images: a completed artwork, a second faint image for you to trace or photocopy for practice, and a final image with only the outline for you to fill in, copying the lines to develop your own technique.

The outlines have also been supplied for you to trace, to copy or print onto paper. Printing a few copies onto paper will give you the scope to practise as many times as you wish. Take your time; first look at the example and the direction the pen line has been drawn and where the weight has been applied. Remember you will be pulling the pen nib towards you, so may have to adjust or rotate the paper position to achieve this. You will also want to move your paper around to find the best position for your hand – however be careful to avoid those areas you have just inked so you don't accidentally smudge them.

First, ink up the nib by gently dipping it into the ink, gently removing any ink excess on the side of the bottle. Place your hand in a comfortable position and begin practising on the paper by bringing the pen towards you, creating a line. If you increase the pressure, the tines will spread slightly apart, so more ink will be applied to the paper. If you apply too much pressure, the tines will move too far apart, however, and the ink will not flow onto the paper correctly. In contrast, once you have started a line, gradually lift your hand back from the paper, this will reduce the pressure and create a thinner line. Whenever possible, draw the pen smoothly towards you or gently sideways for the best results.

Position an inexpensive spare sheet of paper under your drawing hand while you are working. This will prevent any imperceptible greasiness from your hand transferring onto the paper, which will prevent the ink from adhering correctly as you draw and may create a blotchy result. The sheet of spare paper will also help to facilitate a freer sweeping movement, through the paper being able move and glide with your hand as it draws. Again, keep an eye on those areas you have recently inked, to avoid smudging them, this is so easily done! Try and keep the drying ink clear of your hand and the sheet of paper as you move.

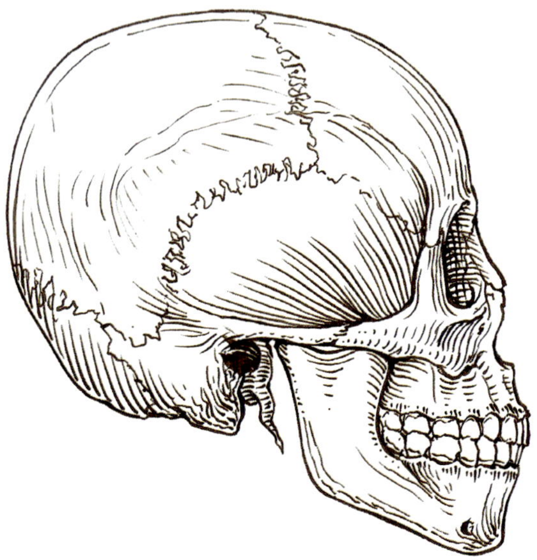

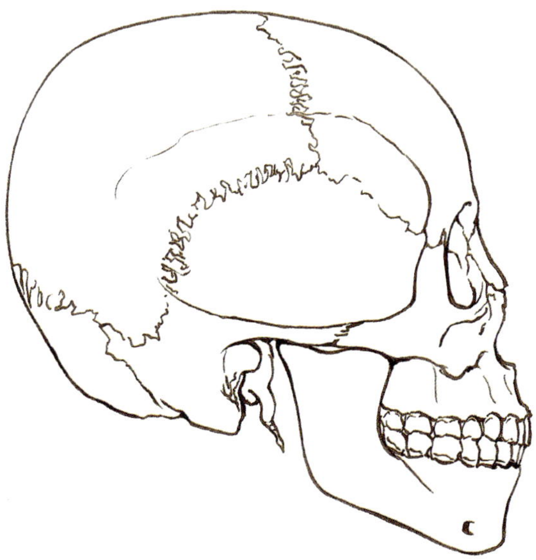

Lateral view of the skull.
First copy the line work of the skull in pencil on the outline version to the right and then trace over the pencil lines in ink.

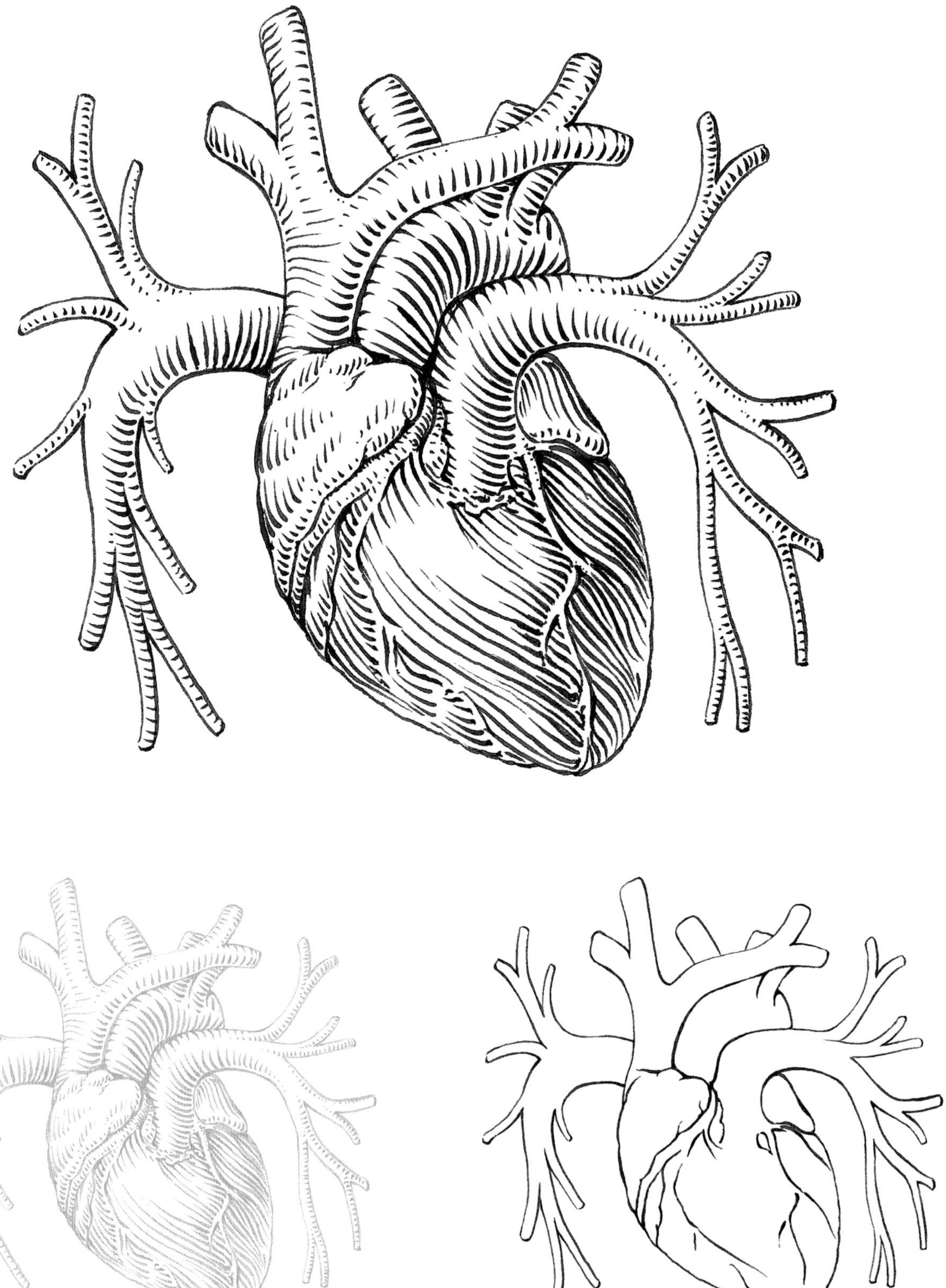

The heart image for practice: following the main artwork, trace over the paler image to gain confidence in developing line shading through curved lines, to completing the simple outline with your own line work.

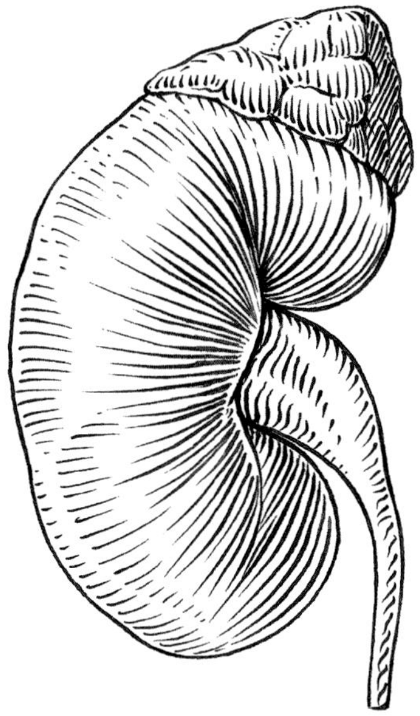

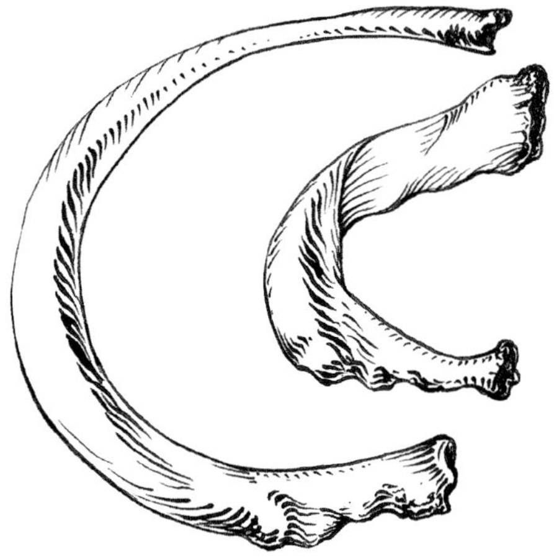

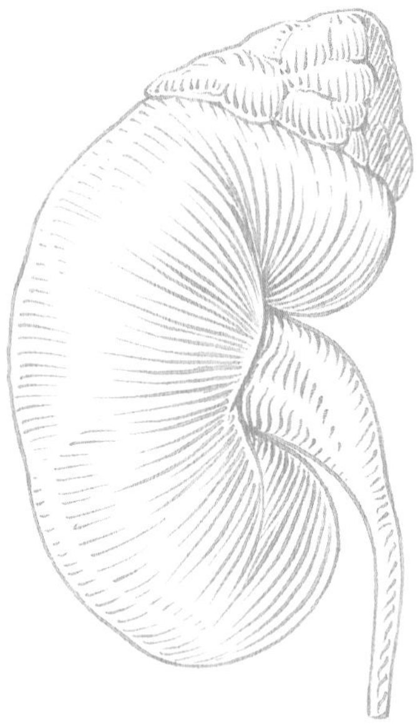

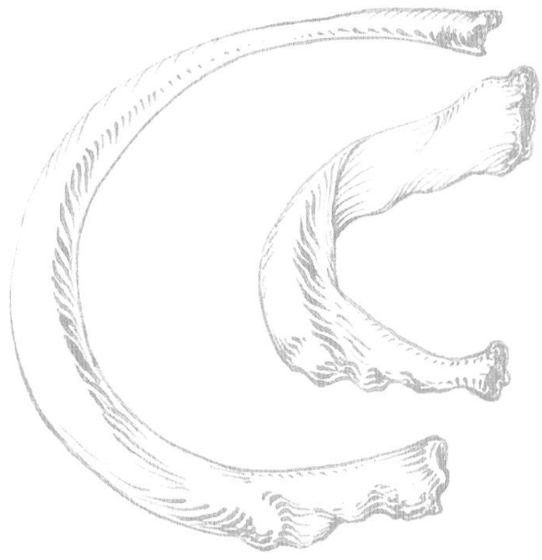

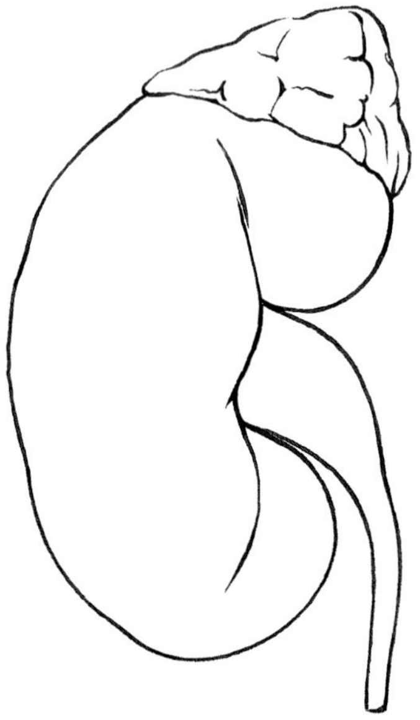

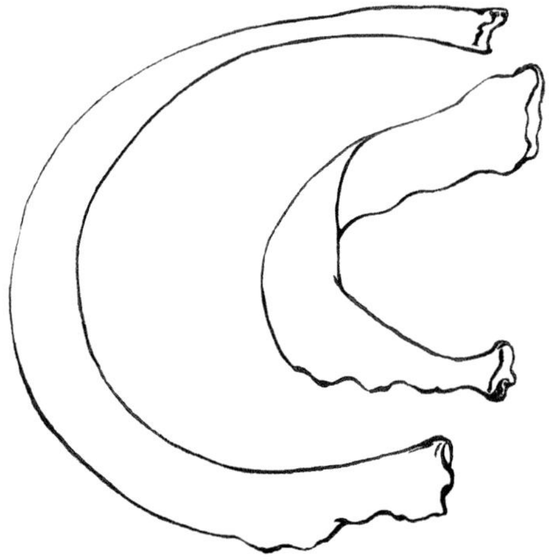

The kidney (left), two ribs (above), vertebrae (right) and the superior view of the sacrum (Far right) are for gaining line work practice. Begin by tracing over the paler image to develop skills in shading with curved expressive ink lines, to completing the simple outline with your own line work style.

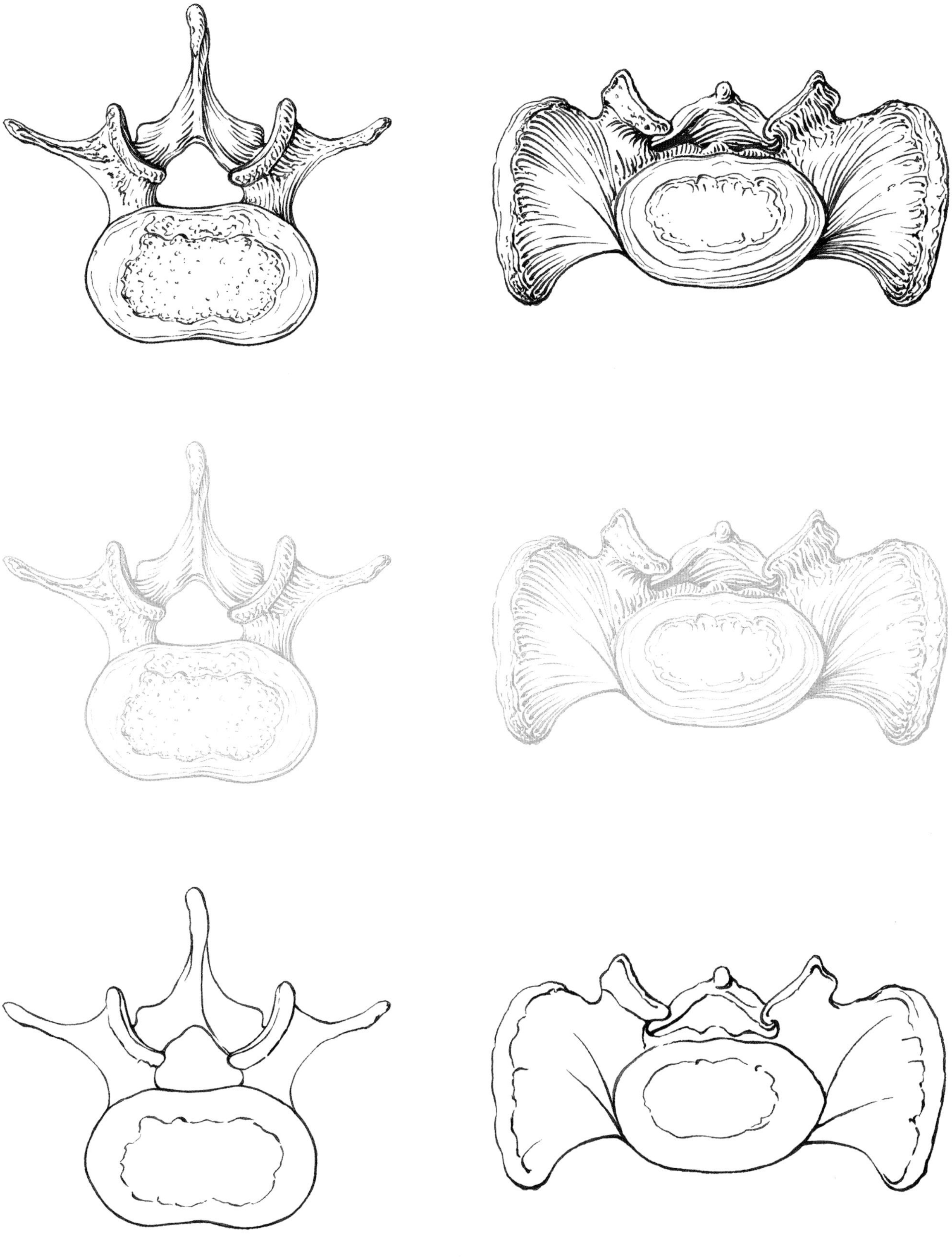

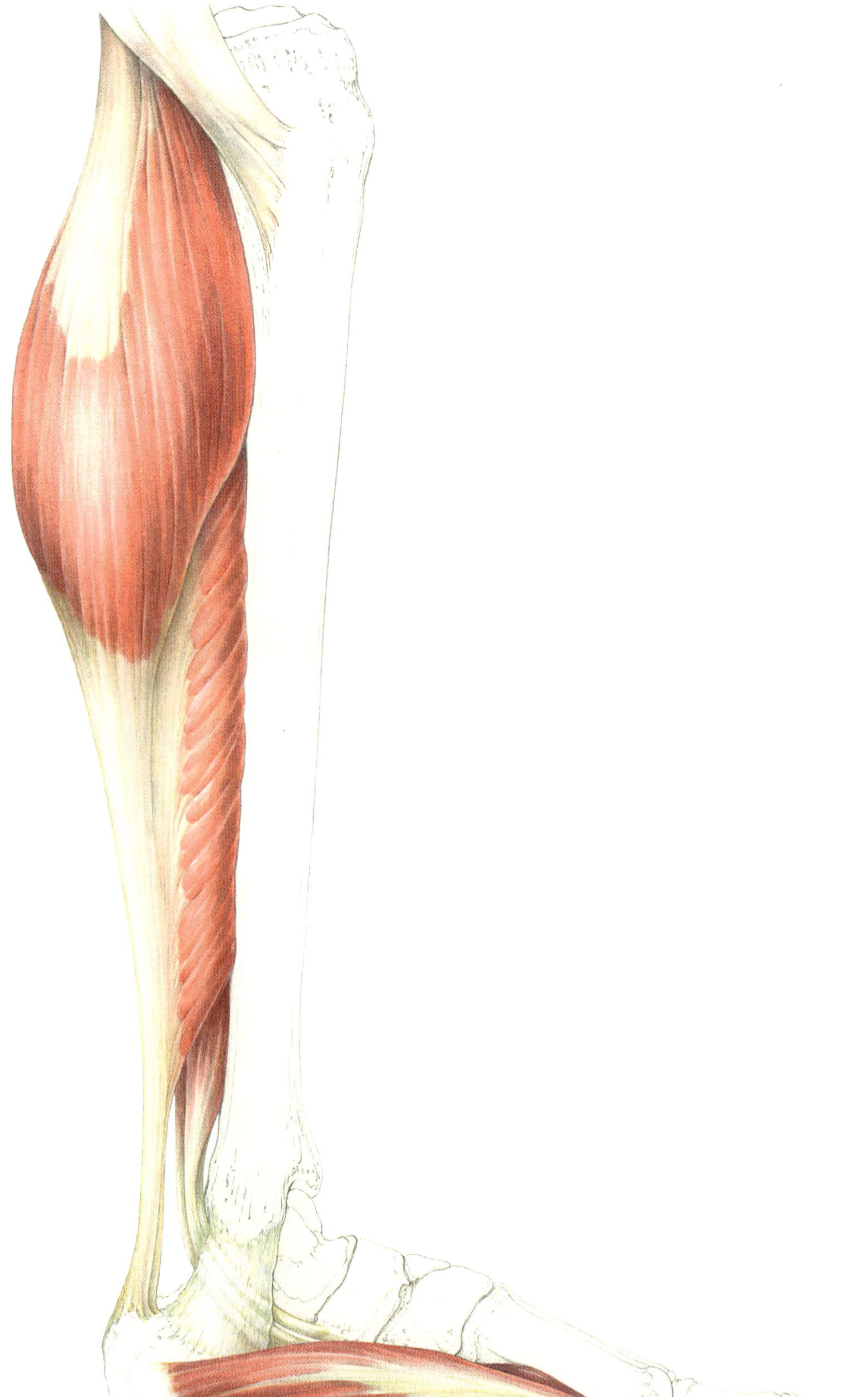

CHAPTER 11

WORKING IN WATERCOLOUR

Working with watercolours is always a delight! This is such a versatile medium, enabling the medical artist to paint detailed, high-quality anatomical artworks. Watercolour has a unique luminous quality, allowing the whiteness of the paper to show through – a quality that is difficult to replicate in quite the same way as any other medium. 'Watercolour' here refers to the traditional form of watercolour pigments, as opposed to gouache, acrylic or chalk paints.

WATERCOLOUR PAINTS AND PIGMENTS

Watercolour paints come packaged in several ways, most commonly found as tubes, pans or blocks of colour. Pans and blocks require water to release the pigment, whereas paint within tubes is kept softer and ready for application – useful where larger quantities of pigment are required. These paints have been pre-prepared for ease of use. Alternatively, pigments can be purchased as finely ground powders, which will need to be mixed and held together with a binder, such as gum Arabic, before being used for painting.

Each paint tube, pan or packet of powder will be labelled with its own identification information, from the colour name, a number indicating the pigment grade and compounds. For watercolours, it is recommended to choose artists' or professional grade paints, as opposed to student ranges, which may be cheaper but invariably a false economy. The artist's ranges will be of higher quality with more finely ground pigments, which will be reflected in the price, however, they will be worth the additional expense.

Each paint manufacturer will have their own specific watercolour range, with colour charts providing the colour name, accompanied by a colour swatch, alongside further information about the pigment's permanence and opacity. Each paint will have a series number indicating the quality of the pigments involved, ranging from series 1 (highest quality) down to a series 5. The pigment grade will be reflected in the cost. For those who wish to experiment further with watercolour pigments, explore the range of ground pigments available or try making your own.

Wherever possible, select colours produced by the same manufacturer because each paint company has designed their paint pigment range to work together. Mixing paints from different manufacturers occasionally causes pigments to split, producing an uneven or blotchy result.

Medial view of the lower leg, showing the gastrocnemius muscle of the calf and abductor hallucis muscle of the foot. Watercolour and graphite pencil.

CHOOSING COLOURS

There is a wide range of tempting paint sets available on the market, but you can get started by simply buying the three primary colours red, yellow and blue, adding to these later to build up the colour palette you need. This approach avoids selecting box sets that may not even include all three primary colours.

Three recommended primary colour options are Windsor Red, Windsor Blue and Windsor Yellow, each producing a crisp, clean result; from these colours you can mix almost any colour you require including a black, created by combining all three primary colours together.

Box sets regularly include white and black pigment options, these are the pigments least used by watercolour artists. Black is a different colour from a dark tone. Mixing the three primary colours together will give you a complementary darker tone to your artwork, as opposed to a ready-mixed palette black, which may not be created from the same pigments and have an overpowering effect. Mixing watercolours provides an endless palette with which to work; creating reference colour swatches is covered in Chapter 12.

With regard to white pigment, remember that watercolour is a transparent medium, usually working on light-coloured or white paper. The whiteness of the paper creates highlights by leaving areas of the paper either free of pigment or covered with a very diluted wash. Overpainting with a white pigment – to lighten an area, for example – will often have the opposite effect and create a more solid, opaque appearance, thus losing that unique translucent quality watercolour is renowned for.

The three primary colours. The selected colours chosen here are from the Windsor range.

Windsor Yellow Windsor Red Windsor Blue

Mixing all three primary colours will create a natural dark or black colour

Developing your Colour Palette

Watercolour is an excellent medium for creating medical art illustrations, the quality and colour palette complimenting the natural colours of the human body. Broadening the range of pigments in your colour palette will give you a wider variety of pigment choices from which to mix warm and cool colours. There are many colours to choose from, so those colours you select will be ultimately down to your personal preference.

Listed are a few suggestions for additional colours to consider including within your palette:

- Alongside Windsor Yellow, consider Cadmium Yellow and Lemon Yellow
- Alongside Windsor Red, consider Cadmium Red and Alizarin
- Alongside Windsor Blue, consider Ultramarine and Cobalt
- Consider additional earthy or opaque pigments: Indigo, Indian Red, Burnt Umber, Raw Umber, Sepia, Yellow Ochre and Raw Sienna

PAPER

For producing quality medical illustrations, a smooth-surfaced paper, often referred to as hot-pressed (HP), is best. For example, try Fabriano, Arches or Sanderson papers, selecting a paper weight between 300gms and 425gms. Paper can be sourced as individual sheets, pads or blocks, each paper having its own unique quality. Buy a selection of papers in different weights and styles and keep a swatch of each type, noting on each the manufacturer, name, weight and style for future reference.

Each artist acquires a preference for a particular paper or two. Equally, a paper that works for one style of painting may not suit another; different papers achieve different results.

Stretching the paper to prepare the surface before painting is recommended for single sheets of water-colour paper. This involves dampening or soaking your paper with water, either on one or both sides, before attaching it to a board with gummed or masking tape and allowing it to dry. Even if the paper bends and buckles during the water application, it will straighten out flat again once dry.

Watercolour paper can also be purchased as sealed block pads, which are the equivalent of stretched paper. When an artwork is complete, simply peel the page from the block.

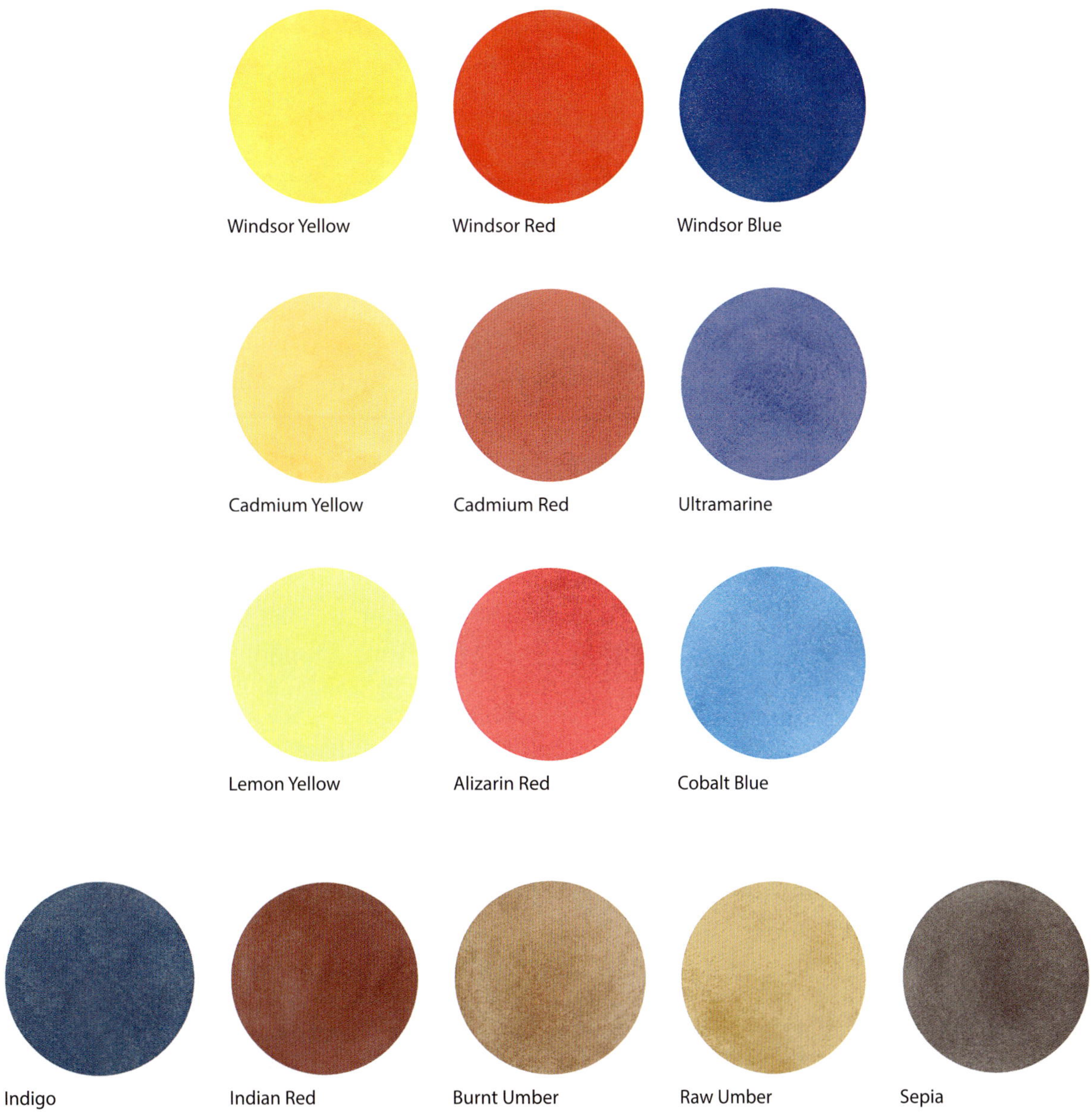

ANATOMY OF A PAINTBRUSH

Tip or toe Where the hairs come to a point
Bristles, hairs or tufts The type of hair will be your most important consideration when purchasing a paintbrush
Belly The plumpest area of the hairs of the brush
Heel The compressed area of the hairs entering the ferrule
Brush sleeve Clear sleeve covering that protects the brush hairs
Sizes Brushes are numbered depending on the width and length of the hairs. The numbering system may vary between manufacturers
Ferrule or neck The metal casing that holds the hairs and joins to the handle. The hairs are glued inside the ferrule
Crimp of the ferrule Where the metal ferrule is crimped to firmly grip the handle of the paintbrush
Tapered handle Usually about 15cm (6in) long. Wooden handles are the most comfortable to hold. The name of the manufacturer and brush size are usually found printed on the handle

The brush 'size' will depend upon the width and length of the bristle hairs

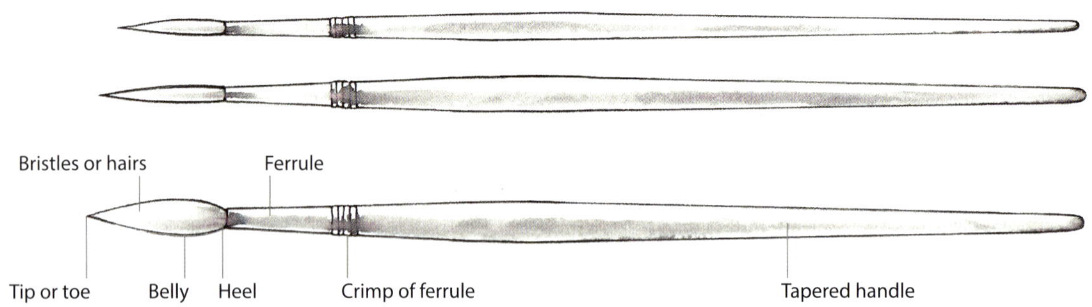

WATERCOLOUR BRUSHES

When working with watercolour, it is recommended to use high-quality, pure sable-haired brushes. Paintbrush hairs may be made from many different animal hairs, including squirrel, mink or horse, each hair type having its own characteristics. Quality brushes will allow the colour to flow freely across the paper. In contrast, coarser haired brushes may be less efficient at holding the paint or allowing it to flow smoothly.

When selecting brushes, always check the hairs before purchasing. Look for brush hairs that come easily to a point. Avoid ones where the hairs are splitting in different directions or have been unevenly trimmed.

Brush sizes range from a 00 size (0000 being the smallest), with very few hairs and perfect for dry brush work, up to thick and wide size 30 for large washes.

Over time you will undoubtedly collect a broad range of brushes in both size and styles, either for different project requirements or personal preference. You will soon discover which brushes you prefer working with.

Begin with three, four or five sable brushes, with sizes between 2 and 10. For example, a set of brushes in size 3, 5, 8 and 10 will cover you for nearly every requirement. Smaller sizes – less than size 4 – are good for detailed work, and larger sizes – size 6 or above – are good for washes and covering larger areas, although a good-quality larger size 6, 8 or 10 with a sharp point will also do very well for detailed work. Note that brush sizes may be graded differently between manufacturers, in both the numbering and the brush length and thickness.

Most importantly, look after your new sable brushes to protect your investment; a good-quality sable brush will last a lifetime if looked after with care. Always clean your brushes after use and whenever possible wait until they are completely dry before placing them inside the roll for storage. When travelling, open the roll once you have returned to your studio to allow the brush hairs to dry completely.

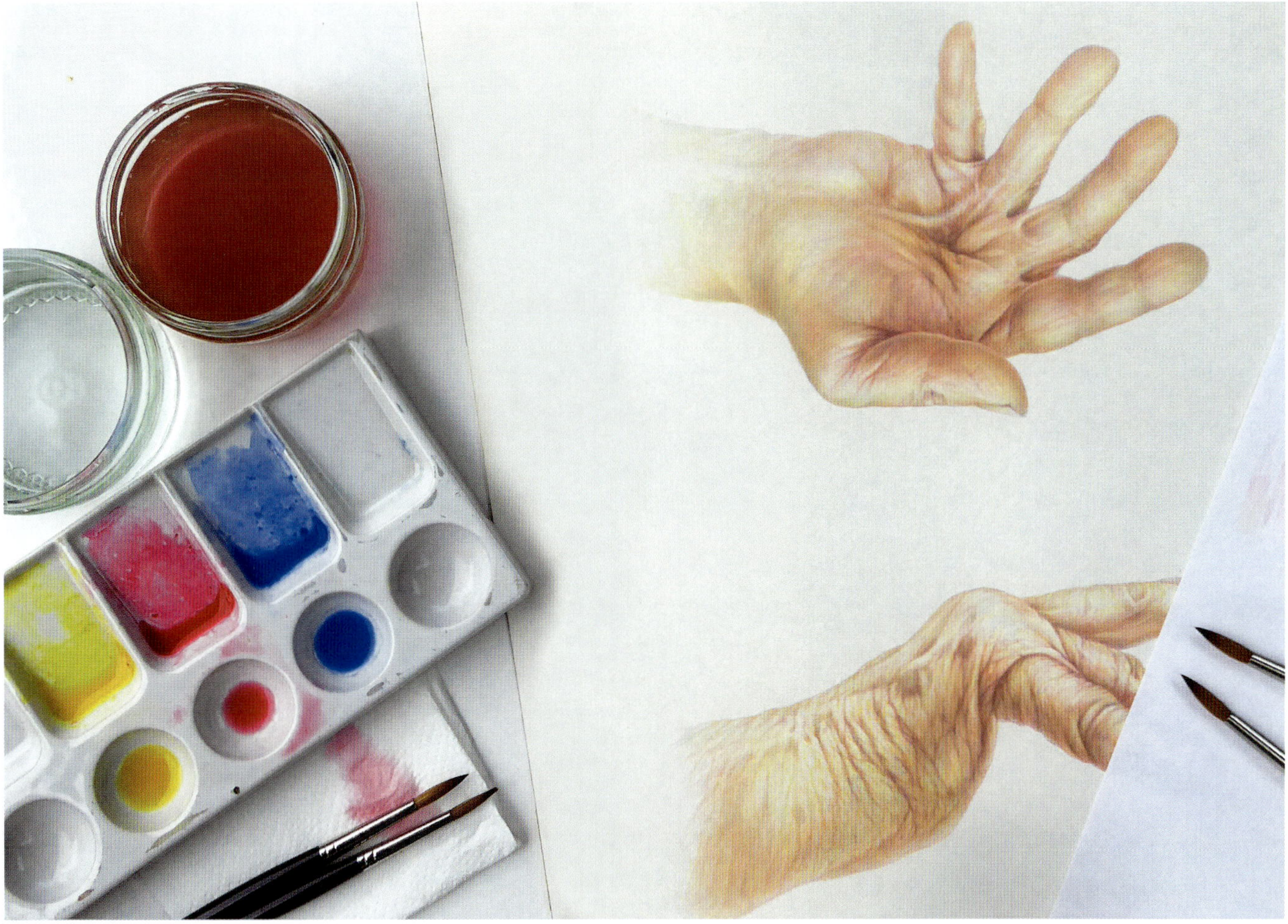

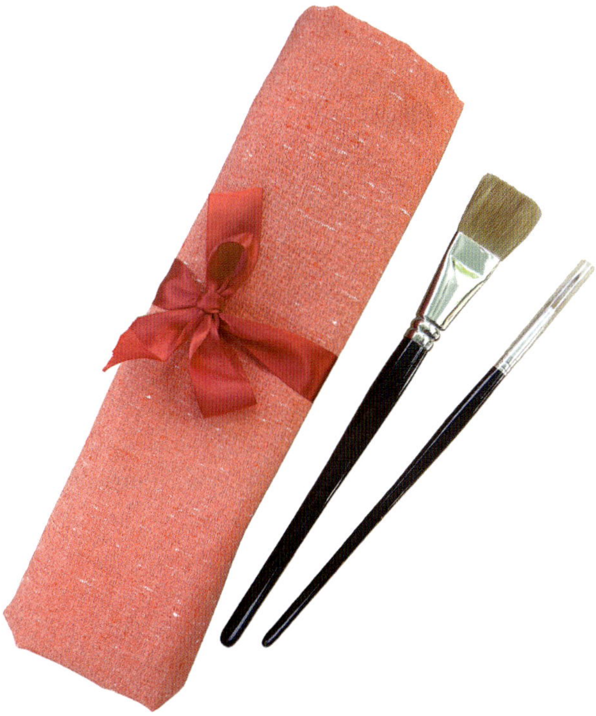

Brushes are supplied with clear plastic sleeves to protect the delicate hairs when purchased. A soft brush roll is ideal for storing brushes safely and is economical to purchase; or you can make your own brush roll if you are handy with a sewing machine (left). A roll will keep the hairs straight and protected, preventing them from becoming bent or out of shape.

PAINTBRUSH CARE

- Always rinse your brushes in clean water after use
- Avoid leaving brushes point down standing in water, which can damage or bend the hairs
- If the hairs dry apart, immerse them in water and gently wipe against the side of your water jar until they reform into a point
- Protect the delicate hairs within their clear sleeves when not being used
- Allow brushes to dry fully in the open air before storing
- Store the brushes between use safely in a roll

PAINTING MATERIALS

Paper Sheets, pads or blocks of watercolour paper
Palette For mixing paints
Paints Pans, tubes or pigment blocks
Brushes A variety of sizes
Two water pots One for clean water i.e. for working with your paint and one for cleaning your brush

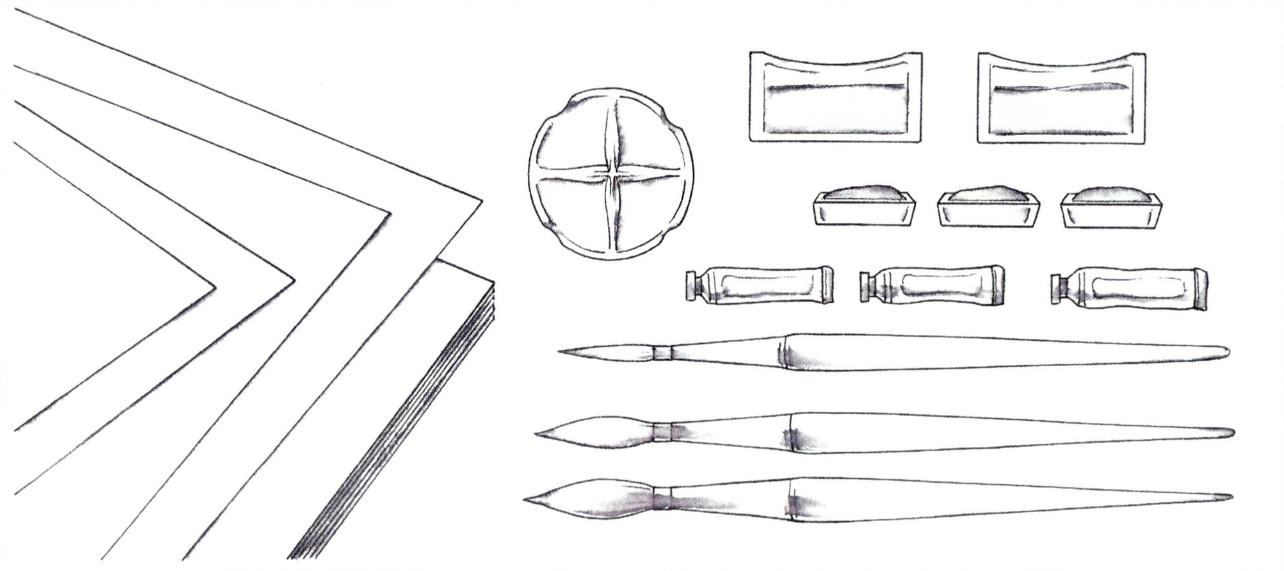

ADDITIONAL ITEMS

Collate the following studio items to begin:

Two pots or jars of clean water One pot will be for diluting and mixing paints, the other for cleaning your brush. Change the water regularly or whenever it begins to become murky. Murky water will create murky paintings!

Water storage If you are working away from your studio, carry a spare bottle of water to have available to change the water if there is no direct access to a tap. Alongside a watertight container to pour the used water into. When travelling, ensure your water bottle has a tight seal and consider placing it within a waterproof sealable bag to prevent any leakages into your art case.

Tissues A packet of strong tissues or kitchen roll will always come in handy.

Paint-mixing palette Ceramic palettes are preferable for watercolour, as the water can move easily within the holding wells and they are easy to clean. Large ceramic palettes can be rather heavy, however there are smaller ceramic dishes available. There are also many lightweight plastic mixing trays available; with these, however, it may become trickier to see the exact colour you are mixing due to the plastic which can become stained over time. Whichever style of palette you choose, ensure at least some of the wells can hold a good amount of water, as you will always need more prepared paint than you think.

WATERCOLOUR TECHNIQUE

Watercolour painting can be approached in one of two ways, or a combination of the two. Either by applying and building up successive layers of individual pigment colour washes onto the paper, or by premixing the pigments on your palette to create the colours ready to apply onto the paper. Both methods can be used to great effect, however layering the paint as individual colours will give you more control. Colour swatch examples for individual pigments and premixing are covered further in Chapter 12. Which approach you choose will depend upon the effect, style and result you are looking for and each artwork may require a different approach, alongside your personal preferred painting method.

Applying Watercolour

Watercolour can be very versatile, and can be used for anything from quick colour note-taking to covering large areas with paint or controlled and detailed work. It can be applied to the paper surface in many ways: loose sweeping washes, to carefully placed controlled strokes, layering or mixing individual colours, or with a dry brush for fine detail. This last technique is when the paint is applied in small quantities with an almost dry brush and nearly dry paint, working on small areas at a time.

Project: Beginning with Watercolour

Aim: To practise painting with a combination of colours. To layer or premix the colours and recording the results to form colour reference charts.

Art materials required:

- Watercolour paints
- Brushes
- Mixing palette
- Two pots of water
- Watercolour paper

Project: Create your own watercolour colour reference charts by applying different pigment combinations.

Take your time when you begin working with watercolour, it is best approached slowly and methodically. You will quickly acquire confidence, gaining speed with practice.

Start by creating individual colour swatches for all the colours in your palette and name each swatch with the pigment colour.

Secondly, layer two pigments one over another, allowing each layer to dry before overlaying the second. Layering will give you more control while keeping your work looking fresh and retaining the luminous quality of watercolour. Mixing colours on your palette can sometimes give a muddier look, especially when several layers of premixed colours accumulate on top of one another. Note the difference below when red has been overlaid on yellow and vice versa.

Thirdly, for comparison, premix colours together before applying them onto the paper; record and note the colour combinations for future reference.

Yellow overlaid on red

Blue overlaid on red

Blue overlaid on yellow

Premixed colour: yellow and red

Premixed colour: blue and red

Premixed colour: blue and yellow

GLOSSARY

Blocks Compressed pigment in individual colours
Cool colours Colours broadly within the blue, green and purple categories of the colour wheel
Dry brush Application of colour with little or no water added to either the brush or the paint
Gum Arabic A natural substance sourced from acacia trees, used as a binder to create watercolour pigments in a prepared usable format, such as in tubes
Lightfast Resistance to fading. Watercolours are graded according to how lightfast they are, with AA being the most resistant
Opaque Letting less light through i.e. the opposite of transparent
Pans Pre-prepared small blocks of pigment, also known as cakes
Pigment Finely ground powder used to make colour
Split When two pigments are not binding together evenly when mixed or when laid on the paper
Stretching paper Soaking paper on one side or both sides with water, before attaching it to a board with gummed tape and allowing it to dry prior to painting
Tubes Prepared pigment in a squeezable tube
Warm colours Colours broadly within the yellow, orange and red categories of the colour wheel
Washes Colour diluted with water and applied with a brush

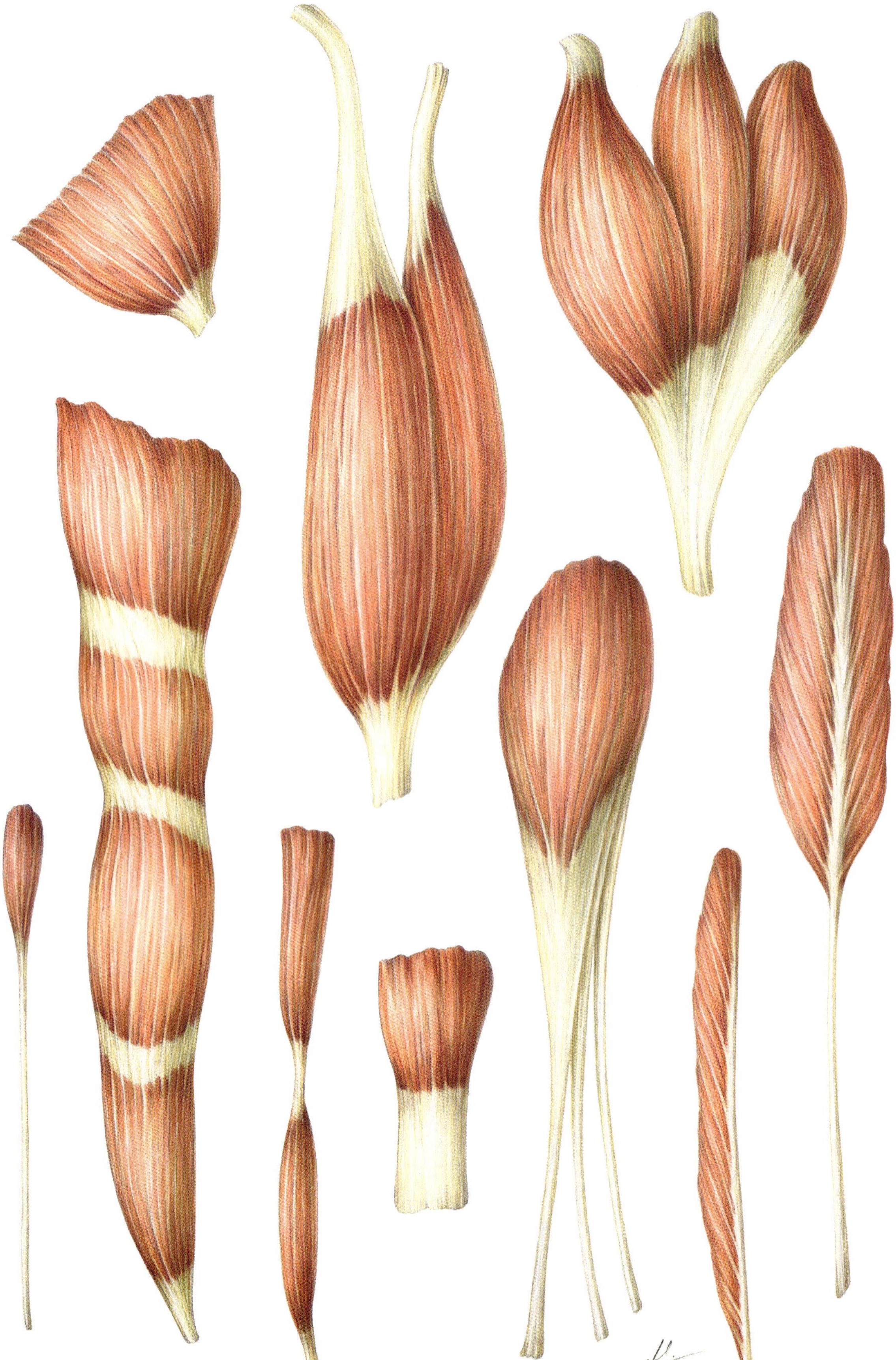

A selection of muscle shapes. Watercolour.

PAINTING MUSCLES

The human body has more than 600 muscles. The muscular system includes muscles, tendons and cartilage, with muscles dividing primarily into three groups: skeletal muscle, smooth muscle and cardiac muscle. Medical artists need to become familiar with these muscle types and how to represent them for anatomical, surgical, clinical and educational publications.

Step by Step: Painting Muscles in Watercolour

Aim: Create a watercolour painting by layering watercolour pigments to build up the muscle form, tone and colour, illustrating two muscles of the head, the masseter muscle and the temporalis muscle.

Art materials:

- Pencils 2H and 2B
- Pencil sharpener
- Putty rubber
- Watercolour paper A3 sheet or pad
- Callipers or measuring device
- Watercolour paints
- Sable paintbrushes
- Two pots of water
- Tissues
- Spare paper

Steps

1. Measure and draw a skull outline from your specimen. (*see* Chapter 9). *Refer* to Chapter 6 for information about measuring devices.
2. Identify the areas where the muscles attach to the lateral side of the skull and jaw bone (mandible) with the aid of an anatomical textbook. This illustration shows the masseter muscle attachment areas in yellow and the temporalis muscle attachment areas in blue. Note the temporalis passes behind the zygomatic arch and attaches to the coronoid process of the mandible, i.e. connecting two bones; and the masseter muscle attaches between the inferior margin of the zygomatic arch down to the mandible, also connecting these two bones.
3. Develop a graphite pencil (black and white) tonal drawing to become your primary reference source for the final artwork.
4. First, dampen the surface of the paper, then apply the first layer of watercolour. It is recommended to choose a yellow pigment to apply first; here, Windsor Yellow has been chosen, creating a light and unifying background colour.
5. Allow your first layer of yellow to almost dry, before choosing the next colour for the second layer – here Windsor Red has been selected.
6. Once your second layer has almost dried, placing your third blue pigment – here Windsor Blue has been chosen – as your final top layer.

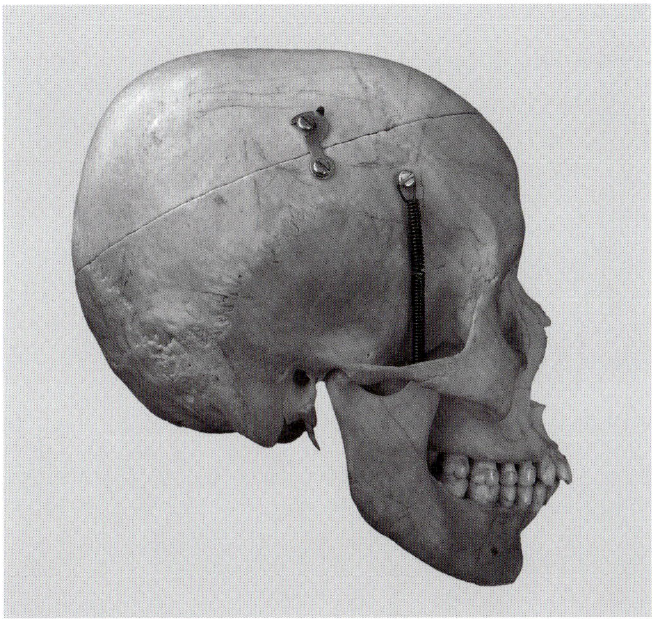

Select a skull for studying the areas where each muscle attaches, linking between the skull and the mandible.

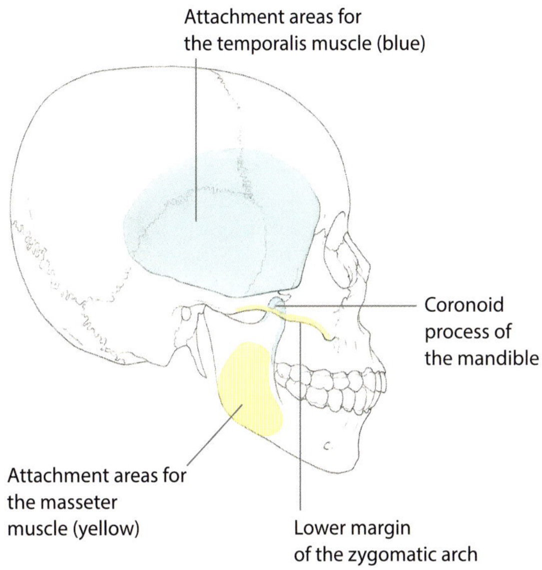

Coloured areas demarcate the muscle attachments – blue for the temporalis muscle and yellow for the masseter muscle.

Steps

1. Measure your skull specimen carefully and prepare an initial pencil outline in conjunction with a good quality anatomical textbook study where the muscles attach for the masseter and temporalis muscles. You will be able to see the slightly raised or ridged areas on the skull, which demarcate the areas of attachment. By gently running your finger over the surface of the skull, you will also be able to feel the subtle changes in the surface texture, which will help you to identify them.
Create a tonal drawing of the muscles, building a reference image from which to base your watercolour artwork.

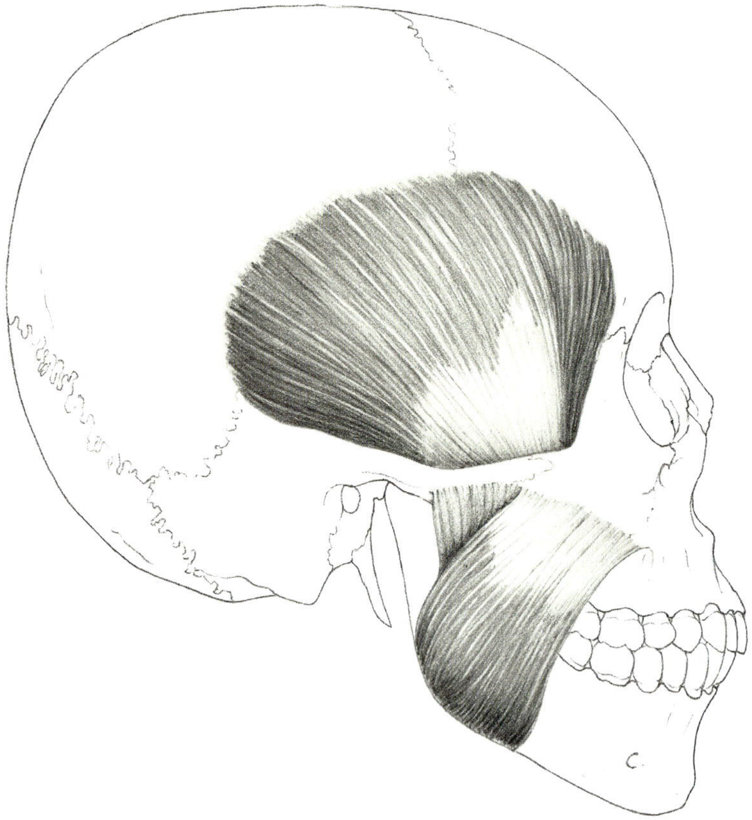

2. First, slightly dampen the surface of the watercolour paper, which will allow the paint to flow more evenly over the surface. If you inadvertently apply too much water, then lightly pat the surface dry with a clean paper towel. Select your yellow pigment and gradually build areas of tone and depth while still keeping to one colour. Once you have established the overall form of the muscle and tendons, then select your second colour, red and repeat the process to continue building the forms.

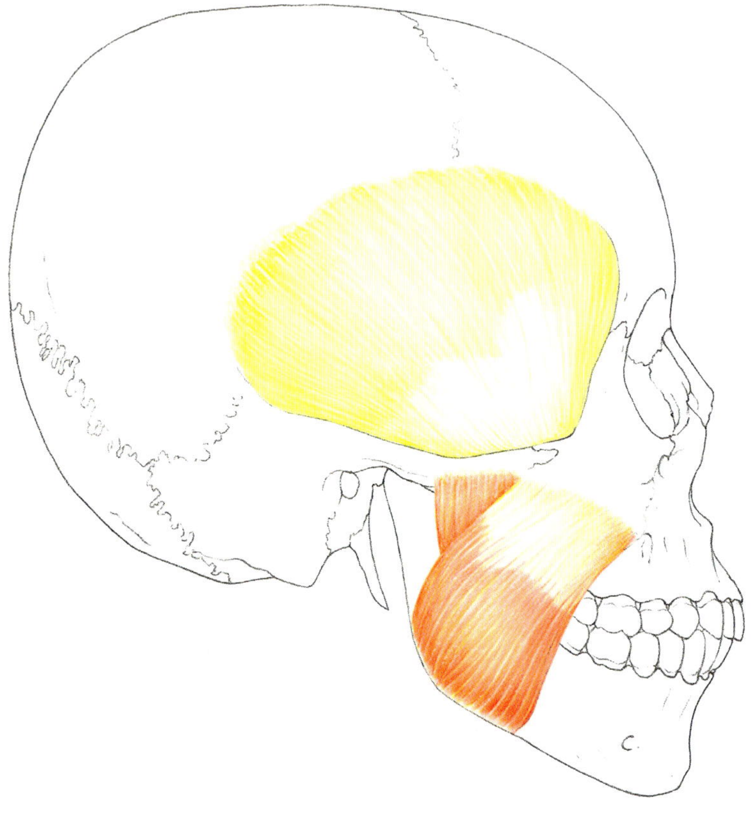

3. To complete your watercolour muscle painting, now choose your blue pigment and selectively place the blue on those areas only of shadow or those areas requiring additional form. This will allow the form created with red to be retained and the yellow beneath to show through unifying your whole image.

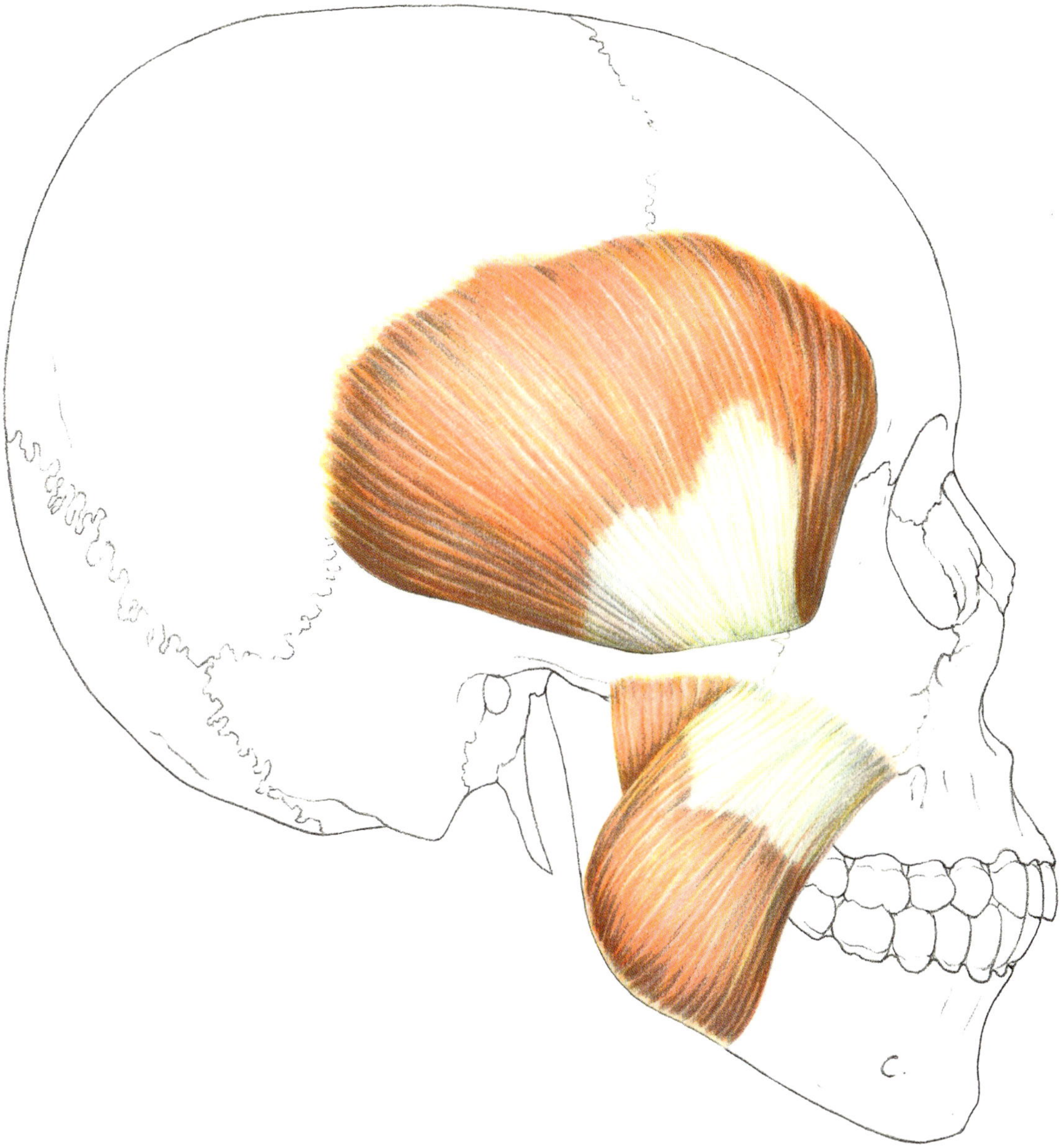

WATERCOLOUR TIP

Very slightly dampen the watercolour paper before applying the first wash either with a brush or a small spray bottle of clean water. A slightly dampened surface will allow the paint to 'sit' on the surface, allowing your first wash to flow more readily over the surface of the damp paper, whereas painting your first layer onto dry paper may cause the paint to soak in too quickly, making it less pliable and harder to blend, leaving dark edges – experiment by painting on both dry and damp surfaces and compare the results.

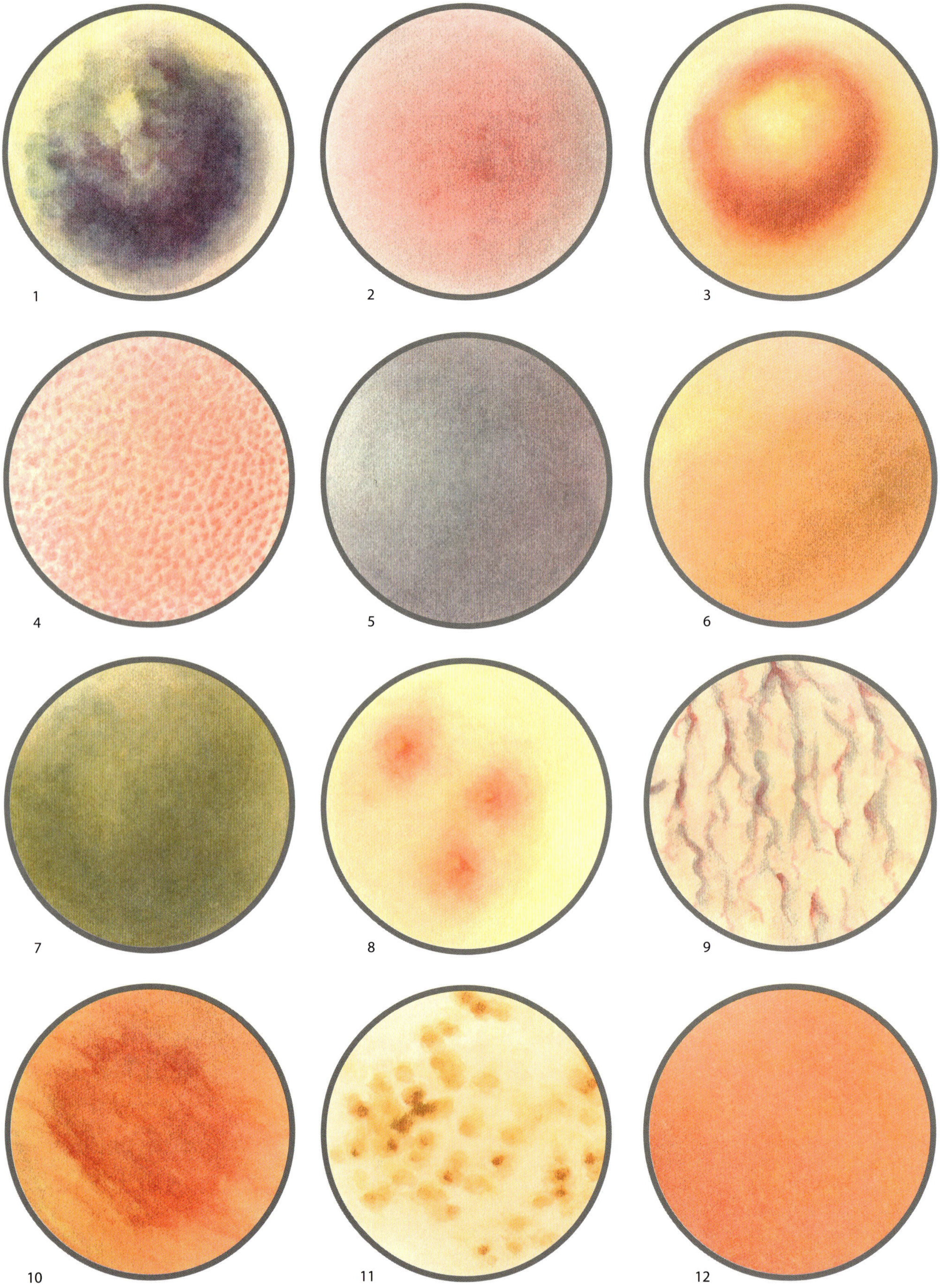
1
2
3
4
5
6
7
8
9
10
11
12

CHAPTER 12

SKIN

Our skin is a marvel! Recording and interpreting our skin into an illustration that reflects our skin's uniqueness, character and charm requires careful observation. When you begin to truly observe skin, the appearance, texture and colour variations are endless. Each clinical subject that a medical artist illustrates becomes a fascinating world of interpretation. As artists, we don't just observe the exterior surface; we also interpret the character beyond those external layers. This section will look at external observable variations through a combination of artworks and photographs and provides an introduction to creating your own watercolour skin colour palette for future reference.

THE NATURE OF SKIN

We all have those little imperfections, whether freckles, pimples or varicose veins. It is doubtful if skin can be ever called flawless; however, some skin imperfections are considered charming or even beautiful, such as freckles. Skin's diversity is endless, from the soft tones of a new-born child to a characterful mature wrinkled and weathered face.

The skin helps to regulate our body temperature, keeping us warm or cool, and contains many sensitive nerve endings. It naturally renews every month, with the dead skin cells flaking off from the top surface layers. Skin is the largest organ system of the body, and is part of the integumentary system. This classification includes the skin itself (with its associated glands and nerves), hair and fingernails. Skin protects the whole body in several ways, providing an outer protective layer for all our internal structures and organs.

Skin can be affected by many conditions, ranging from acne and dermatitis to severe life-threatening skin conditions such as necrotising fasciitis. Skin conditions may also be caused by an underlying issue affecting an internal organ – for example jaundice is a disease of the liver giving the skin a distinct yellow colour.

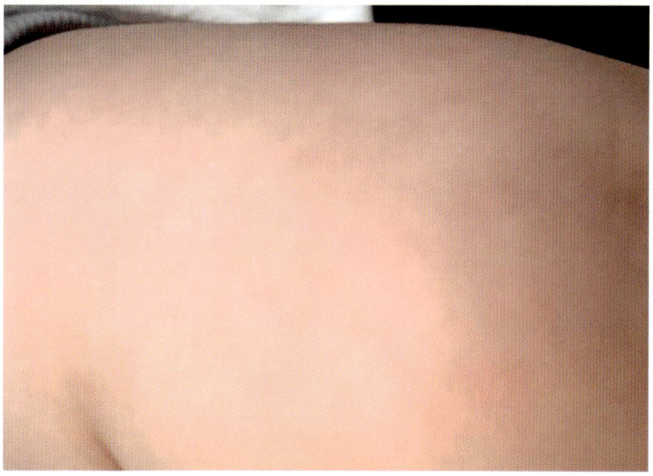

A new-born baby's skin is smooth, supple and soft. The skin's outer layer, the epidermis, is thicker when young containing more fat and collagen.

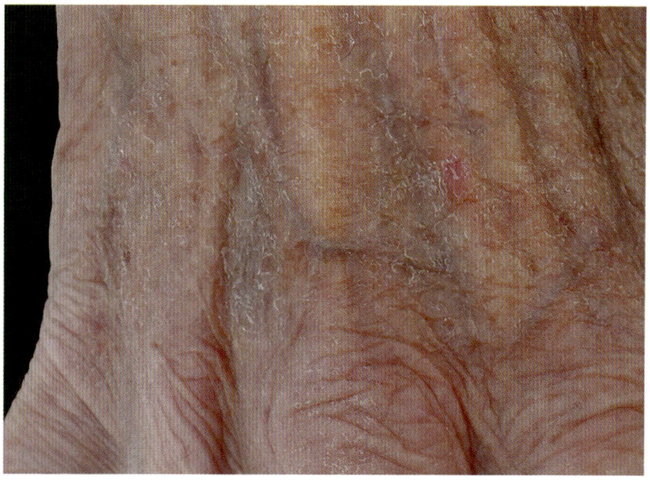

As we age, our skin becomes thinner, fragile and more translucent; forming an uneven surface due to the loss of fat and structure within the layers.

Twelve skin condition in watercolour (left). 1 Bruise. 2 Inflammation. 3 Inflamed insect bite. 4 Rash. 5 Cold. 6 Hot flush. 7 Jaundice. 8 Small insect bites. 9 Superficial blood veins. 10 Allergic reaction. 11 Freckles. 12 Sunburn.

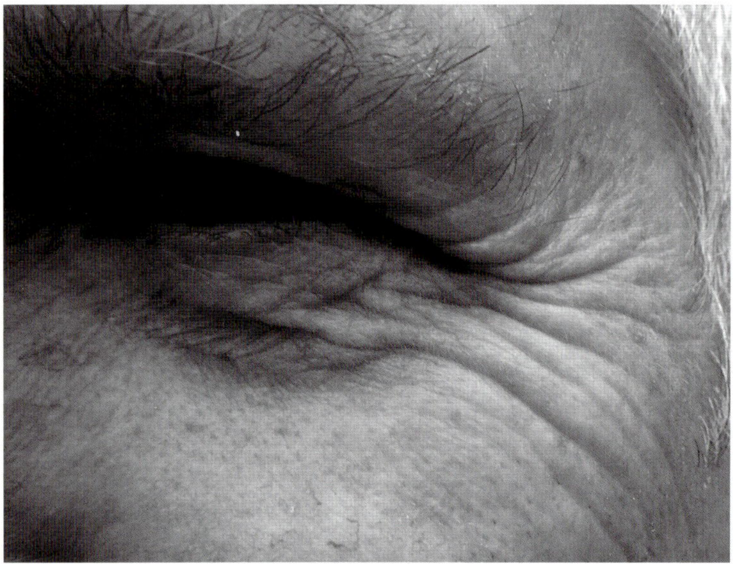

The face has many muscles and wrinkles develop around the eye when we smile. Smiling also involves muscles around our mouth, cheeks and eyes, collectively known as the muscles of facial expression.

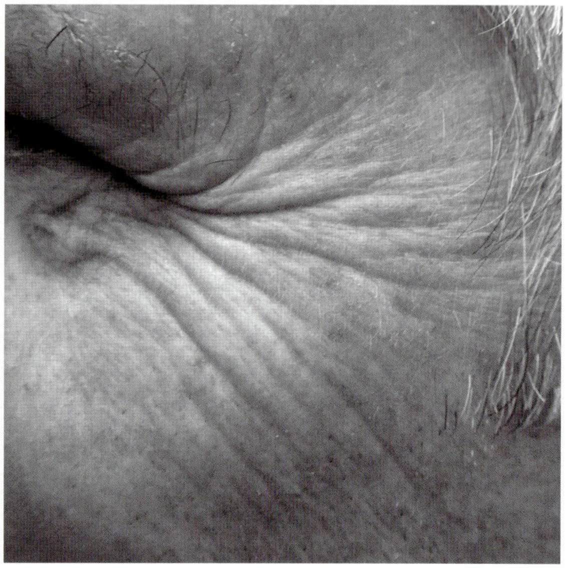

Lateral view of the upper cheekbone area around the eye, forming the wrinkles commonly known as 'crow's feet'.

For clinicians, observing skin conditions may be a factor in determining whether further clinical tests are required for diagnosis and treatment. Observing our outer layers is important not just for clinicians but also for artists. The medical artist will need to observe variations in shape, texture, colour, tone and lighting to portray the skin faithfully in illustrations and artworks.

Our skin changes constantly in colour and texture. The skin can appear reddened from sun- or windburn, or even an annoying insect bite, or paler with a blue tone if we are cold. We appear 'less red' when we are cold, because the body has withdrawn the blood from the surface of the skin to prioritise keeping the inner organs warm. When studying skin, look beyond the individual limbs and observe the body as a whole.

The two images below show differing facial conditions, from a pair of naturally occuring moles to brown areas commonly know as 'sun spots, which often increase in size and number with age and are frequently associated with regular sun exposure.

The images (opposite top right) show two different skin conditions which have occurred on the face for comparison. They have caused very different blistering effects, though both are visible.

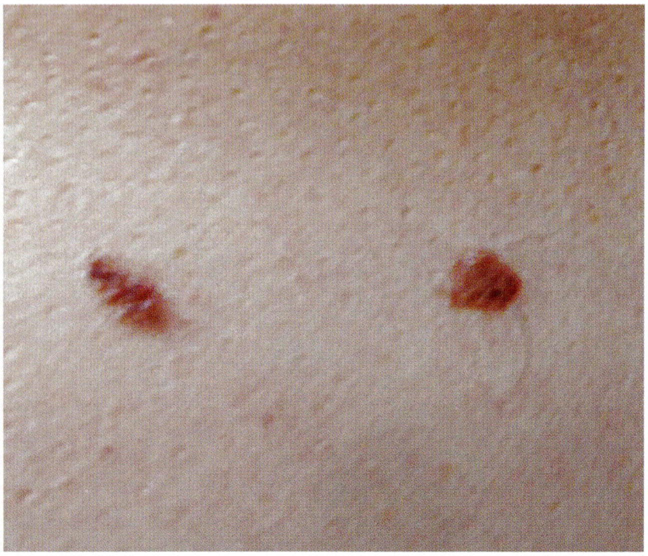

Two small moles. Moles may vary significantly in size, form and colour.

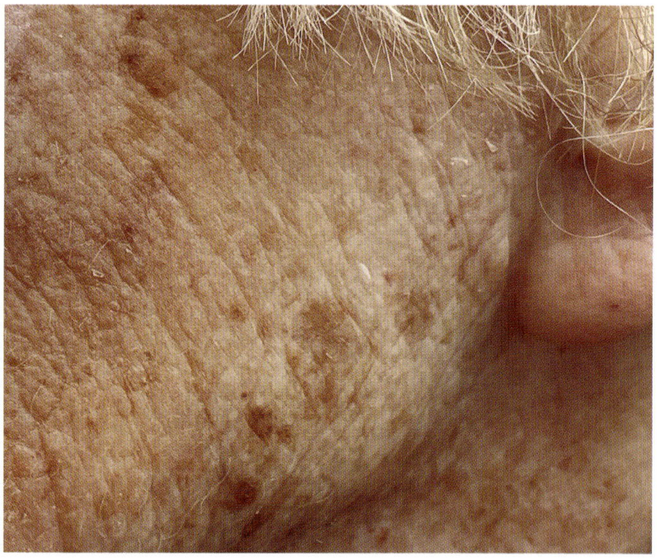

Exposure to the sun over time may cause discolouration to the skin in the form of irregular darker patches, called sunspots.

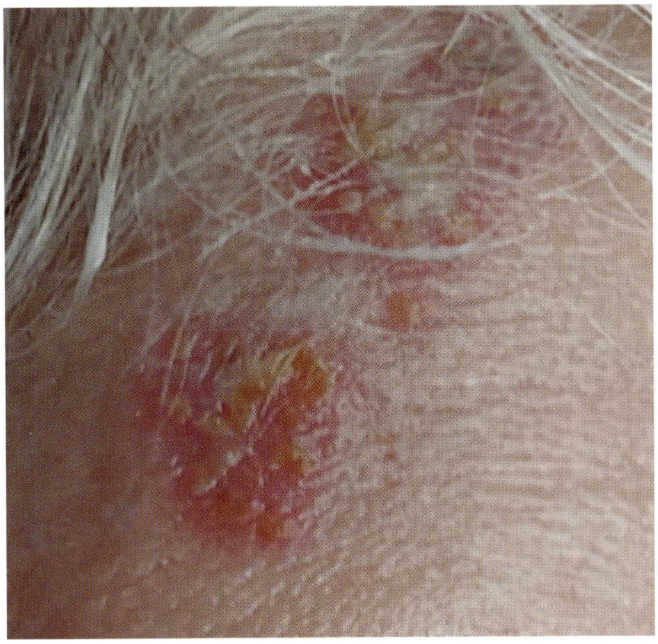

Shingles is an unpleasant and often painful nerve condition, causing raised blisters in the area served by the affected nerve. Here the line of blisters had followed the path of the nerve across the forehead and down towards the eye.

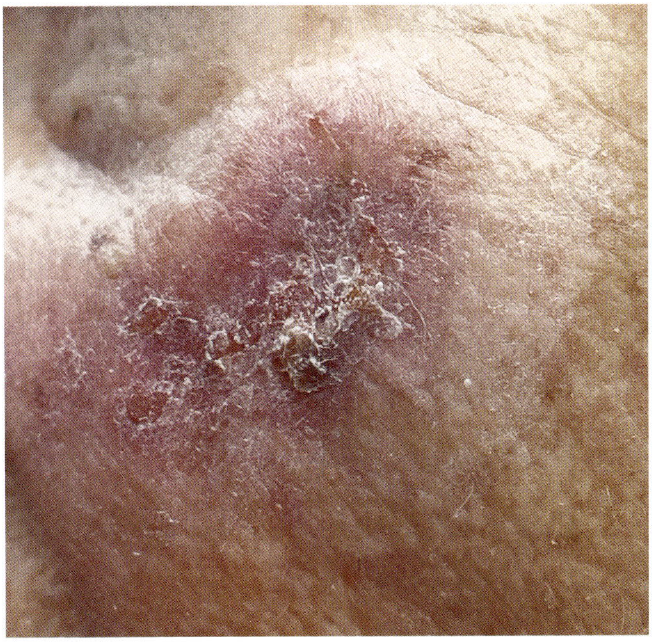

An area being treated for the presentation of a pre-basal cell carcinoma, where the sun has damaged the lower layers of the skin's epidermis. Sun damage occurs on those areas frequently exposed to the sun, as for example on this cheek.

Bruising

Bruising is due to bleeding into the skin, which may happen for many reasons, usually accidental, for example colliding with a corner of a table! Or an underlying clinical condition. The image examples below show how a bruise will produce an array of different skin colours as the body repairs itself after the original 'trauma' reaction, gradually returning to the normal skin colouring over time. Occasionally, a scar may remain from the impact or injury.

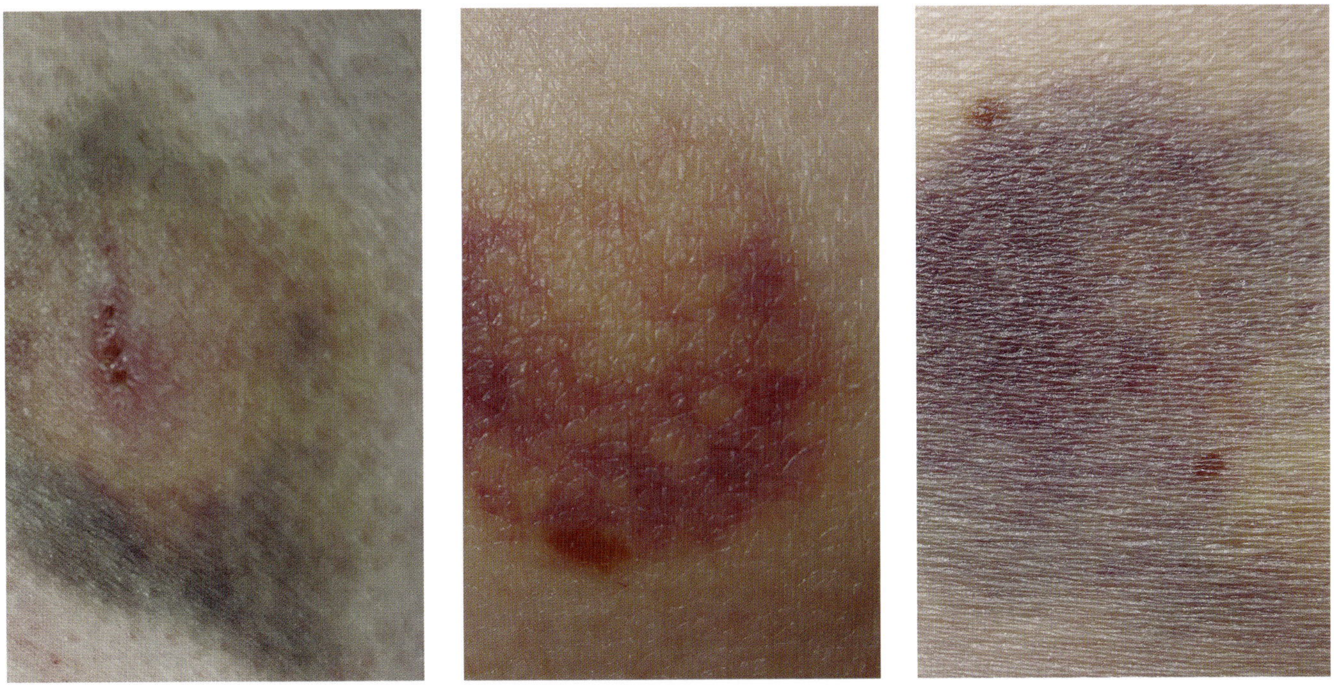

Bruising to the skin can change colour significantly over time, as the healing process within the tissue layers occurs.

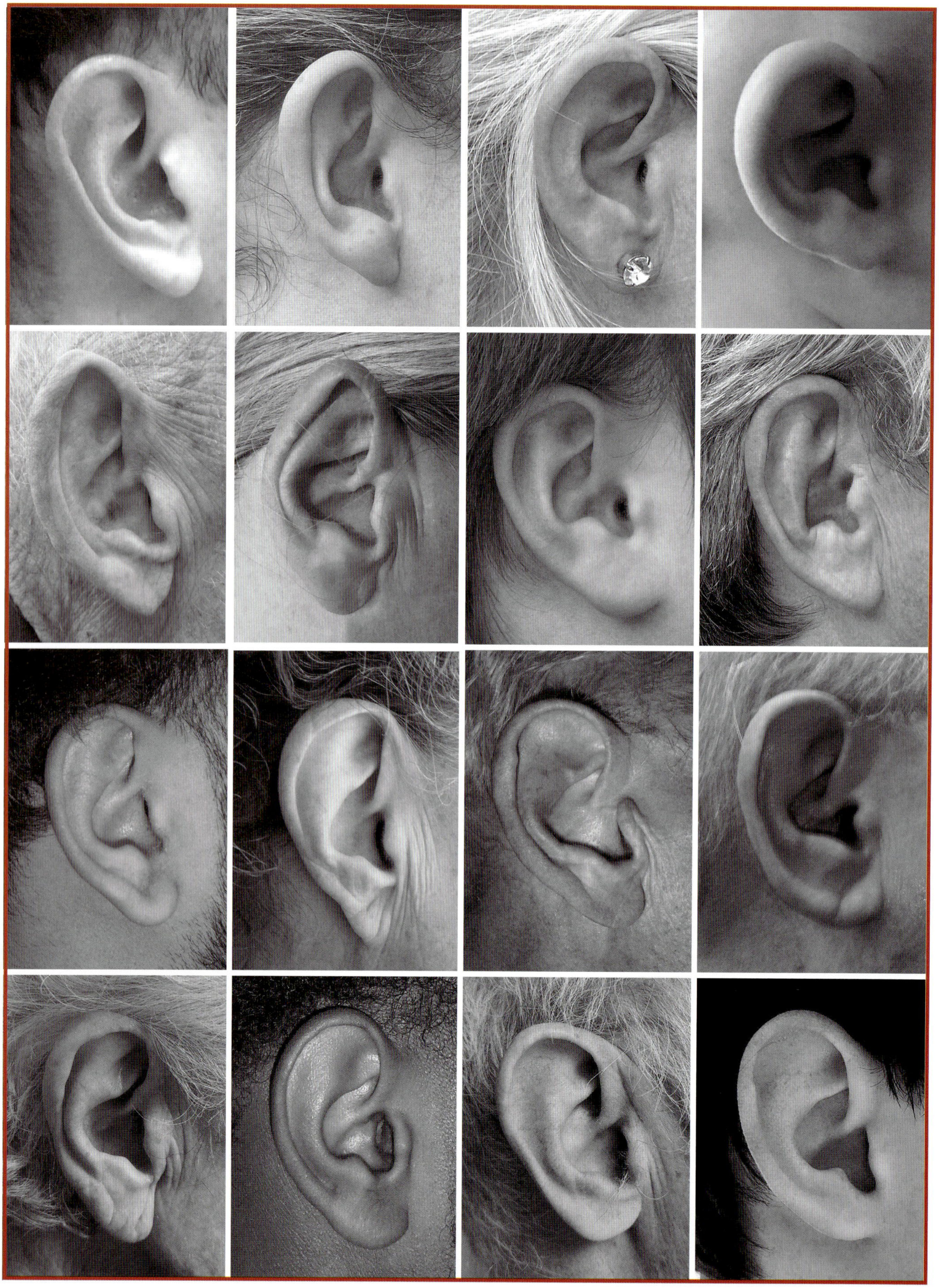

Project: Your Own Skin

Aim: To observe and record varied skin tones.

Art materials:

- Sketchbook
- Graphite pencils – 2H to 4B
- Coloured pencils – Yellow, Red and Blue

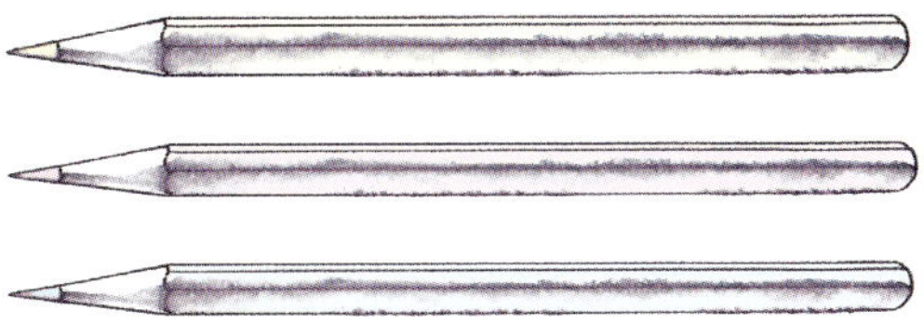

- Watercolour paints
- Paint brushes
- Mixing palette
- Two pots of water
- Arches watercolour paper HP 300gms

Project: Look closely at your skin, or a partner's, relative's or close friend's, always checking for their permission first. An ear may be a good skin example to observe initially. Take written and colour notes in your sketchbook, closely observing the skin type, the colour and, if possible, how does it feel. Is the skin hot or cold? Does the skin feel rough, smooth, or wrinkled? How is the skin reacting at this moment in time? Is the skin shiny, matt, waxy, dry or flaky? Look closely at the formation of the folds, the curves and areas of depth or in shadow. Take notes over successive days, observing any skin change, both in colour and texture. Record and illustrate each subtle change.

Recording in coloured pencils is a convenient and quick method if watercolours are unavailable. Continue with the three-colour method, combining the three primary colours, yellow, red and blue pencils (left). Begin by laying down yellow pencil tones, gradually overlaying with red pencil to give warmth and detail, then finally add blue pencil tones to create form and shadows, for a subtle skin tone drawing.

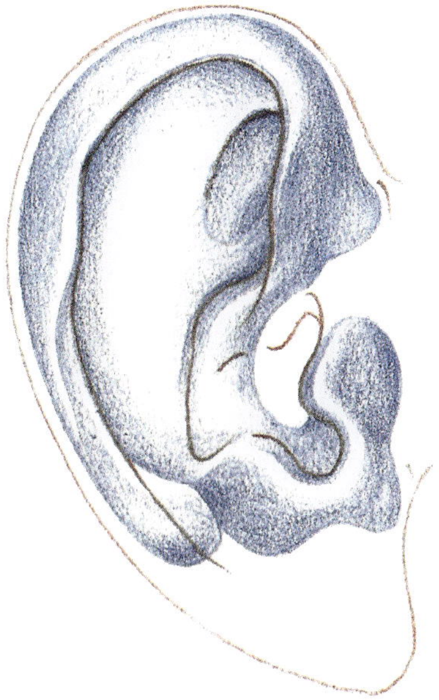

Ears are a complex structure. The outer shape is supported by the internal folds of cartilage, shown shaded in blue pencil above.

The structure of the ear is covered further on page 38.

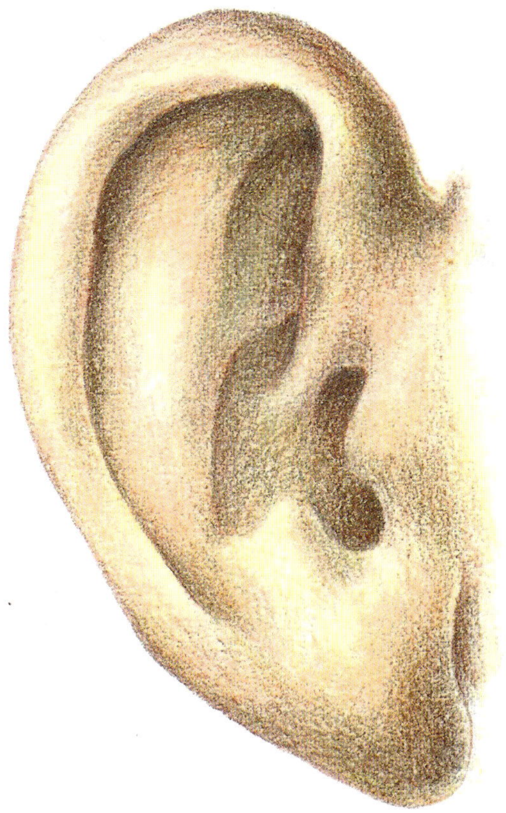

Every ear is different. The sixteen examples (left) show the wide variety in each individual shape and form. No two ears are exactly the same.

PAINTING SKIN TONES IN WATERCOLOUR

Medical artists are often required to record skin conditions. Skin is translucent, making the translucent qualities of watercolour an ideal art medium in which to replicate the many subtle variations of skin tone and features, to illustrate the clinical features required accurately. Observation of a patient's skin tone is an important external feature to consider in relation to a patient's medical condition. Their skin can reflect whether they are hot and flushed, i.e. with a temperature, or pale, cold and clammy, or even presenting with a hint of yellow undertone, perhaps indicating an underlying condition such as jaundice.

Painting realistic skin is relating more than one single colour – there are highlights, reflections, reflected light, shadows and cast shadows each forming variations in colour and tone. When beginning, it is advisable to limit your palette to just three colours – yellow, red and blue – and to become familiar with their complementary colours (refer to the colour wheel below). This will give you the basis for all the tones you require. By changing one or more of the primary colours for a similar shade, for example, switch one red pigment and choose a different red option. Red is also a good balancing colour for your artwork if you find it has gone too yellow or too blue. Carefully overlay a light wash of colour to a small area or over the whole artwork to change the emphasis and tone as required.

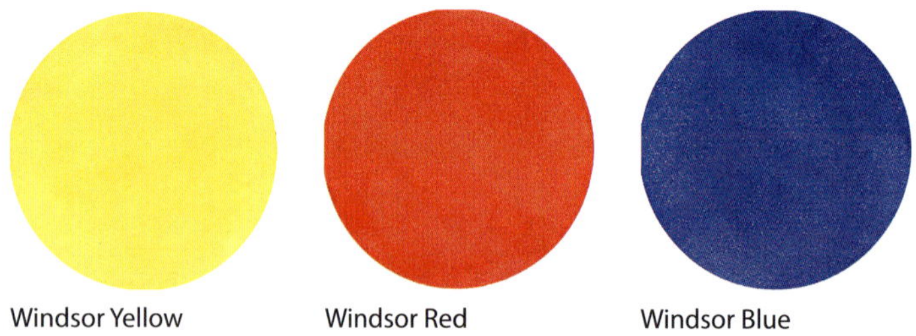

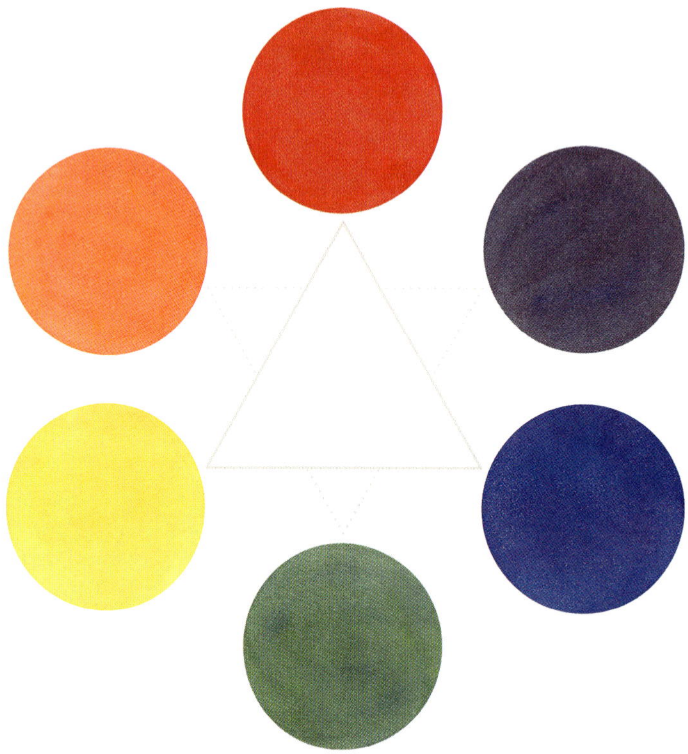

The traditional colour wheel.
Between each of the three primary colours – yellow, red and blue – will be those colours achieved by mixing the two adjacent primary colours to create a third colour. The colours positioned opposite to each other diagonally across the wheel, are considered to be their complementary colours.

CREATING COLOUR CHARTS

Creating your own colour charts will give you an excellent reference from which to choose colour combinations that work for you in different situations. Are you looking to create a pale or darker tone, or is the skin tone warm or cool?

When building your colour charts or preparing artwork, remember watercolour will always dry paler than when first applied. It is straightforward, however, to build up further layers by applying more paint if you wish to make an area darker.

Begin with a pale yellow wash and then build up layers of red and blue from the primary colour selection, choosing either a warm or cool palette of colours depending upon the result you require. This will give you more control and help to keep the beautiful translucent quality of skin tones.

Gradually vary the quantities of each colour to see all the possible variations. If you add more primary red paint pigment, the skin tone will be warmer, whereas if you use a cooler Alizarin Red pigment, the overall tone will appear cooler. If you change your first mix by adding more blue pigment the effect will also appear cooler or toned down. Experiment and try different combinations of red, blue and yellow to create a broad range of complementary skin colours, from light to dark tones and warm to cool colours.

You can expand your colour range by replacing one of the three primary colours at a time, for example, changing Windsor Red to Alizarin or Windsor Blue to Indigo or Ultramarine. Ultramarine may cause a splitting of the colour combination when premixed – this colour works better overlaid as a single unmixed colour.

Create colour charts with the paints in your own palette for future reference. Vary the quantities of each pigment either as overlaid layers of colour or premixed colours on your watercolour paper.

The chart here demonstrates the range of colours achieved by changing one colour at a time. Charts can be extensive and run to many pages; these are just a few samples to start you off. When you create your own charts, label and note along each row with the colour combination you have used. This will be invaluable when you wish to recreate similar skin tones in the future.

The skin chart shows that you will see some tones are darker than others. This can be achieved by adding more pigment to your mix, especially more blue pigment. Blue also works well for shadows and darker areas; just remember paint dries lighter than when it's first applied.

The following additional watercolours were premixed with Windsor Red, Yellow and Blue to create the skin colour sample chart: Alizarin Red, Indian Red, Yellow Ochre, Indigo and Ultramarine.

Project: Colour Reference Charts

Aim: To mix watercolour combinations to create gradated colour charts for future reference.

Art materials:

- Watercolour paints
- Brushes
- Mixing palette
- Two pots of water
- Pencil
- Arches watercolour paper HP 300gms in block form

Project: Create your own skin colour reference charts, by varying the pigment combinations and proportions from your palette. Examples are shown on the following page.

Five additional colour options for creating colour swatch mixes.

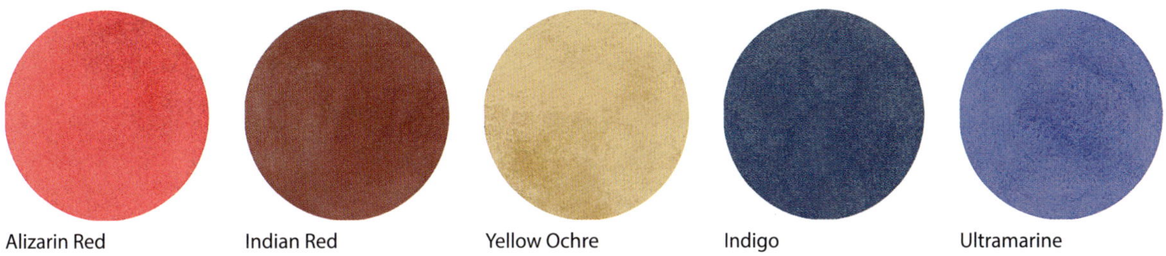

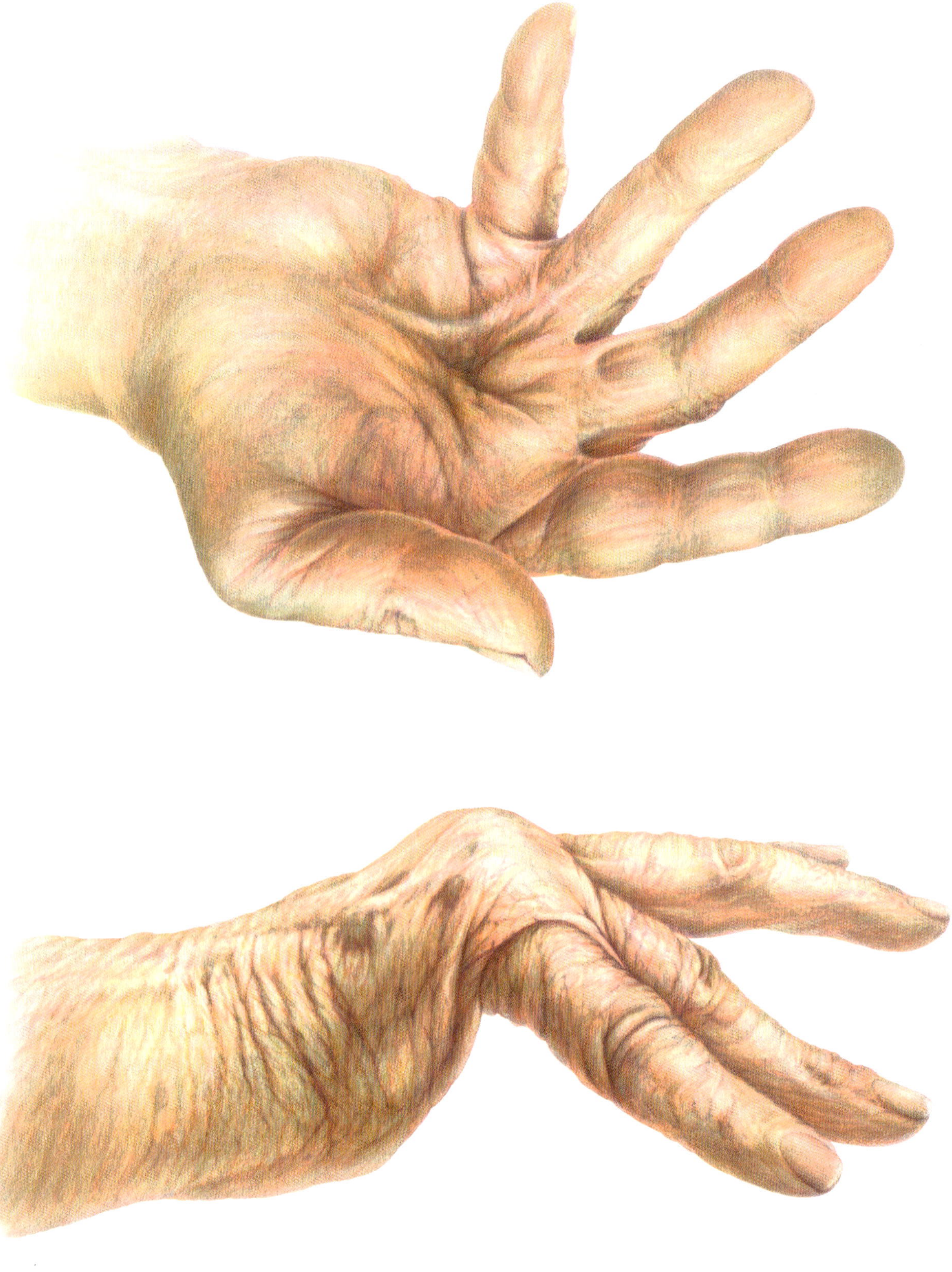

Dupytrens contracture of the right hand. Watercolour.
Skin may thicken abnormally in the palm of the hand and cause one or more fingers to contract or tighten, curling them towards the palm.

Skin Colour Swatches

These skin colour swatch examples have been created by mixing a combination of the three primary colours alongside a selection of additional colours in varying ratios, keeping to three colours within each mix. Create your own colour charts by mixing each colour combination in turn and in varying proportions, noting the colours you have used beside each swatch. These charts will become invaluable reference resources when planning skin tones. Over time, you will accumulate many charts while experimenting with all the colour options available – the colour variations are endless! Store these reference swatches in an art folder, box file or similar storage to keep them clean and safe.

Row 1
Windsor Yellow
Indian Red
Windsor Blue

Row 2
Yellow Ochre
Alizarin Red
Indigo

Row 3
Windsor Yellow
Alizarin Red
Windsor Blue

Row 4
Yellow Ochre
Indian Red
Windsor Blue

Row 5
Yellow Ochre
Indian Red
Indigo

Row 6
Windsor Yellow
Windsor Red
Ultramarine

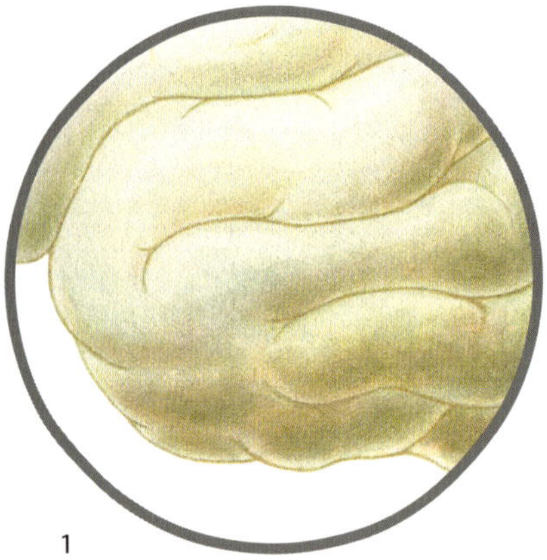

1

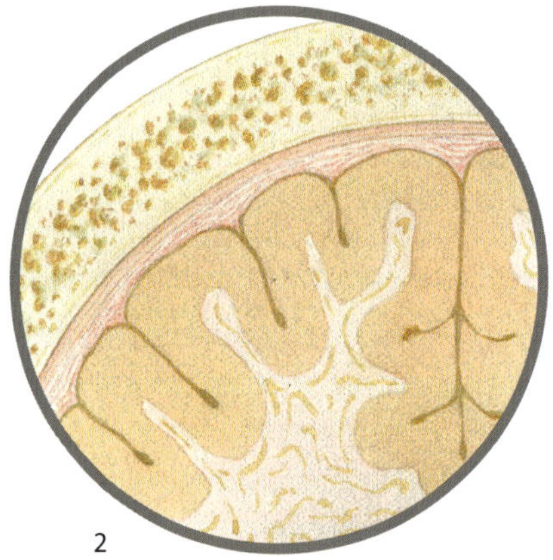

2

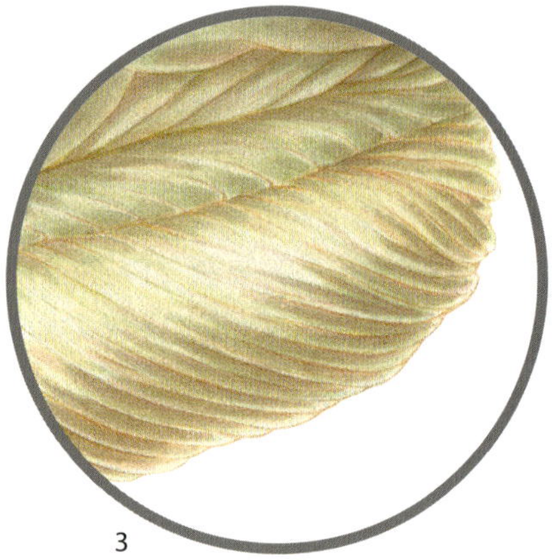

3

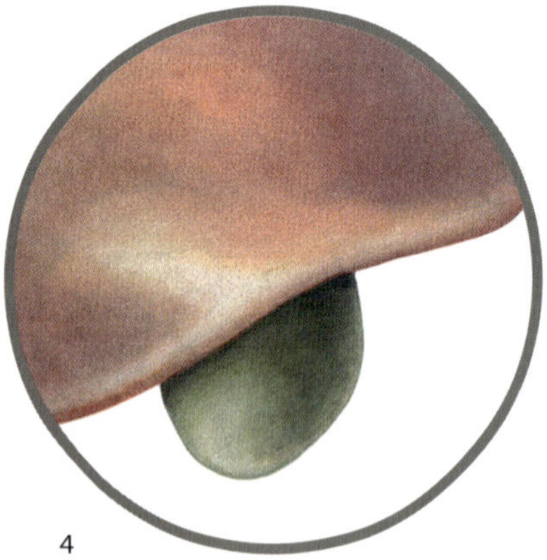

4

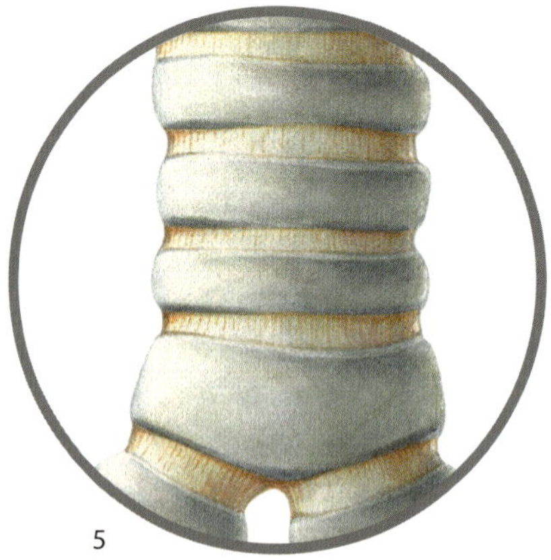

5

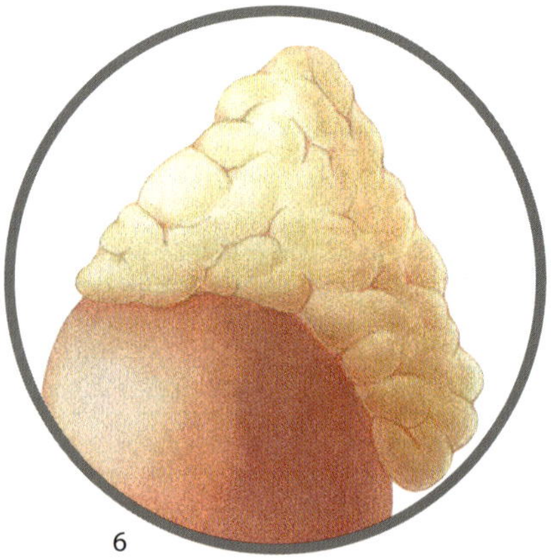

6

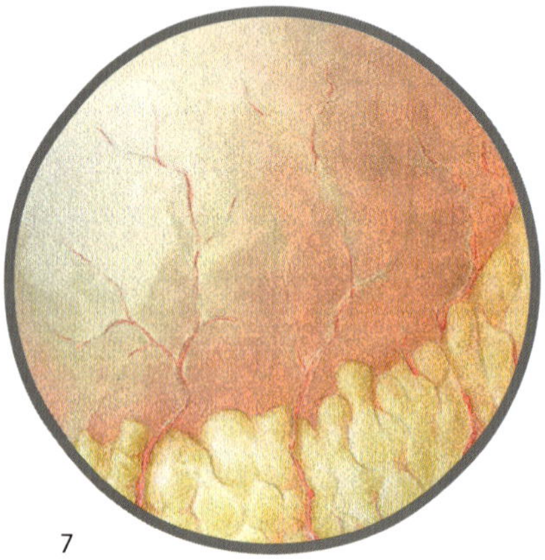

7

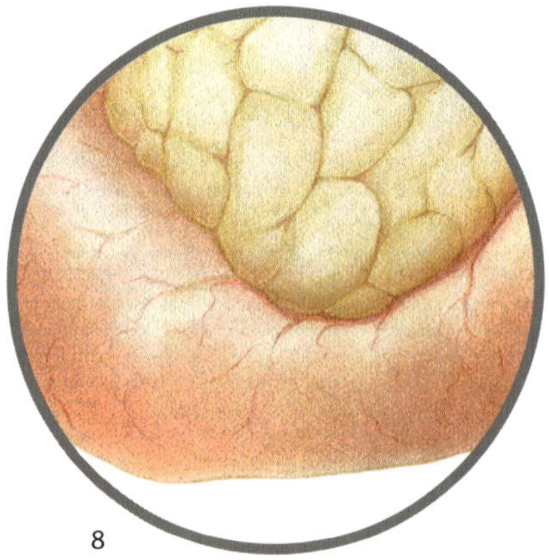

8

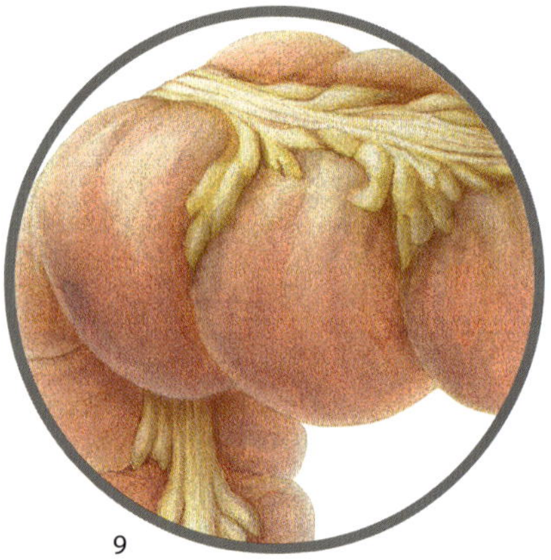

9

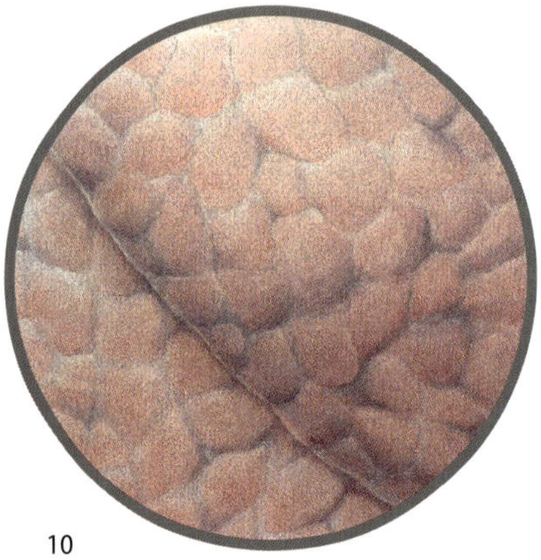

10

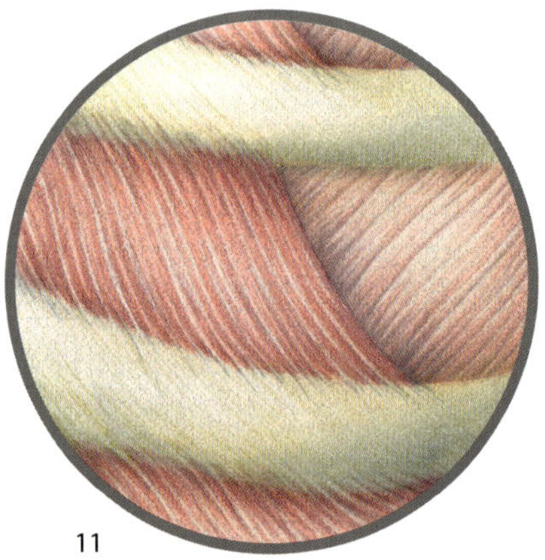

11

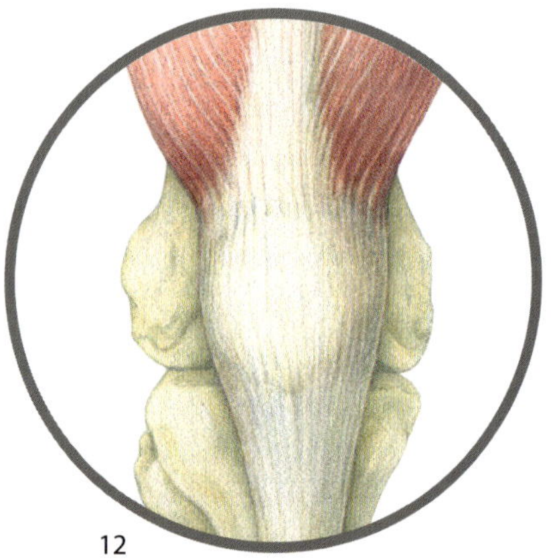

12

CHAPTER 13

CONVENTIONS IN MEDICAL ILLUSTRATION

The body has an amazing 78 organs, including the brain, heart, liver and intestines, all of which are subjects a medical artist will be asked to create artworks for either patient information, leaflets, educational charts, textbooks, technical information and, online apps, etc.

Here we will look at a variety of anatomical structures and the regular conventions used within illustrations for their representation in both colour and line work. Ink line drawings have been included of the same structures to provide a useful cross-reference (*see* also Chapter 10).

There is a sample step-by-step project illustrating an anatomical specimen for practice – a kidney. This example demonstrates how a range of art media can be used, beginning with an initial graphite line pencil drawing, developing into a pencil tonal artwork, thirdly progressing with the pen and wash technique and concluding with a watercolour illustration to complete the set.

COLOUR CONVENTIONS

For medical artists, the intrinsic elements of the human body have become represented in standardised colours, style and format. This enables the reader or viewer to recognise each anatomical element with ease. For example, arteries are shown in red tones (representing the oxygenated blood leaving the lungs) and veins in blue tones (representing the darker, deoxygenated blood returning via the heart to the lungs) and nerves in yellow. If an illustrated text took a different approach, for example, the arteries in blue and the veins in red, this would cause significant confusion and potentially lead to serious consequences in misinterpretation of the information. Medical artists are expected to use the current conventions to create consistent and reliable illustrated material for the public and clinical settings.

Twelve anatomical representational watercolour illustrations.
1 A portion of the left cerebral surface of the brain, lateral view. 2 Frontal cross-section through the cranium (skull), revealing lobes and fissures of the brain. 3 Lateral view of the exterior surface of the cerebellum. The cerebellum lies in the posterior fossa. 4 The inferior margin of the right lobe of the liver, with the gall bladder (in green) below. 5 Bifurcation of the trachea (windpipe), showing the annular ligaments between the tracheal cartilages.
6 Adrenal (suprarenal) gland above the right kidney. 7 Lower portion of the stomach, showing the edge of the greater omentum and its attachment along the edge of the stomach. The omentum is a fold or peritoneal flap covering and connecting the stomach to the other abdominal organs. 8 The duodenum (small intestine) and head of the pancreas. The duodenum is the first section of the small intestine from the stomach. The pancreas is important for digestion, creating enzymes that help break down food. 9 The colic flexure and transverse section of the colon (large intestine). The large intestine often has many small fatty appendices called epiploicae. 10 A fissure separating lobes of the right lung. 11 External and internal intercostal muscles, giving flexibility between the ribs. 12 Ligaments of the patella. The medial and lateral rectus muscles sit above the knee, and the tendon of the rectus femoris muscle runs centrally between these muscles to the patella. The patella ligament is attached inferiorly to the tibia.
The corresponding ink line images can be found on Page 92.

The four artworks on the left show the regular colour and style conventions used within medical illustrations. With monochrome comparions drawn in sepia ink on the right.

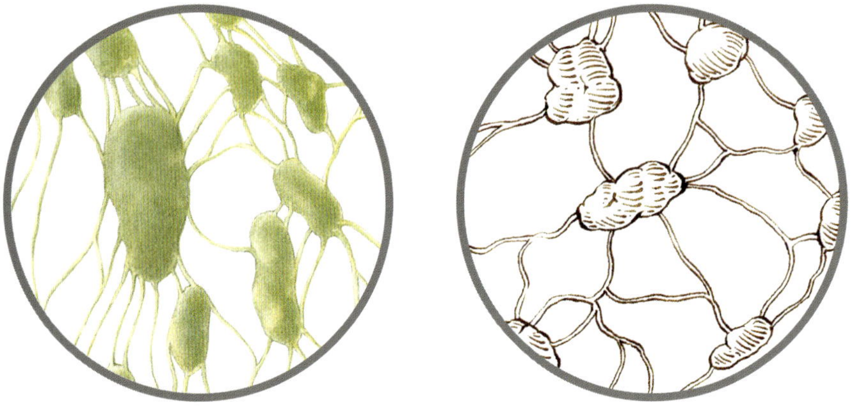

1. The lymphatic system is usually represented in soft blue/green hues.

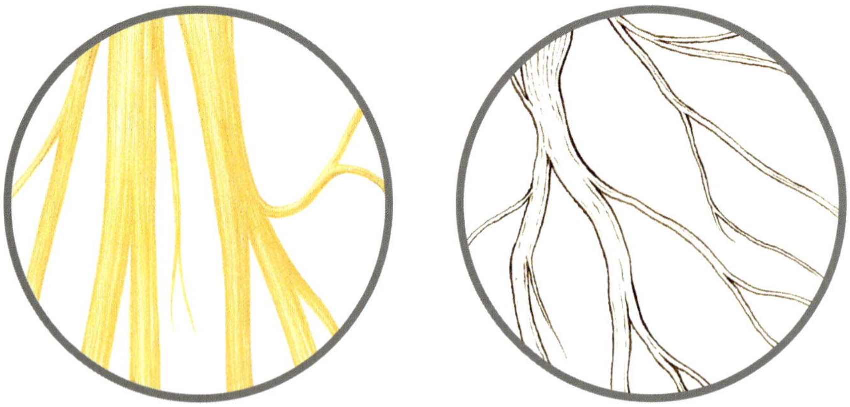

2. Nerves are usually represented in yellow with limited shading or form.

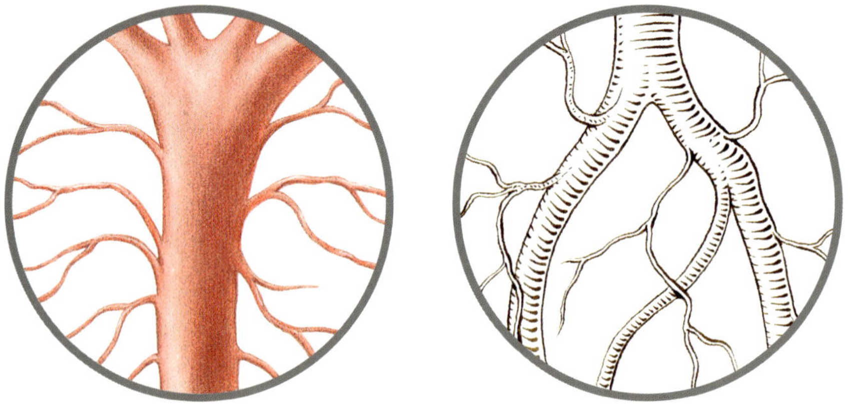

3. Arteries are represented in red and shaded to reflect their cylindrical shape, due to their thicker and muscular vessel walls.

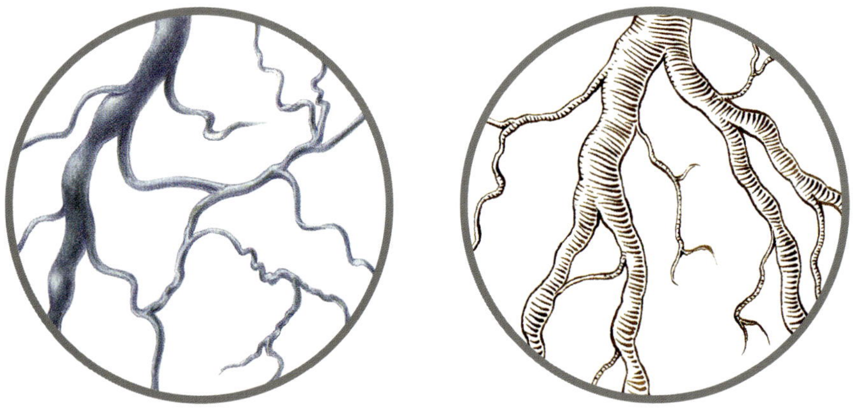

4. Veins are represented in blue, with a more flattened and irregular appearance due to their thinner vessel walls and internal valves.

The regular colour conventions are as follows:

The lymphatic system is usually represented in soft blue/green hues.
Nerves are usually represented in yellow with limited shading.
Arteries are represented in red and shaded to reflect their more cylindrical shape. Arteries need a thicker wall than veins because they have to withstand greater pressure from the blood when pumped from the heart.
Veins are represented in blue, with a more flattened appearance due to their thinner vessel walls.
Muscles are usually coloured with a red hue, consider combining red with a deeper red.
Tendons are rarely coloured but left nearly white, with just the fibrous structure being represented with delicate blue/grey or ochre shading, depending on the colour scheme of the artwork.
Fat is usually yellow, consider using a deeper yellow, aim for a colour similar to mature cheese! Fat is often globular in shape.
Bones' outer surface is often represented in soft grey or ochre tones. The inner bone marrow of long bones tends to be represented yellow in colour, due to the high fat content, while the inside of flat bones is represented in dark pink and red hues due to marrow being the main area where red blood cells are made.

Illustration versus Real Life

There are accepted interpretations for published works, for both line and colour artwork, which may not be quite the same as seen in real life. However, most elements are represented by their perceived 'normal' colour and texture. You may also come across museum specimens or illustrations in texts drawn from such specimens that do not reflect the 'true' colour of a 'live' specimen. Furthermore, no two artists will view and interpret the colours of a specimen in the same way. In published works, the bright colours that are naturally seen in real life are often toned down. The colour palette chosen may also reflect the designer's decision, with a colour scheme chosen to be more visually appealing.

Suppose you are researching a particular colour reference to be as accurate as possible, there are now numerous online images and videos covering just about every subject you can think of in relation to human anatomy, alongside published works to guide you as to the shape, colour, or texture.

WORKING FROM A REAL SPECIMEN

Obtaining Specimens

An excellent way to begin practising illustrating anatomical structures, shape and textures is to obtain one or more specimens from your local butcher. Most butchers will be happy to supply organs such as kidneys and hearts for educational purposes. If you specify that they are for your study and request that they leave the surrounding fat and vessels in place, i.e. not trimmed. Specimens may be purchased for a nominal sum.

It is recommeneded to purchase a minimum of two specimens of each item. One specimen can remain whole for you to study the external features, concentrating on the outer shape and texture, while the other specimen can be sliced vertically (in half) to enable you to study and draw the intricate internal structures. Your local butcher will have the skill with sharp knives to do the latter for you. Trying to slice a somewhat slippery small item with inexperienced hands at home is not advisable!

Pre-order the items from your local butcher, keep them in a fridge or freezer until you use them. Plan your study and drawings while they are still fresh. Consider the weather; a cooler day is preferable, and working early in the morning before the ambient temperature becomes too warm. Specimens can deteriorate quite quickly on a hot day. Although you can place them back into the freezer for another day, defrosted specimens often lose elements of their shape, character, and even colour, so studying these while they are fresh is always best.

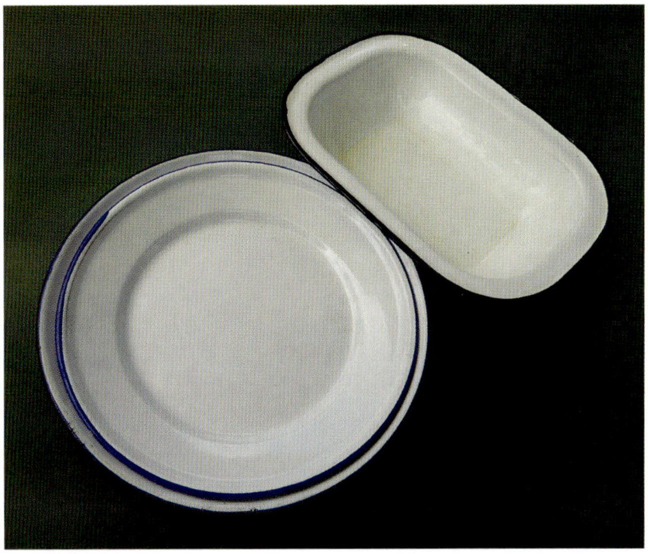

An enamel plate or pie dish are ideal for placing your fresh specimens on ready for drawing.

Keep one or more spare plates or bowls in your studio reserved just for this purpose. You can then keep these plates quite separate from those in your kitchen. Old, enamelled metal plates or pie dishes are ideal and easily obtained either new or second-hand.

Step by Step: Kidney Anatomical Study

As a medical artist, you may be asked to record specimens, although this is now less common as it used to be. However, it is still important to practise recording from accessible specimens such as this kidney and knowing how to record colours and textures accurately is a very complimentary skill, with many adaptable uses.

Aim: To develop your skills in accurately recording an anatomical specimen.

Art materials:

- Black fibre-tipped pen
- Rigid perspex or glass sheet with a grid of 1cm squares pre-marked onto the surface. If you choose glass, then ensure you choose glass with rounded edges so you avoid cuting yourself. Glass with smoothed rounded edges can be purchased from a glazier outlet
- Cloth for cleaning the perspex or glass after use
- Enamel plate or bowl, with supports if required to hold the perspex/glass sheet above the specimen without touching it

Project: The human body has two kidneys, one on each side of the body, positioned posteriorly on either side of the spine within the abdomen and may present at different heights and in shape. This example uses a lamb's kidney, purchased from the local butcher, presented with the areas of fat surrounding the kidney still attached.

Firstly, and importantly, spend a few moments just studying the kidney specimen, then touching it gently to feel the different textures. Carefully pick up the kidney, noting its whole weight of it in the palm of your hand, feel the smooth surface texture of the body of the kidney and study its overall rounded form. Observe how this compares to the lumpier surface and texture of the fat. The kidney and fat have very different colours and textures, the kidney being smooth, glistening and dark, and the fat globular, pale and matt. You may also be able to see several blood vessels alongside the ureter, on the medial side or inner curve of the kidney. The ureter is a tube which takes the waste product urine from the kidney to the bladder.

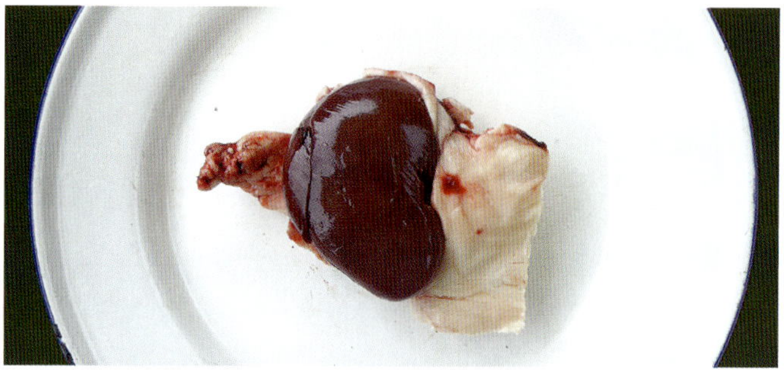

A fresh lamb's kidney placed on a white enamelled plate.

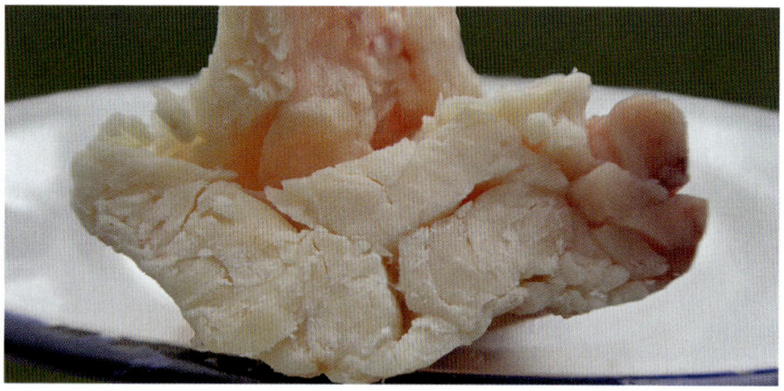

Study the texture and structure of the fat. This image shows the cut area of the fat revealed in cross section. Compare the colour and texture to that of the kidney itself.

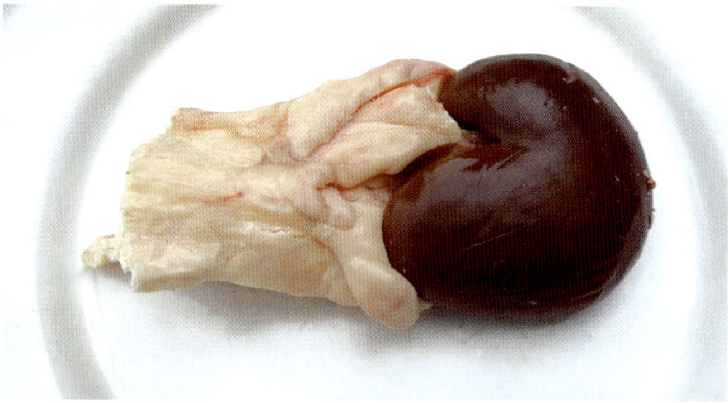

This second kidney example shows the form and shape may differ from kidney to kidney. The left and right kidney will not be exact reverse copies of each other either.

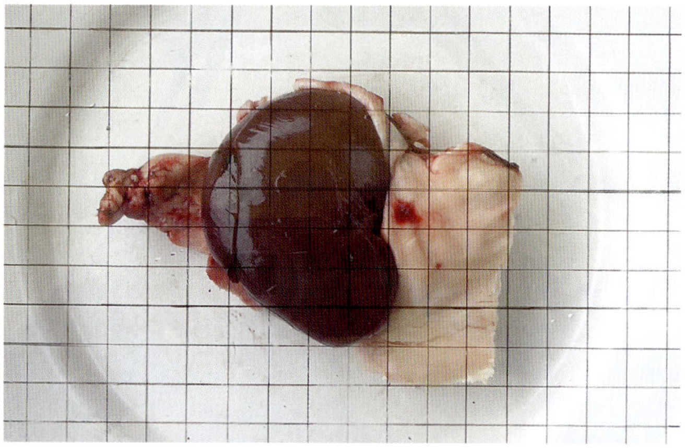

A grid of 1cm squares has been marked onto a sheet of hard clear plastic. The sheet has been secured between two pieces of mount card for extra support. The sheet can then be carefully drawn on with a pen.

Place the glass or rigid plastic grid just above the specimen but without touching it. If the glass or plastic touches or presses onto the kidney, this could distort the shape of the specimen. The method described below is a quick and accurate way to record an outline drawing of the specimen of its actual size. This is referred to as being the 'same size', often abbreviated to SS. While tracing the specimen, also take notes in your sketchbook of any key anatomical details, textures or colour variations you may need to refer to later. Specimens are perishable, so accurate recording of the colours and structure while the specimen is still fresh is important. Even after a short time, the colours and textures may begin to change.

Once traced, your outline image can be transferred onto cartridge or watercolour paper. At this stage, check all the details are accurately represented, using callipers or another hand-held measuring device if required (*see* Chapter 6).

Steps

1. Set up your studio drawing position and check the direction of your light source.
2. Place the kidney on the plate or bowl, and ensure the clear sheet is clean before you begin.
3. Measure the overall length and height of the specimen, including the fat, then mark ink dots on your plastic or glass as a guide to work within these dots.
4. Place your clear sheet over the dish holding the specimen. A bowl is ideal because the sheet can rest comfortably on the raised sides of the bowl. If you use a plate, you may need to raise the sheet up higher by one or more supporting blocks placed on either side of the plate, as shown below.
5. For drawing on the clear plastic or a sheet of glass, a fibre-tipped or drawing pen will both work well. The line drawing can then be easily wiped away and the glass left clean after you have finished.
6. To begin drawing, position yourself comfortably, with your head directly above looking down onto the specimen, move slowly across the grid, tracing with the pen – a process called mapping. Use your original marker points on the sheet to keep your position steady.
6. Finish tracing the outline of the kidney or chosen specimen onto the clear sheet and note down any further details for future reference.
7. Once you have completed your drawing, transfer this onto cartridge paper, where you can then finalise a tonal pencil image of the specimen, adding any additional structure, form and anatomical details.
8. To prepare a coloured artwork, trace your original pencil drawing using a standard tracing method.
9. Finally remember to clean the ink from the surface of the clear sheet and safely store any glass, ready to use again.

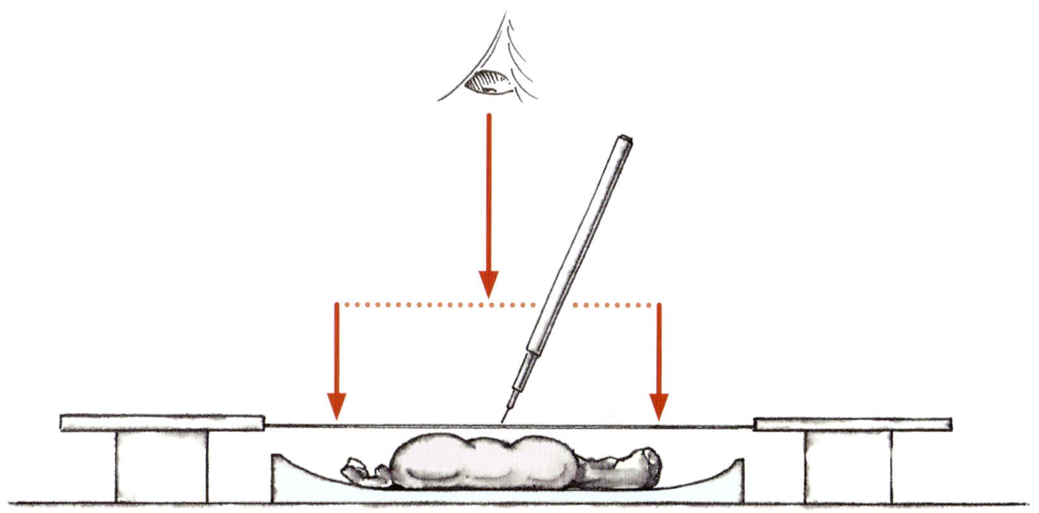

How to map the outline of your specimen. The top single arrow represents your eye position and view, which will move from side to side as you move across tracing the specimen, while keeping the same distance above your specimen. The two parallel arrows below indicate where you will place the outer specimen markers on the clear plastic sheet and then draw with your pen between those marked points.

Step by step: Kidney Specimen Study in Different Media

Aim: Developing skills in observation and accurately recording an anatomical specimen, here shown with a kidney specimen, using four different mediums and art techniques.

Art materials used:

- Graphite pencils: range 2H to 4B
- Putty rubber
- Black water-soluble pen
- Three water brush pens: fine, medium and large
- Watercolour paints: Windsor Yellow, Red and Blue
- Watercolour sable brushes: sizes 4, 6 and 8
- Arches watercolour paper HP 300gms in block form

Project: In this project, you will build a set of accurate illustrations observed directly from a fresh kidney specimen through four stages, beginning with an initial detailed and accurately observed pencil outline, developing the outline into a pencil tonal artwork adding form and depth. Continuing with the pen and wash technique for an intuitive and natural three-dimensional interpretation of the form, followed by a final full-colour watercolour artwork to complete the set, developing your skill in observation through the four stages. Each method provides techniques to collate accumulative information for your future reference.

Steps

1. The first step is to develop your traced image (*see* previous project) into an accurate pencil outline, carefully measuring and noting any elements of the kidney and surrounding tissues and adjusting your original drawing as required. It is always worth spending time on this initial stage to ensure all the elements are accurate before embarking on tonal or colour work. Change pencil weights as necessary to give your initial image more form.
2. Develop your pencil outline into a tonal drawing, adding depth, form and detail. Change to a softer pencil for areas you require to be darker in tone.
3. A quick method of recording, especially if you are having to work at speed, is by using ink pen and wash (*see* Chapter 14). Water-soluble ink pens, used in conjunction with a water brush pen with an integrated water reservoir attached, are ideal. This combination will prove useful for many situations where you may not be able to take pots of water with you for painting with watercolours. First draw outlines with the pen, then use the water brush pen to 'pull' and 'wash' the ink into the shadows to create tone, depth and form.
4. Develop your kidney drawing into a full-colour artwork. Here watercolour has been used, layering the three primary colours: red, yellow, and blue. Layering using a limited colour palette (as opposed to mixing with many colours from a palette) will give you a fresh and reflective artwork. If you are in a museum or other setting with a small travelling art kit, then watercolour pencils used in conjunction with a water brush pen are a useful alternative.

Project: Specimen Study Practice

Aim: To observe and accurately record further anatomical specimens of your choice to develop your recording skills.

Art materials:

- Graphite pencils: range 2H to 4B
- Putty rubber
- Black water-soluble pen
- Three water brush pens: fine, medium and large
- Watercolour paints: Windsor Yellow, Red and Blue
- Watercolour sable brushes: sizes 4, 6 and 8
- Arches watercolour paper HP 300gms in block form

Project: Obtain one or more of the same specimen subject, or obtain a variety of different specimens from your local butcher to provide further practice of the techniques outlined above. Begin each project in the same way as for the kidney specimen step by step. First study the specimen carefully, feeling the weight and looking closely at all the external features and structures. Observe the difference in texture between the muscle, vessels and areas of fat. Measure the external shape, taking notes in your sketchbook on the form, structure, texture and colours in preparation for a complete full-colour artwork.

Steps

1. Observe the specimen closely and prepare an accurate graphite pencil outline, carefully measuring the kidney length and width. Continue measuring the surrounding tissues. Choose pencils grades ranging between 2H to 4B. Apply varying pencil pressure to create graded lines and change the pencil weight as necessary to give your image outline form and depth.

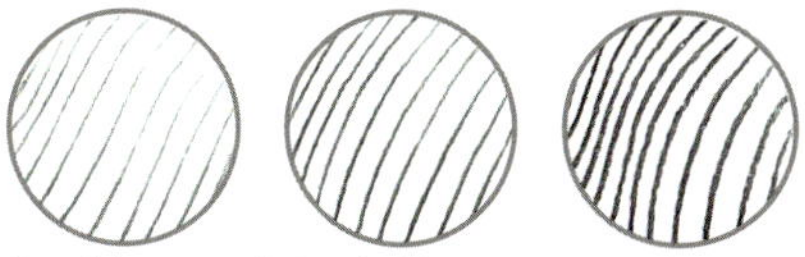

Graphite pencil: Graded lines creating form B, 2B and 4B.

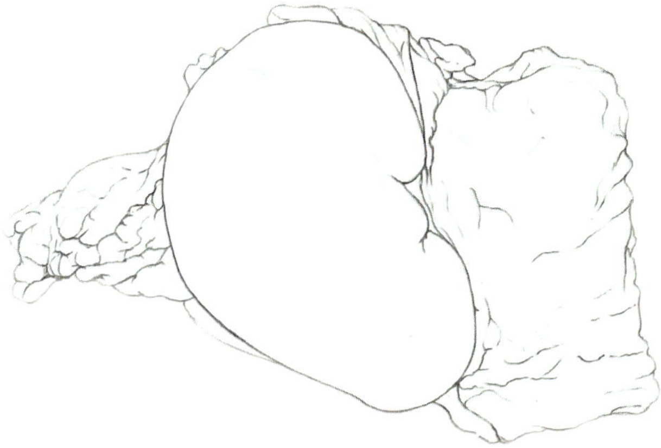

2. To create a tonal drawing of the kidney specimen, either trace your graphite pencil outline from Step 1 onto cartridge paper, or work into your outline to develop the tonal drawing. Apply varying pencil pressure to create tonal shades, gradually building up the darker areas by selecting the B grade pencils and leaving the highlights with limited or no shading, working on the image as 'a whole'.

Graphite pencil: Tonal shading B, 2B and 4B.

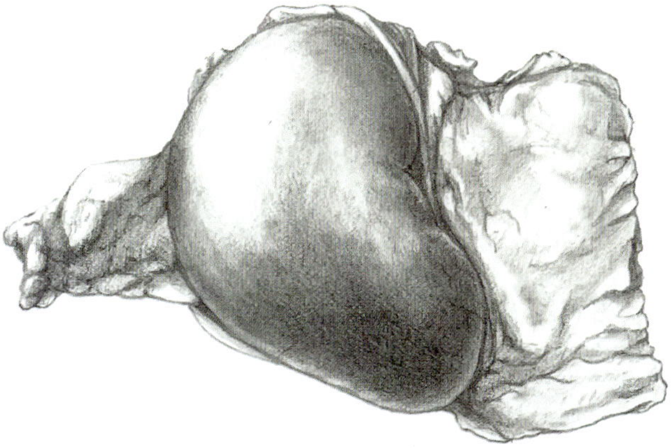

3. To create a pen and wash tonal image of the kidney specimen, first trace your graphite pencil outline from Step 1 onto watercolour paper. Similarily with pen and wash, a soft tonal image can be created through this technique. Pen and wash gives a subtle hint of colour and tone. Draw with the black water soluble pen and then over wash the water brushes spreading the ink into soft tonal forms.

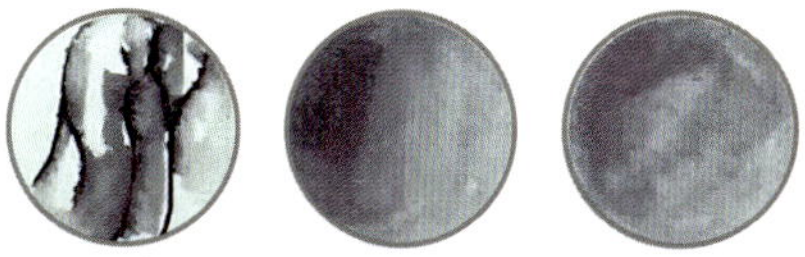

Pen and Wash: Black soluble pen line and washes.

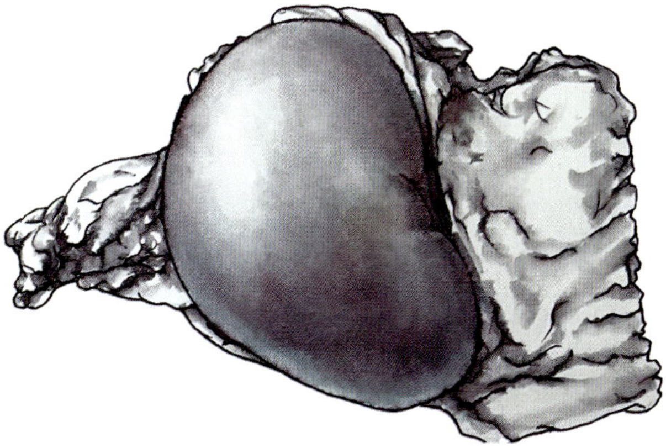

4. To create a full colour painting trace your graphite pencil outline from Step 1 onto watercolour paper. First select the yellow pigment and begin by painting the first layers of tonal washes. Secondly select red and build further layers to gradually build the overall form. Finally select blue for the final layers, including for the darkest areas, remembering to leave the whiteness of the paper for the light and highligted areas.

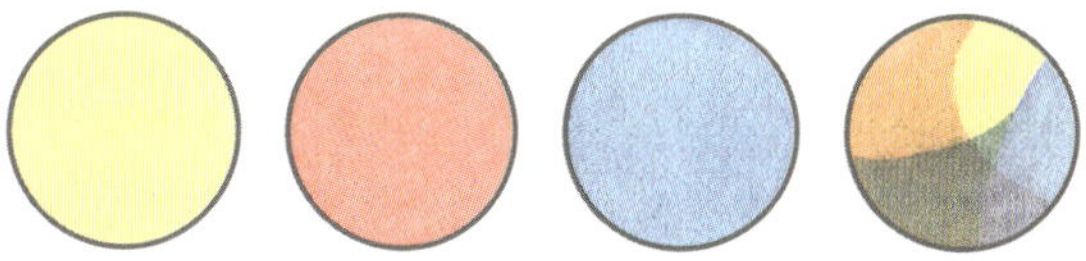

Watercolour: Yellow, red, blue and overlaid colours for comparison.

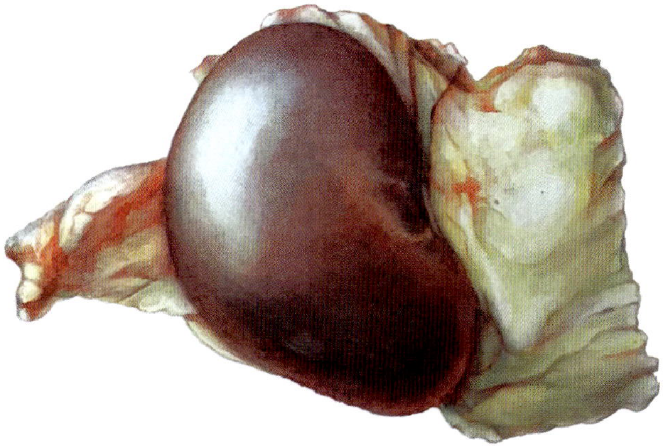

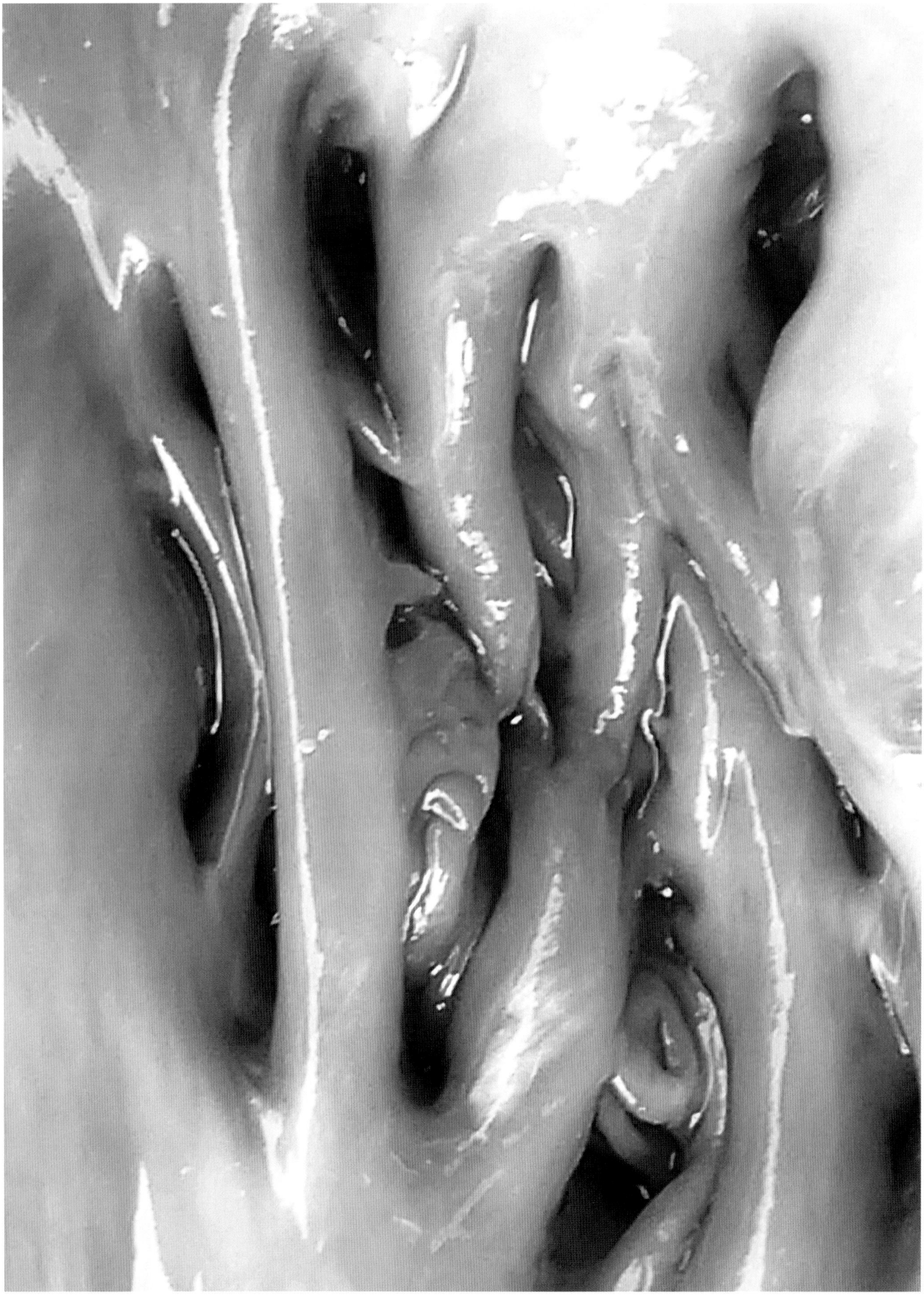

CHAPTER 14

PEN AND WASH TECHNIQUE

There are moments when an artist instinctively needs or wishes to record the first impressions – either the turn of the light, the highlights, fleeting shadows and a movement – or capture the solidity of the whole form. In this and many other situations, medical artists need to make their illustrated records quickly and efficiently, so knowing which media are available to them and which will work best in the circumstances is essential. The pen and wash technique, working with soluble-ink pens and water brushes, is a very versatile and expressive medium ideal for recording the natural forms of the human body. This medium creates a soft tonal effect with a subtle hint of colour from the diluted ink. It allows you to record tonal and three-dimensional aspects of your subject efficiently, capturing light, shade, form and the fine details of the subject you are working from.

For medical artists, recording the vitality and three-dimensional form of a specimen is equally as important as recording the minute, closely observed details. Those initial impressions, captured in swift pen and wash, record the form and essence of the subject, which are needed to create the follow-up illustrations back in the studio. The artist can then pull together a combination of detailed drawings, sketches and handwritten notes to form a final completed artwork.

Using pen and wash is quick and does not require much equipment, so is ideal in settings with limited workspace or a venue that does not allow watercolour paints and water pots, for example.

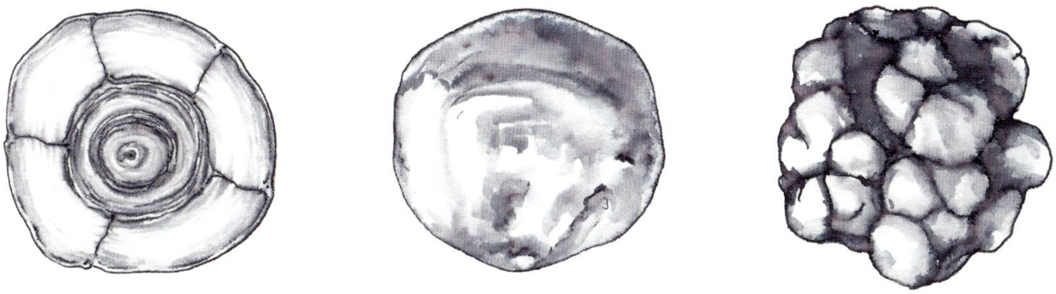

Kidney stones.
Left: cross-section. Middle and right: external views.
Pen and wash.

Papillary muscles of a lamb's heart.

Always check with the museum or venue before you visit as to which art materials you may take with you, as some have specific restrictions; *see* Chapter 4 for further information on visiting museums.

A black water-soluble pen, used in conjunction with a selection of water brushes, makes for a very portable and convenient medium. Both pens and water brushes are readily available from stationery and art suppliers.

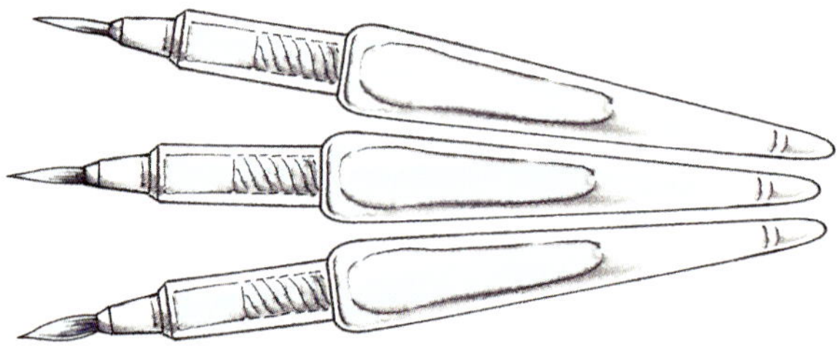

Water brush pens are available in several sizes, with fine, medium or large options. The brush pen can be unscrewed into two sections to allow the water cavity to be refilled. The cavity holds a good amount of water, which is usually sufficient for the artwork required. Ensure the water cavity is full before you begin.

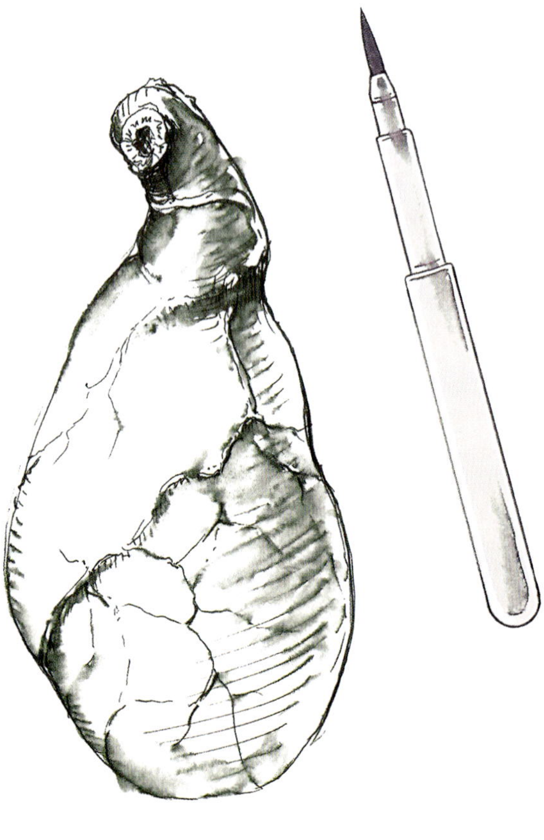

Gall bladder sketch. Pen and wash.

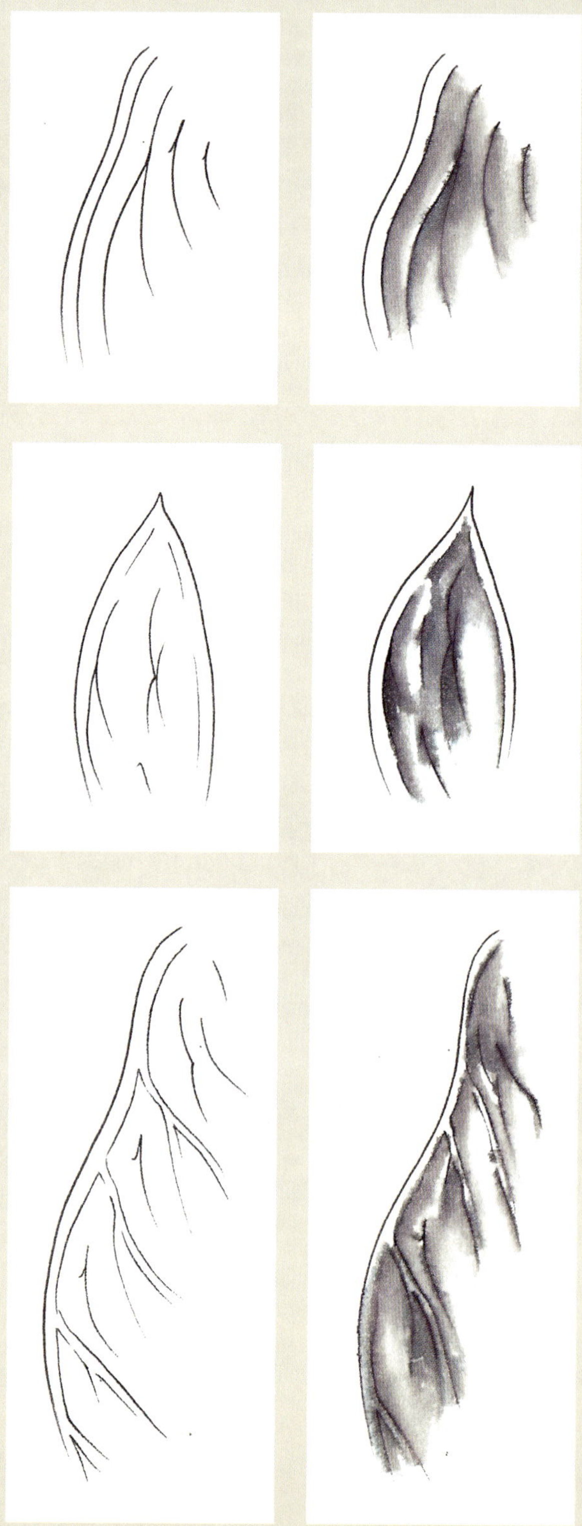

- Draw a variety of outlines and shapes with the water-soluble pen.
- Taking the water brush, wash over or between the lines, pulling the ink towards those areas you wish to create shaded tonal layers.
- If you wish to only pull the ink into a limited area, ensure the water does not cross over the line to the either side.

WORKING FROM A SPECIMEN

Medical artists may be asked to record and take notes from a clinical procedure or record a fresh specimen; in both cases, they will have a limited time frame in which to work. Pen and wash provides artists with a quick and versatile medium for making records, including light, shape and form. The project below allows you to practise your technique without rushing, so take your time to observe and develop your pen and wash skills.

Working from fresh specimens, however, does impose some time constraints because the specimen will start to deteriorate and, on a warm day, perhaps even start to smell strongly. Obtaining more than one specimen from your butcher is therefore recommended so you may carry on working from a second specimen if required.

Project: Heart Study

This project allows you to build your skill in working at speed, while concentrating on the light, shape and three-dimensional form of the specimen. It begins with a detailed and accurately observed pencil outline, progresses to the pen outline, then building tone and form to lead to a completed pen and wash artwork with an instinctive and natural feel. The watercolour paper used here is Archers 300gms paper in a block pad. These pads are versatile and portable for watercolour techniques, removing the need for stretching paper on board.

Project: Follow the same preparation for the kidney specimen, using a lamb's heart or a similar specimen from the butcher. It is advised to begin this project early in the day, to allow plenty of time to draw the specimen while it is still fresh and in good daylight. Set up your working position and place the heart specimen on a plate, ready to begin. First, begin by really studying the specimen: note the overall shape, feel the weight of the heart in your hand, look carefully at all the different features, from the thickness of the heart muscle, to where are the main blood vessels, to how the smaller external heart vessels curve around the external features, passing under and through the surface between areas of fat.

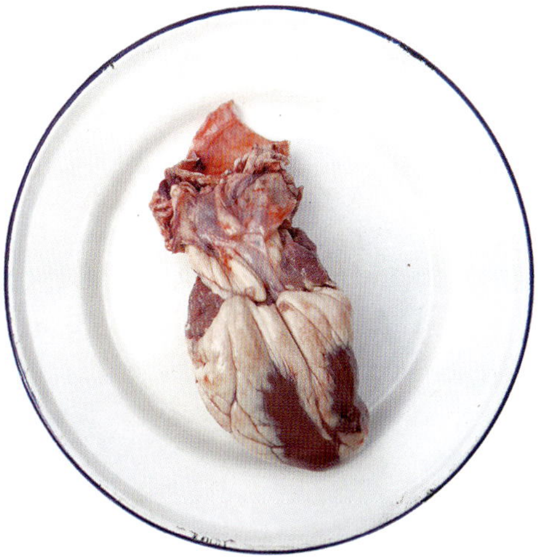

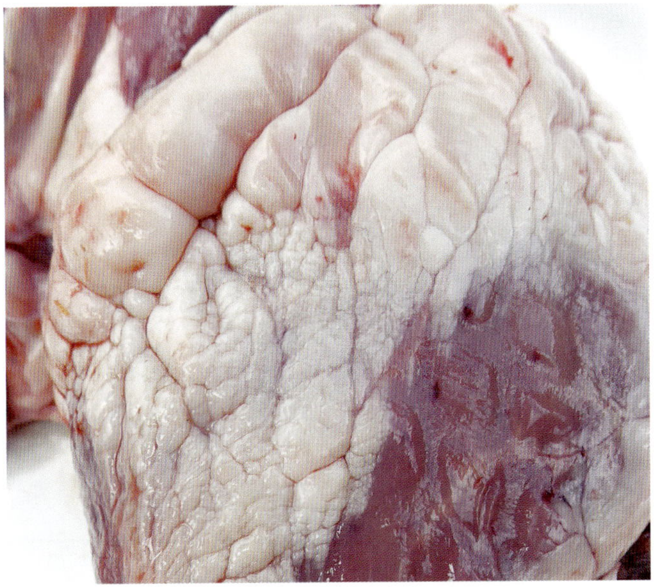

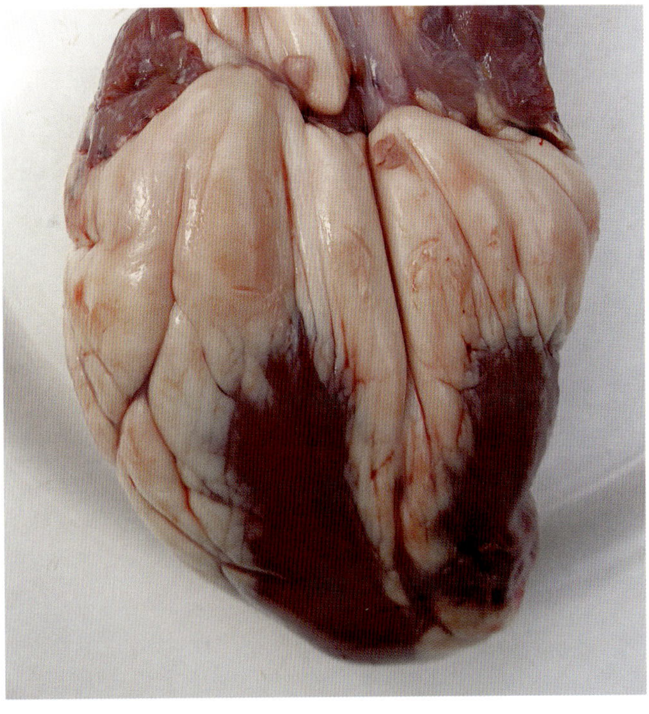

The external shape of the heart will be different when viewed from each side, reflecting the inner anatomical heart chambers and structure. Rotate the heart in your hand and observe these variations. Identify the areas of heart muscle – the dark red areas – and the direction these muscle fibres follow. Make plenty of notes by sketching small, detailed areas of the heart, gradually collating a series of comprehensive notes and sketches to prepare for your final artwork.

Step by step: Heart Specimen Study in Pen and Wash

Aim: Developing skills in observation and accurate recording of an anatomical heart specimen. First recording a detailed pencil drawing, through to developing the form and structure with the pen and wash technique.

Art materials:

- Graphite pencils: range 2H to 4B
- Putty rubber
- Black water-soluble pen
- Three water brush pens: fine, medium and large
- Arches watercolour paper HP 300gms in block form

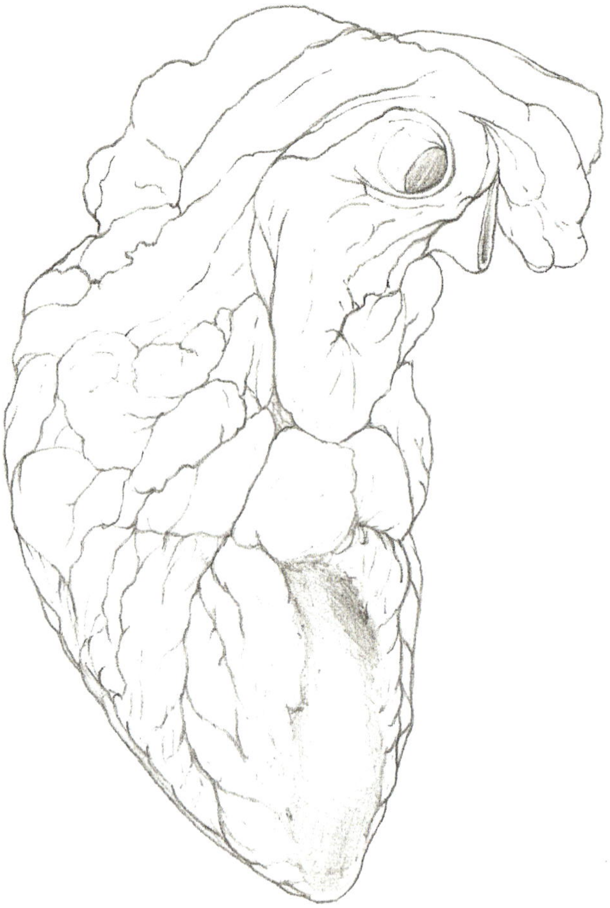

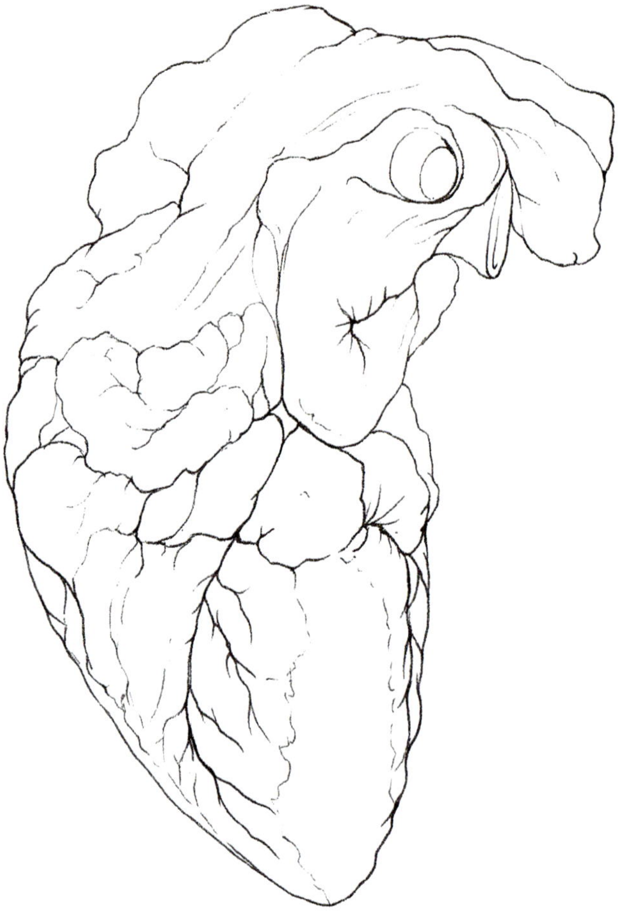

Steps

1. The first step will be to observe, record and create an accurate pencil outline of the specimen. Measuring the whole and individual parts carefully and noting any significant features. Measurements can be taken by the finger-and-pencil method or, with practice, by eye alone. It is always advised to spend time on this initial stage to ensure all the elements are accurately recorded before embarking on the next stage.

2. Transfer your completed pencil drawing onto the watercolour paper. Graphite transfer paper is designed for tracing down and is a very useful addition within your studio toolkit. The transfer paper can be easily cut into smaller sections depending on the size of your artwork. To begin your ink wash artwork, first draw over the outlines and all the key structures and features with the soluble black ink pen.

Project: In this project you will create an accurate illustration of a heart specimen obtained from the butcher. To observe and record the external features of the anatomical specimen quickly and efficiently, focusing on the form, light, shade and depth. Begin by drawing a detailed and accurately observed pencil outline.

Within the initial outline, develop a tonal artwork by adding form and depth with the pen and wash technique, building layers of additional tone as required. This technique allows for a instinctive interpretation of the natural form, forming a very useful approach for recording especially when speed is required.

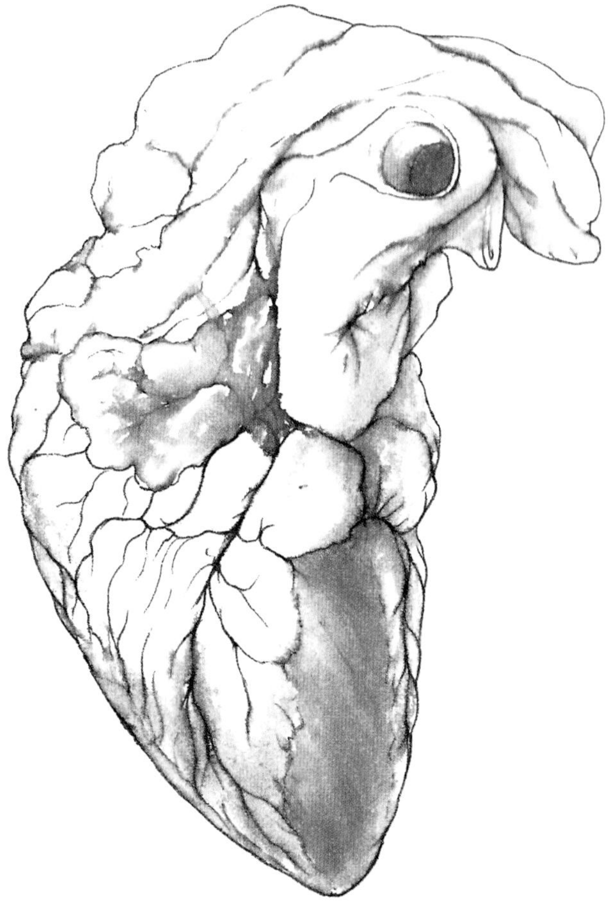

3. First select a medium sized water brush pen, using the water brush pen to 'pull' and 'wash' the ink lines to begin building the depth and form of the specimen. Concentrate on those areas that are in shadow, forming these into darker tonal areas, then gradually work towards the lighter or highlighted areas, or where reflective light occurs.

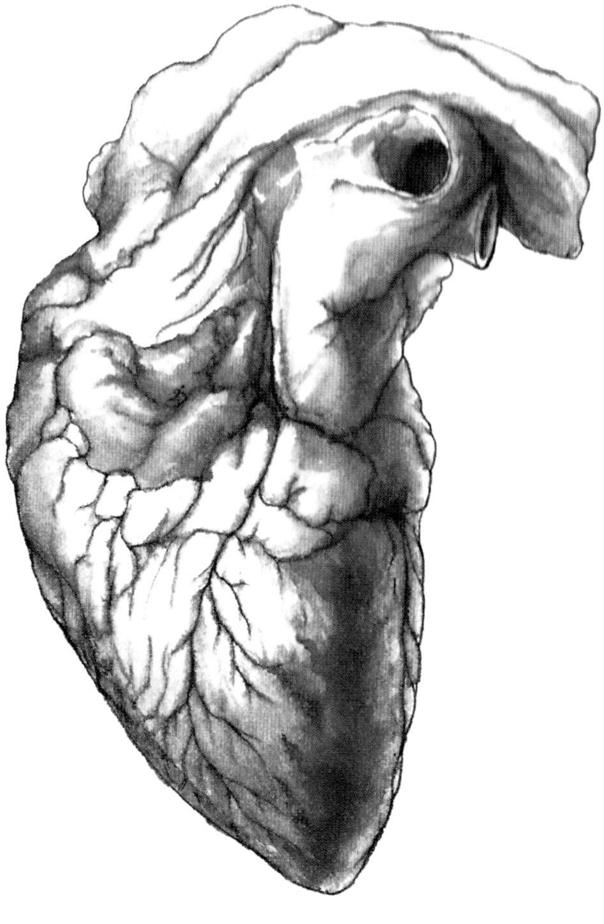

4. Work across the entire specimen, building your artwork up 'as a whole'. Continue adding more areas of tone and gradually focusing on the specific anatomical details. With the pen continue working back into the artwork to deepen tonal areas as required, finally developing your heart drawing into a full and detailed tonal pen and wash artwork.

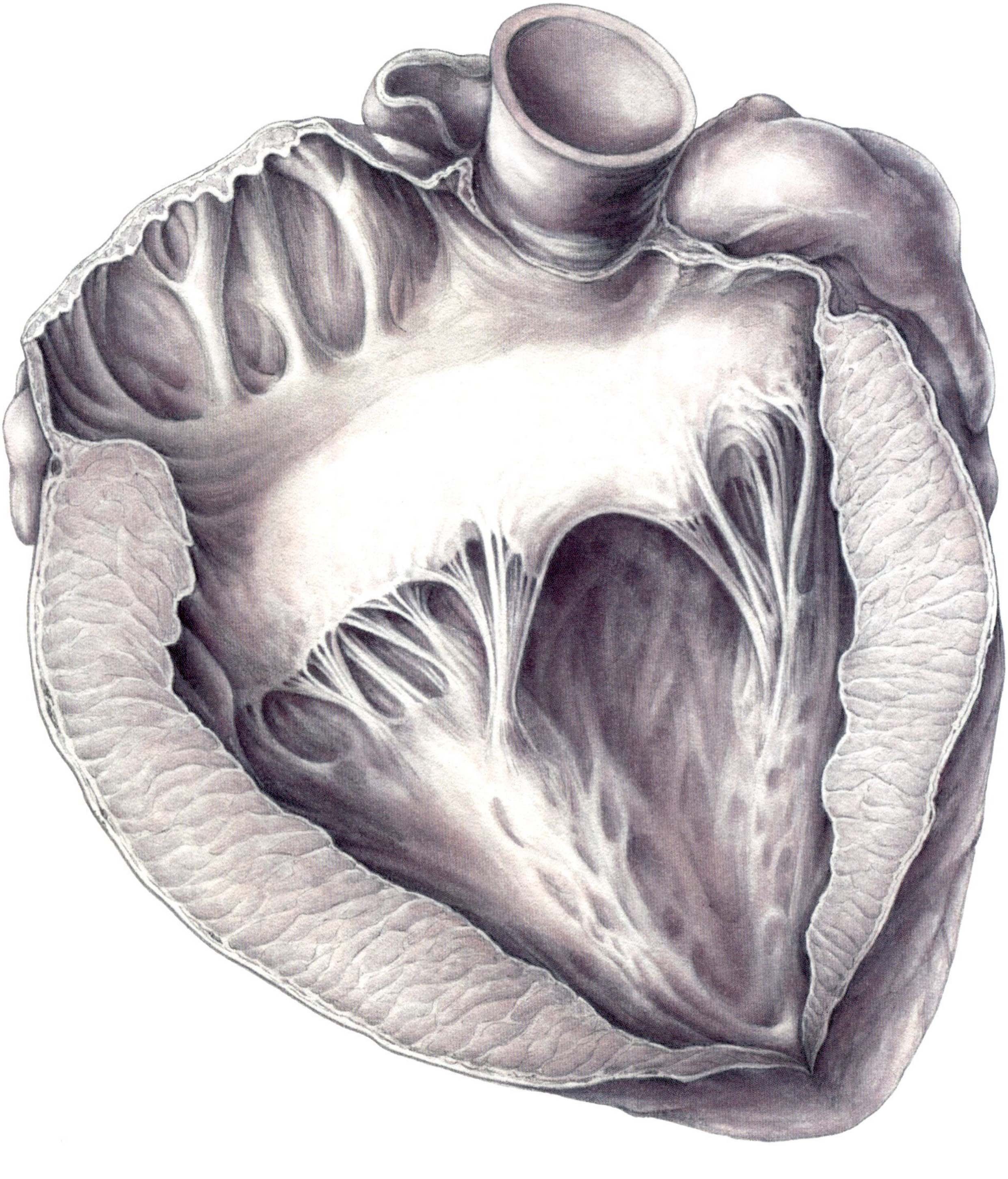

Cross-section of a pig's heart specimen. Pen and wash.

Project: Anatomical Heart Study

Aim: To further develop observational skills of anatomical structures.

Art materials:

- HB pencil
- Cartridge paper 220gms
- Black water-soluble ink pen
- Three water brushes: fine, medium and large
- Arches watercolour paper HP 300gms block form

Project: Obtain one or more heart specimens from your local butcher; this example is a lamb's heart. Ask the butcher to prepare the specimen in cross-section, opened cut across the ventricles and valves to reveal the inner structures. It is best for the butcher to slice the specimen for you, as this can be difficult to do yourself. The internal structures of the heart appear delicate and yet belong to one of the most powerful organs, responsible for pumping blood around the body. Spend time observing then recording all the intricate features.

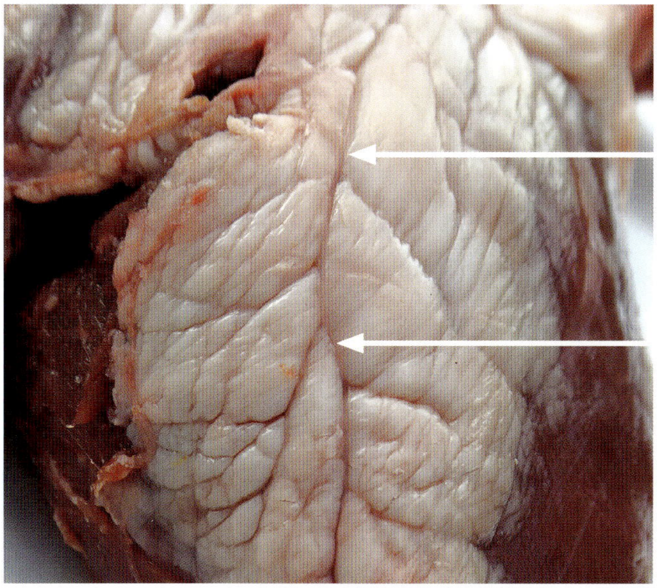

Note the direction and route which the smaller arteries take across the external surface of the heart. These vessels follow a path down, around and through areas of extrenal fat, creating a groove called a sulcus. These vessels create a charactistic feature over the surface of the heart.

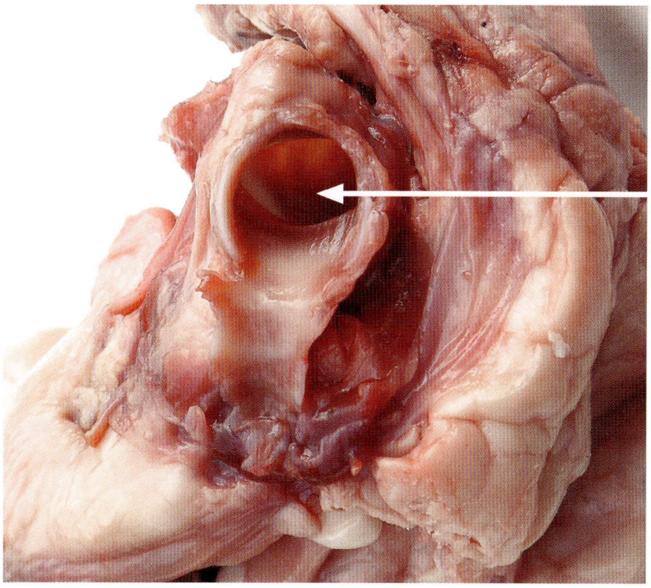

Note the largest blood vessel in the body, the aorta, leaving the heart from the superior aspect. This vessel can easily be identified for being large and round, with thick walls to support the blood vessel under pressure as the blood leaves the heart to be pumped around the body.

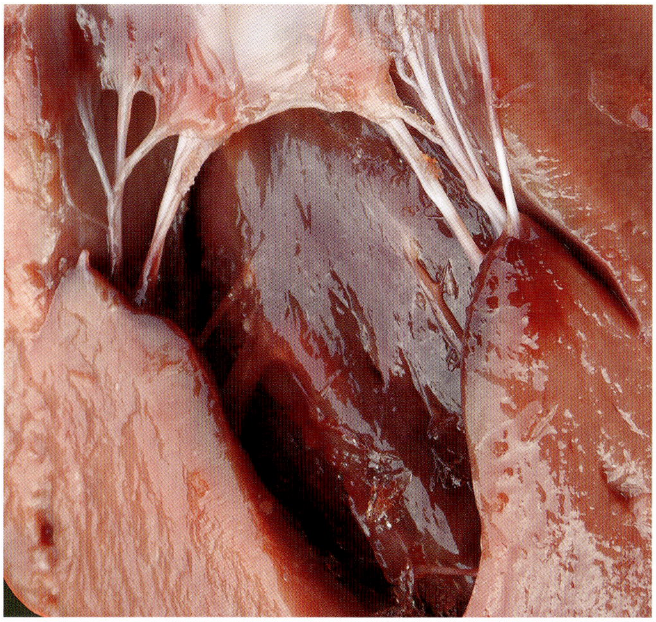

The valve and chordae tendineae are opened to reveal the thin yet strong valve tissue. Note the thick muscular wall of the heart.

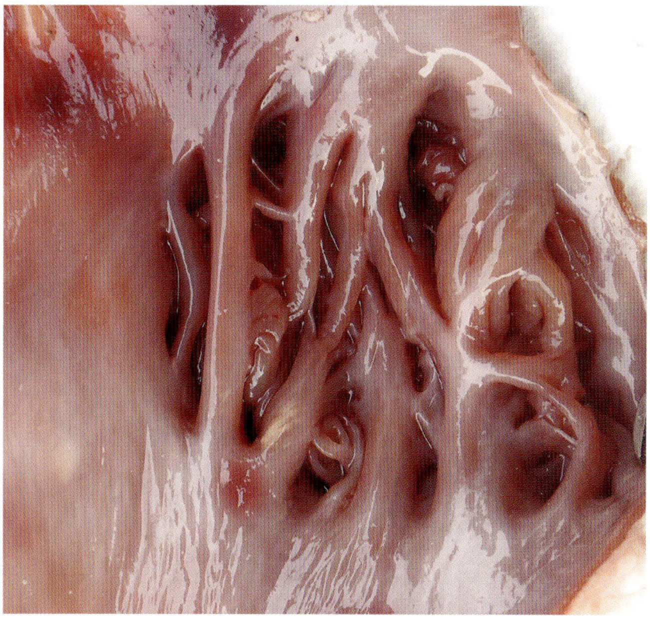

The intricate network of the valve and papillary muscles.

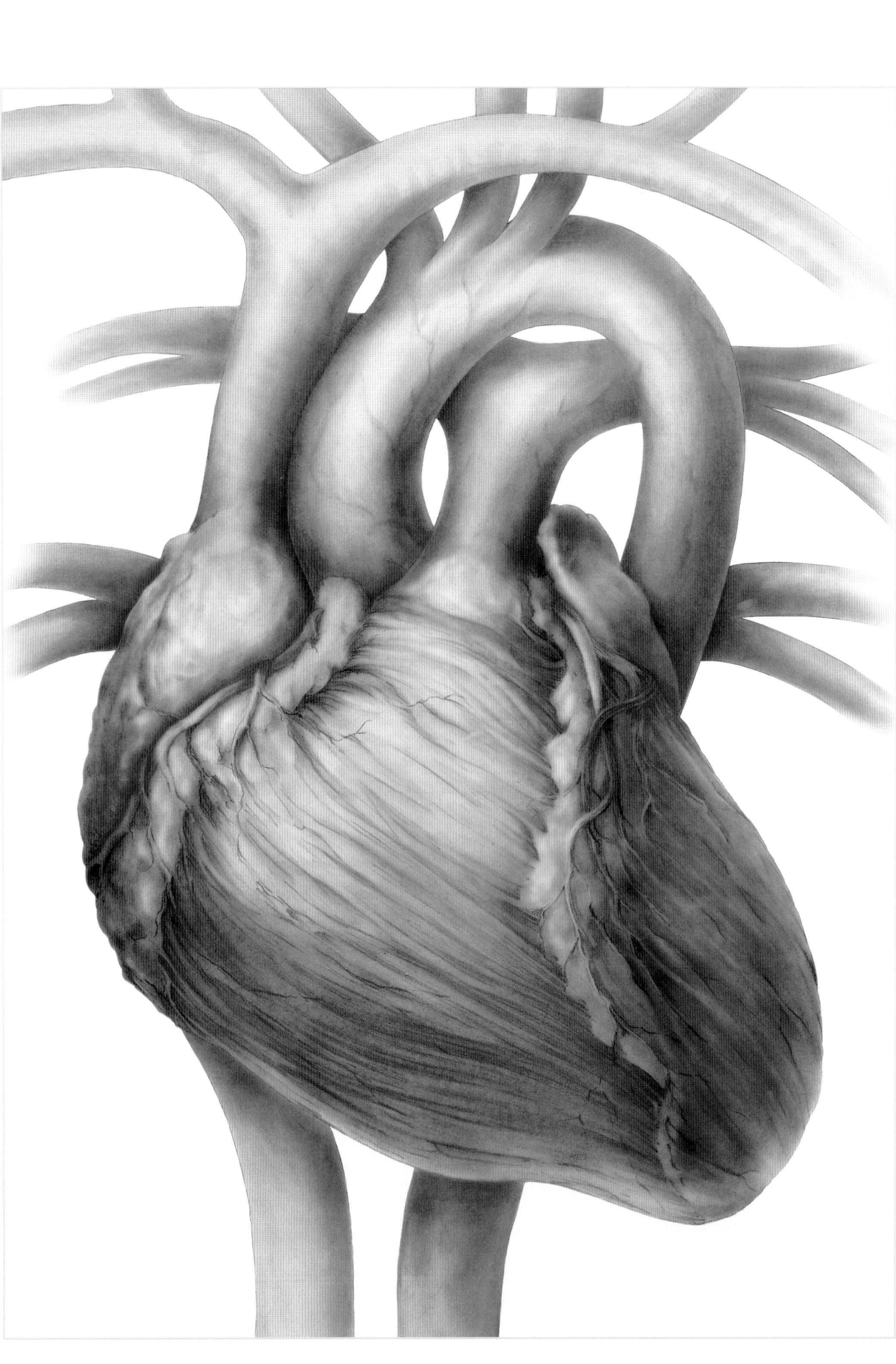

CHAPTER 15

ADVANCED TECHNIQUES

Medical artists use a plethora of different media and techniques. This chapter will look at two slightly more unusual ones, firstly drawing with carbon dust and secondly with silver point, both are established techniques that are now enjoying a revival, with each method used to create their own distinctive look and feel.

Finally, medical artists are often commissioned to illustrate surgical procedures, which is a specific anatomical and technical area studied within a medical art postgraduate programme. This chapter provides a brief introduction.

CARBON DUST TECHNIQUE

Carbon dust has been widely used among medical and scientific illustrators since the twentieth century and was the preferred medium of American medical artist and illustrator Max Brödel. This technique is still taught today and has seen increased popularity due to the soft, detailed and rich ethereal qualities this medium can create. The carbon pigment is very fine and may be purchased in powder form or as a stick or pencil. The pencils create a velvety matt black.

The carbon-dust technique combines two methods, drawing with carbon pencils and applying dust washes with a brush, which are then manipulated with stumps, a chamois, or lint-free cloth. The artwork results in rich tonal renderings with a strong tonal value range.

Precision highlights can be created with highlighting by lifting out specific areas with a cloth, for example, or scratching out with a scalpel.

SILVERPOINT TECHNIQUE

Silverpoint refers to a technique where lines are drawn onto a prepared paper or board, which has been prepared with a layer of chalk or gesso that creates a smooth surface on which to work. Lines are drawn with a thin metallic rod typically of either copper, silver, tin, lead or gold, held within a holder called a stylus, although other similarly pointed implements may also be used. Silverpoint gradually builds up the artwork by drawing successive lines with light to medium strokes or by cross-hatching. The resulting illustrations are subtle and delicate, with the fine metal stylus enabling highly detailed work.

This technique will not create very dark tones, nor can marks be readily altered once placed (depending upon the ground used on the surface of the paper), so this is not a technique commonly chosen by beginners.

Historically past masters have favoured this technique in creating both their underdrawings and artworks.

Below is an example of kidney stones drawn with a thin silver wire rod on silverpoint drawing paper.

On the following page a squamous cell carcinoma presenting on the back of the hand was drawn using a thicker silver wire rod.

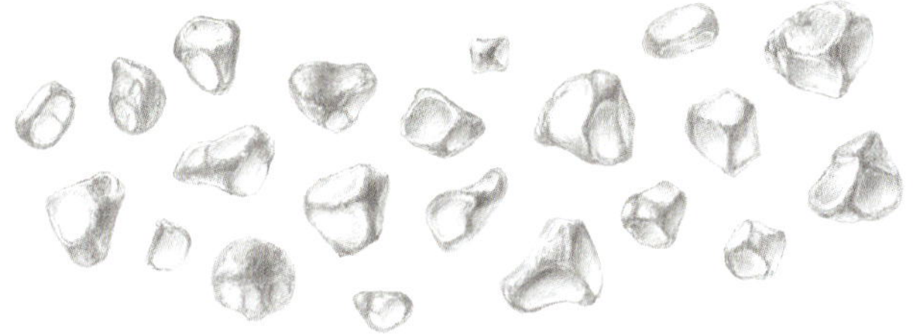

Anterior view of the heart. Carbon dust on board.

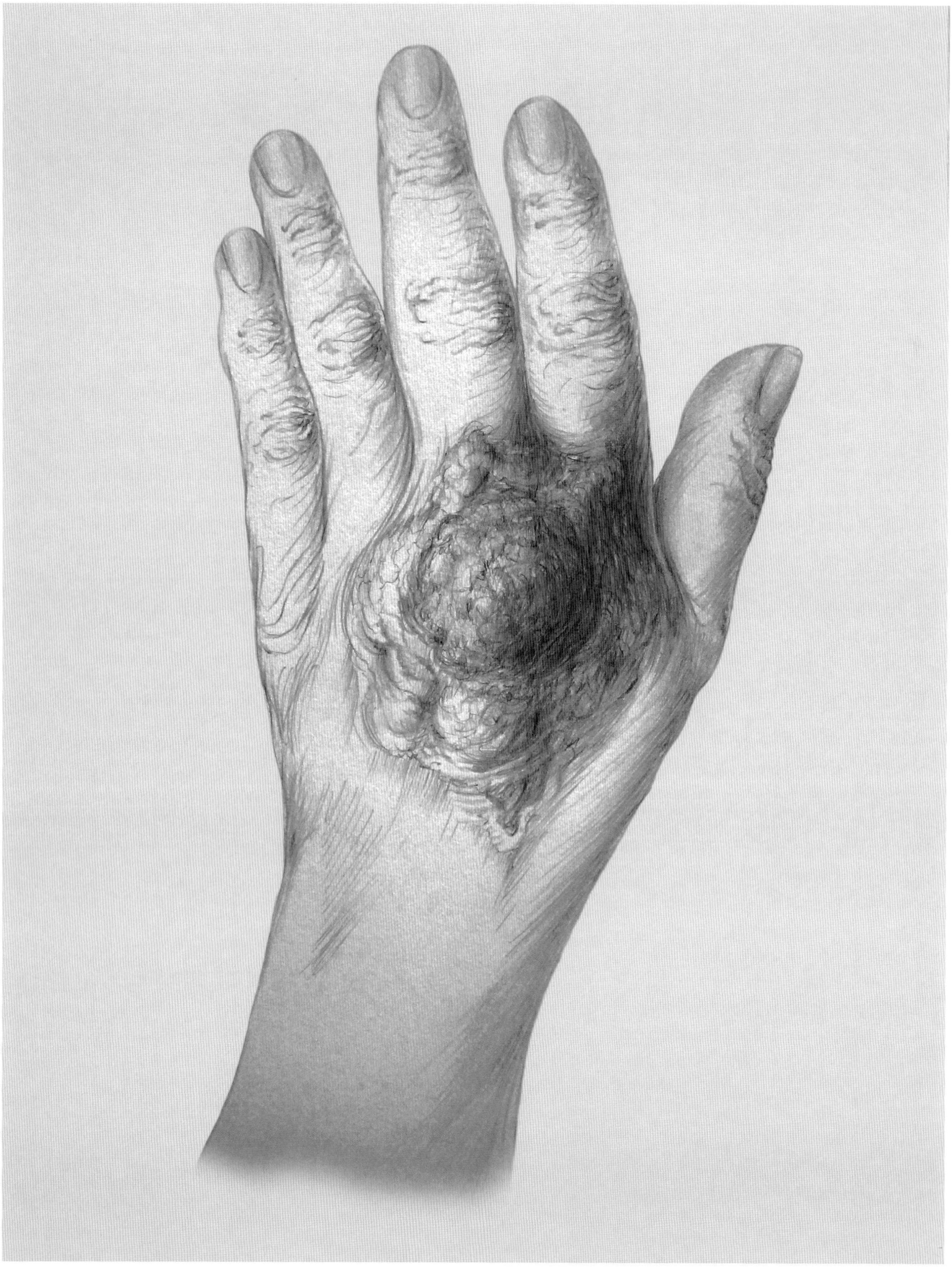

Squamous cell carcinoma presenting on the back on the left-hand. Silverpoint.

ILLUSTRATING SURGICAL PROCEDURES

Illustrating surgical procedures is often the mainstay of commissioned work for professional medical artists. This is an exacting area, that requires a good anatomical knowledge and the ability to work comfortably within clinical settings.

Whether the resulting illustrations are intended for patient information or an indepth surgical textbook, the initial approach will be the same. The artist will ask many questions, beginning with 'who will be the audience for these illustrations' and 'what will be their main purpose'. Will this be a stand-alone image or form one within a series of illustrations?

Unlike many complex medical illustrations where each detail is carefully observed and recorded, surgical illustration often only retains those specific areas of detail that are required to focus the eye and reader's attention onto the pertinent features being illustrated; with all unecessary information excluded. For example, an operating procedure there may be many hands holding clamps and retractors at different stages, unnecessary folds of cloth and extraneous features which would be omitted.

Medical artists will constantly asking themselves – what is the main purpose of each artwork. Providing clear information is often referred to as creating a functional artwork. In this example illustrating an Achilles tendon tear, the two circular inserts focus only on the tendon tear itself and the subsequent repair, showing the planned procedure to rejoin the two ends of the tendon together after the torn edges have been debrided (a process for removing the torn fragments) facilitating the natural repair process. Adding only minimal features to the artwork, such as directional arrows or elements of colour. By keeping each stage uncluttered and instructional are key elements in producing high-quality and effective surgical illustrations.

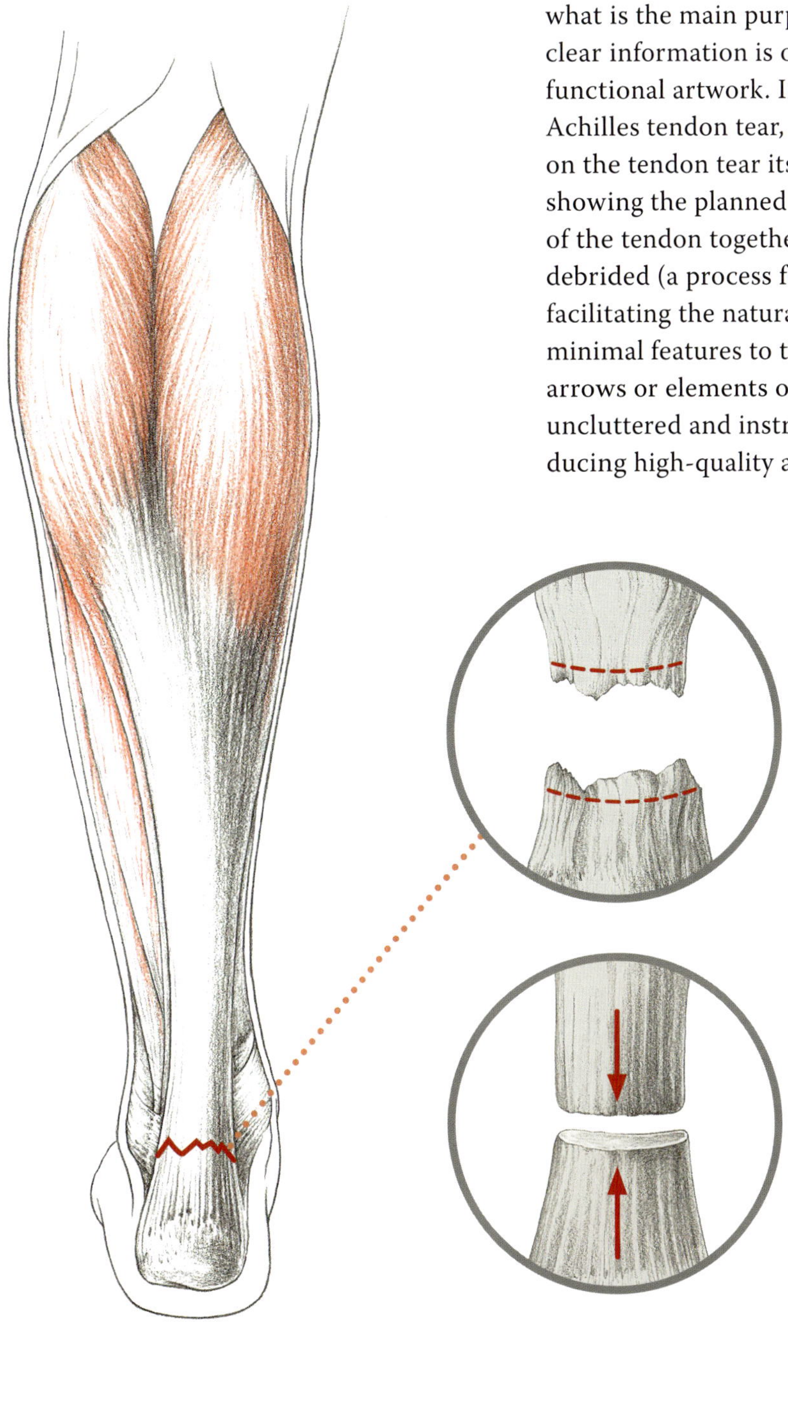

Posterior view of the lower left leg, showing a positional tear distally of the Achilles tendon (left).
With two stages shown for the surgical repair, firstly removal (debridement) of the torn tendon sections, followed by the two portions shown being drawn together to complete the repair.
Graphite and coloured pencils on cartridge paper.

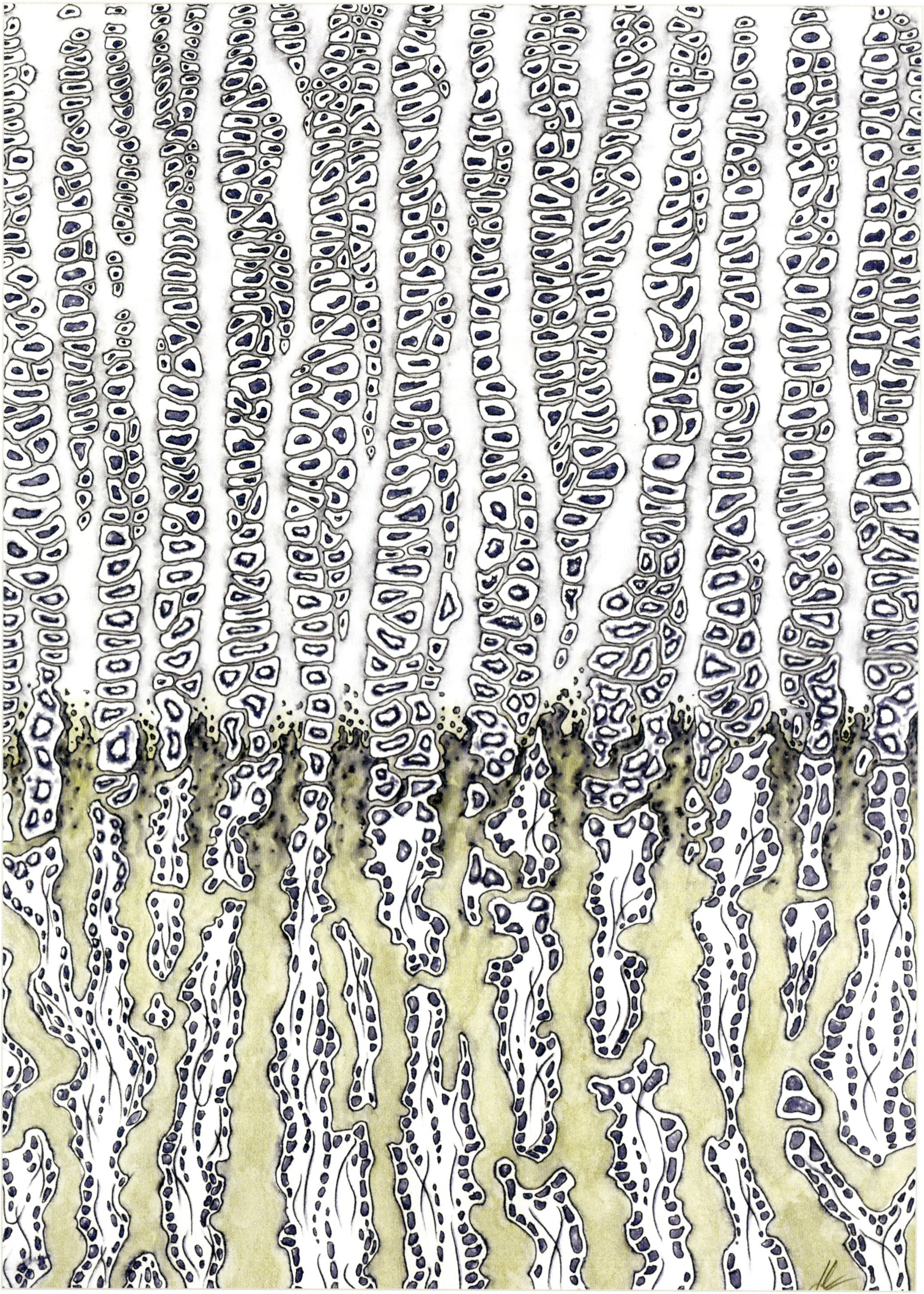

APPENDIX I MEDICAL ART COURSES AND ASSOCIATIONS

Medical art is an inspiring and specialised career. If you have an enquiring mind, a keen observational eye and excellent drawing skills, this fascinating career path really does give you a 'world is your oyster' scenario. Due to the technical nature of medical art, practitioners require a postgraduate or a master's level in training.

Medical artists, illustrators and designers are required to produce a wide range of work, becoming skilled in many different media and digital programs, as well as editorial, printing and technical working knowledge. Medical art requires skill in producing a range of work, including original artworks, illustrations and diagrams, digital art, 2D animations and 3D modelling. Artworks are designed for various purposes, from detailed anatomical illustrations in medical textbooks to healthcare and patient information. Therefore, medical artists are often linked to many allied medical professions, such as forensic, archaeological and healthcare fields, through membership of related professional associations.

MEDICAL ART COURSES

Medical Artists' Education Trust – Postgraduate Programme in Medical Art

This specialised self-directed postgraduate programme is designed to provide students with the skills and techniques used by contemporary medical artists and illustrators, and is taught by medical art professionals.

This course begins with a comprehensive one-year Advanced Foundation Programme (Part 1), whose principal constituents are direct observational skills and traditional art techniques, exploring an array of objects and observing light and shade, tone and texture, alongside studying natural history and osteological specimens. Students who successfully complete this concentrated one-year foundation programme progress onto Part 2 of the Postgraduate Programme, aiming to provide medical artists with a broad set of technical skills and knowledge for a career in visual communication within medical education, combining draughtsmanship with animation, 3D and graphic design. The course is based in London, UK. Students who successfully complete the programme are eligible to become professional members of the Medical Artists' Association of Great Britain.

The Medical Artists' Education Trust became a charity in 1997 and celebrated 25 years in 2022. It held an exhibition of students artworks and producing an accompanying celebratory publication.

Open Days

The Medical Artists' Education Trust hold online course information open events twice a year for prospective students. These are highly recommended for everyone considering a future career in medical art. These events include an overview of the course curriculum, submission requirements and reviews for individual portfolio content, presentation and career advice.

Bone development. The lower coloured areas represent the bone ossification, creating a darker band called an ossification plate. Pen and wash.

Application Process

All medical art courses will require a portfolio submission of your original artwork, with each having its own application requirements and process. Ensure you check the requirements and format for your portfolio submission and only include artworks which are appropriate for each application. Check your contact details are current and correct, and if any details change between the time of application to interview, which may be several months, be sure to let them know.

Applications and portfolio presentations may be divided into two stages, with candidates being asked to submit an initial online portfolio with their application form. Followed by shortlisted candidates being invited to attend a further online or an in-person interview, which will include a complete presentation of your portfolio of artwork to the application board or committee.

Portfolio Requirements

The course will require a portfolio presented to a high standard that demonstrates draughtsmanship in observational drawing, rendering form, tonal values, light and shade, texture, proportion and perspective, including examples of colour and mixed media. You may be required to include examples of graphic design where artwork, images and typography have been integrated and are appropriate for their intended audiences; this is an area that is especially important within the healthcare sector.

Life drawing examples will be required, drawn from your own direct observation of a life model or person, in a mix of pencil, tone, and colour examples. You will be expected to continue life drawing while attending the course. There is further information on preparing a portfolio later in this chapter.

Keep the following points in mind when compiling your portfolio:

- Check the portfolio application requirements for the course you are applying and collate the necessary artworks.
- Select your best pieces and those that are relevant to the application.
- Keep your artworks and portfolio content current. You may need to spend time creating one or more new pieces of work specifically for your application.
- Date your artworks, so the interviewing panel know when they were created. Dates can be written

MEDICAL ART COURSES

In the UK

Medical Artists' Education Trust, London
Postgraduate Programme in Medical Art
Three-four years (part-time) Postgraduate programme
www.maet.org.uk

Glasgow University, Scotland
MSc Medical Visualisation and Human Anatomy
One year full-time course
www.gla.ac.uk/postgraduate/taught/medicalvisualisation

Liverpool John Moores University, Liverpool School of Art and Design, Scotland
MA Art in Science
One year (full-time) or two years (part-time)
Postgraduate course
https://lsad.co.uk/programmes/ma-art-in-science/

University of Dundee, Scotland
MSc Medical and Forensic Art
One year full-time course
www.dundee.ac.uk/postgraduate/medical-ar

Worldwide

University of Illinois at Chicago, USA
Biomedical Visualization MSc
MS degree Two years full-time curriculum
https://ahs.uic.edu/biomedical-health-information-sciences/admissions-and-programs/ms-in-biomedical-visualization/

Johns Hopkins University School of Medicine, Baltimore, Maryland, USA
Medical and Biological Illustration
Departmnent of Art as Applied to Medicine
MA Two years full-time accredited graduate program
https://medicalart.johnhopkins.edu/

Rochester Institute of Technology, USA
MFA Medical Illustration
Two years full-time postgraduate course
https://www.rit.edu/study/medical-illustration-mfa

University of Toronto, Canada
Master of Science in Biomedical Communications MScBMC
Two-years full-time graduate course
https://bmc.med.utoronto.ca/

Further undergraduate and graduate courses

The Association of Medical Illustration
The AMI maintain a comprehensive list of undergraduate and graduate courses for the USA, Canada and Europe:
https://www.ami.org/medical-illustration/enter-the-profession/education

discreetly in pencil on the corner or the back of the artwork.

- Ensure that the artworks being presented are all your own work.
- Where an example has been created specifically for the portfolio to show a style format, let the panel know beforehand.
- Include sketchbooks and selectively include one or more projects showing your work process through to completion.

The above points will also be applicable for an online portfolio application. For an online portfolio, ensure the pages and links are easy to navigate through, flowing smoothly and importantly check that any URL links are active. Include your name and qualifications and include any links which will further showcase your work. There are many online templates to choose from, or you can create your portfolio design.

PREPARING YOUR PORTFOLIO

Time spent collating and presenting your artwork, whether as a physical portfolio or for an online format, will always be time well spent. Above all, enjoy developing a portfolio that highlights your strengths and skills.

A smart and tidy portfolio presentation is essential, whether you are presenting sketchbooks, a traditional portfolio, or a folio of mounted artworks. For a physical portfolio, ensure the sleeves are clean, and mark- and dust-free. If you are updating portfolio images, previous artworks may leave a residue on the inside of the sleeves, so gently wipe these clean. Artwork within each sleeve should fit squarely, ideally being a standard size, such as A4, A3 or A2. If an artwork is smaller than the page, then mounting onto a clean sheet of card or window mounting within card, provides a smart presentation. When you create a window mount, i.e. a 'window' within a sheet of card, your artwork should be attached squarely and with care to the reverse side of the cut card.

Bevelled-edge card mount cutters are readily available to purchase at art stores or online and are supplied as a combination of a cutting ruler and angled blade device. The ruler has a designated raised ridge for the blade fitment, which slides along the ruler to cut into the card. With a little practice, you will achieve professional cut card mounts for presenting your artwork. To make a card cut mount, first lightly mark in pencil the area to be removed on the reverse side of the card. Place the ruler along these pencil lines, then carefully cut through to the front of the card from the reverse side, following one line at a time creating a clean-cut bevelled edge card mount for your artwork.

Once it starts taking more than one slide along to cut through the card, it's time to replace the cutting blade. These can be easily removed and replaced.

Always dispose of your used sharps, scalpel or card-cutting blades safely in a dedicated sharps container, which are designed just for this and always yellow in colour. When the containers are full or no longer needed, they can be disposed of professionally at a designated local community waste collection site. Disposal may be free or incur a nominal charge, with some residential areas offering a home collection service. Medical art departments and design studios will have their own containers available and be responsible for their disposal.

MEDICAL ART AND ILLUSTRATION ASSOCIATIONS

Medical artists have worked in the field of medicine for many years before the first associations were formed, either within hospitals or as independent artists in their own right. Artists eventually came together to form the following associations for collaboration and unifying the training for the next generations of medical artists.

The following associations were formed:

1945 Association of Medical Illustrators (AMI) USA

1949 Medical Artists' Association of Great Britain (MAA)

1986 Association Européenne des Illustrateurs Médicaux et Scientifiques (AEIMS). European schools are also based in Liverpool, Lucerne, Maastricht and Zurich

1989 Institute of Medical Illustrators

1997 Medical Artists' Education Trust (MAET)

2009 Biological and Medical Art in Belgium (BIO MAB). University of Antwerp Art Researches Science International Collaborations (ARSIC), formerly known as ARS, was founded in 2014.

APPENDIX II GLOSSARY

Artists will regularly come across terms relating to print and publishing, often referred to by their abbreviation. A selection of frequently used terms are listed below.

A, B and C series Most countries follow this paper size system (for example A1, A2, A3 and so on) so they are universal across the world
Artwork All images, photographs and illustrations designed for printing and publication. Sometimes called the 'original'
Bleed Print that runs beyond the trim marks of the paper and will be trimmed off
CYMK Acronym of the four-colour printing process: C – cyan, Y – yellow, M – magenta and K – keyline (black)
Crop Where an image has been edited or reduced in size from the original
Crop marks Lines placed onto the page edges to show where the document or print item will be trimmed
DPI Dots per inch. A unit of measurement which usually refers to the image resolution of printed images. For example, 300dpi means there are 150 × 150 pixels per inch in the image; this is the standard resolution for high-quality printed images
Dummy A single sample copy of a book, leaflet or an artwork, produced to show the client an idea for the finished product before printing large quantities
First edition The first published version of a work
Font The style of letters used in printed texts
Format Size, proportions, font and style of the text for a book or other reproduced materials
Giclée An archival fine art digital printmaking process
Greyscale The image presented in tones of black (no colour)
Halftone The breakdown of an image into small dots to simulate the look of continuous tones. Greyscale images need to be broken down into halftones to be exposed onto the screens for screen printing
Header Information that appears at or across the top of each page, for example a running title or page number
Imposition The arrangement of each page in sequence then reads consecutively once printed
Landscape The page or image is oriented in a horizontal position
Layout The design plan for a book, page or publication clarifying the arrangement of text and images
Mock-up A test example of a plan or design, often made for presentations
Pantone colour A universal standardised colour system to enable designers and printing companies to reproduce exactly the right colour
Portrait The page or image is oriented in a vertical position
PPI Pixels per inch. This is a unit of measurement of image resolution that usually refers to digital images; 72–96ppi is the average for digital online images
Proofing To check completed works before printing. This is an important stage to check your work, design, copy and colours are correct
Register marks Marks used as reference points to accurately position images or text onto the paper ready for printing
Reprint editions Second or subsequent editions of a publication
RGB Red, green, blue – the primary colours combined to produce the colours on electronic screens
SS Same size
Trim The line through which a printed work is cut to produce the final size. Trimming through the bleed area for a clean, sharp edge around the image or design
Transparency How opaque an image is. Flatten your transparency to CYMK for printing
Typography Everything related to the text or the design. The printer will want to know the layout of any text, images, along with colour and style

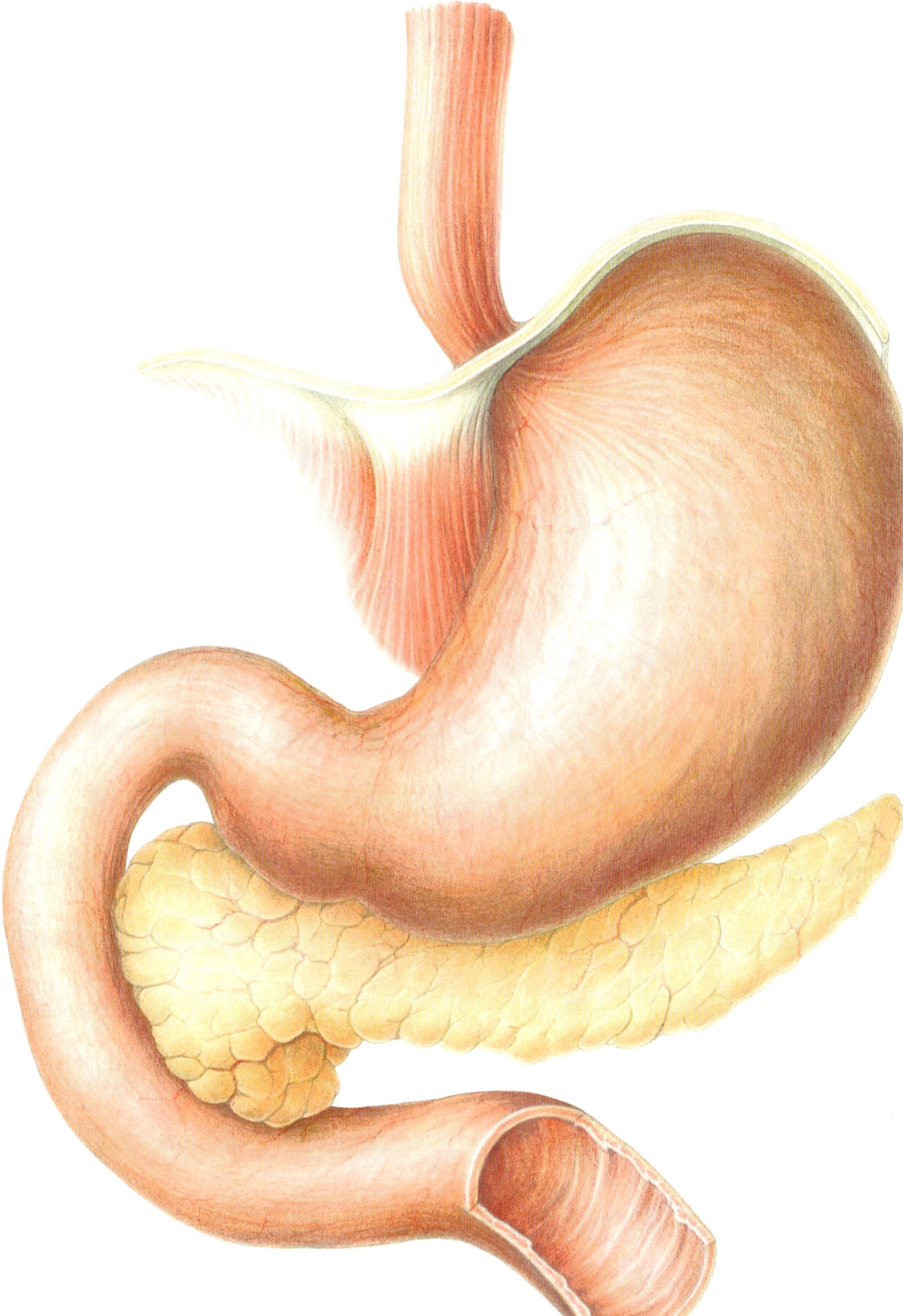

The stomach, pancreas and duodenum. Watercolour and coloured pencil.

APPENDIX III WEBSITES

Websites for institutions and universities offering medical art courses, *see* Appendix I.

Associations, Societies and Official Bodies

Association Européenne des Illustrateurs Médicaux et Scientifiques (AEIMS)
www.aeims.eu

Association of Medical Illustrators (AMI), USA
https://ami.org

Biodiversity Information Standards (TDWG)
www.tdwg.org
Formerly known as the Taxonomic Databases Working Group (TDWG), this international organisation was formed to promote data sharing. Two of its more widely used data standards are the Darwin Core for primary biodiveristy data and the Audiovisual Core for images and video of organisms.

Biological and Medical Art in Belgium (BIOMAB)
https://medinart.eu/biomab_the-official-website-of-biological-and-medical-art-in-belgium/

Institute of Medical Illustrators (IMI)
www.imi.org.uk

Medical Artists' Association of Great Britain (MAA)
https://maa.org.uk

SAA
www.saa.co.uk
The UK's largest community of artists, offering tutorials and workshops as well as artists' supplies.

Art Supplies

L Cornelissen & Son
www.cornelissen.com
Art supplies, specialising in unusual and hard-to-find items. In London and online.

Jackman's Art Materials
www.jackmansartmaterials.co.uk
Own-brand paints and art supplies.

Winsor & Newton
www.winsornewton.com
Reputable brand for art supplies.

Databases

Museum Data Service
www.museumdata.uk
An online database collating over 100 UK museum collections, with over three million records.

The Global Biodiversity Information Facility (GBIF)
www.gbif.org/what-is-gbif
An online database for museum and collections. A free online and open database for anyone in the world, with content from the larger natural history museums worldwide.

The National Sciences Collections Association (NatSCA)
www.natsca.org
UK natural science collections.

Museums

UK

Bethlem Museum of the Mind, Kent
https://museumofthemind.org.uk

George Marshall Medical Museum, Worcester
www.medicalmuseum.org.uk/

Horniman Museum and Gardens, London
https://horniman.ac.uk/plan-your-visit/

London Museums of Health and Medicine
www.medicalmuseums.org
Website covering 27 health and medical museums, collections and libraries across London, including the BDA Dental Museum, Hunterian Museum at the Royal College of Surgeon's, St. Bartholmew's Pathology Museum and the Science Museum.

Museums Association
www.museumsassociation.org/
Membership provides free and discouted access to over 900 museums in the UK.

The Museum of Medicine and Health, Faculty of Biology, Medicine and Health, University of Manchester
www.bmh.manchester.ac.uk/museum

National Museums Scotland, Edinburgh
www.nms.ac.uk/national-museum-of-scotland

Oxford University Museum of Natural History, Oxford
www.oumnh.ox.ac.uk

Thackray Museum of Medicine, Leeds
https://thackraymuseum.co.uk

The Old Operating Theatre Museum and Herb Garret, London
https://oldoperatingtheatre.com
A historic surviving example of an operating theatre.

The Wellcome Collection, London
https://wellcomecollection.org

Europe
Charité Museum of Medical History, Berlin, Germany
https://bmm-charite.de/en

Musée d'histoire de la médecine, Paris, France
https://u-paris.fr/musee-de-lhistoire-de-la-medecine/

Museum Vrolik, Museum of the Human Body, Amsterdam, Netherlands
www.museumvrolik.nl/en/

Pauls Stradins Medicine History Museum, Riga, Latvia
https://mvm.lv

Riga Stradins University Instituite of the History of Medicine, Latvia
http://am.rsu.lv/en

USA
National Museum of Civil War Medicine, Maryland
www.civilwarmed.org

National Museum of Health and Medicine, Maryland
https://medicalmuseum.health.mil/

There are many more national and local museums across Europe and around the world, with the majority being open to the public and/or have online resources.
This selection provides a starting point from which to explore the amazing range of collections, museums, libraries and resources available to you.

APPENDIX IV FURTHER READING

FURTHER READING

MAET, Medical Artists' Education Trust, Educating Artists for Medicine since 1997. (MAET 2022) Available via: www.maet.org.uk

Anatomy Textbooks

Abrahams, P.H. Spratt. J, Loukas. M, and Schoor A., *Abraham's and McMinn's Clinical Atlas of Human Anatomy* (Elsevier 8th Ed 2019)

Leading anatomy and clinical text.

McMinn, R.M.H. and Hutchings, R.T., *A Colour Atlas of Human Anatomy* (Mosby, London, 1998)

Probably one of the most useful and popular reference books, with clear photographs; especially strong on bony skeleton information, with a life-size edition available.

Wilson, K.J.W OBE and Waugh, A., *Anatomy and Physiology in Health and Disease* (Churchill Livingstone 8th Ed. 2000)

An accessible text on human biology and physiology.

Aeillo, L. and Dean, C., *An Introduction to Human Evolutionary Anatomy* (Academic Press, London, 1990)

A clear and concise text with many illustrations, covering the evolution of human anatomical development.

Agur, A.M.R. and Dalley, A.F., *Grant's Atlas of Anatomy* (Lippincott Connect, 2020)

A core anatomical text since 1943.

Cameron, J. and Brown, W.A.B., *Identification of Human Teeth* (Joanna Cameron, 2022)

A set of tooth identification cards and posters.

Dean, C. and Pegginton, J., *Core Atlas of Anatomy*, vols 1, 2 and 3 (1995)

A concise set of anatomy texts: Volume 1: The Limbs and Vertebral Column; Volume 2: The Thorax, Abdomen, Pelvis and Perineum; Volume 3: The Head and Neck.

Gray's Anatomy – The Anatomical Basis of Clinical Practice. (Churchill Livingstone, 42nd edition, 2020)

Probably the best-known anatomy text, aimed primarily at medical students, physicians and surgeons. First printed in 1858 and is now on its 42nd edition. The text was originally written by Henry Gray and illustrated by Henry Vandyke Carter, London.

Terminology

Oxford Concise Medical Dictionary, 9th ed (Oxford University Press, 2014)

This is the current online version.

Art History and Techniques

Barnett, R., *The Sick Rose – or: The Disease And The Art Of Medical Illustration* (Thams and Hudson 2014)

Clayton, M. and Philo, R., *Leonardo da Vinci Anatomist* (Royal Collection Enterprises 2012)

Crosby, R.W. and Cody, J., *Max Brödel – The Man Who Put Art Into Medicine* (Springer-Verlag 1991)

Dirix, T., *In Search of Andreas Vesalius – The Quest For The Lost Grave* (Lannoo Campus 2014)

Gill, R., *Basic Rendering – Effective Drawing for Designers, Artists and Illustrators* (1991)

Available to download at https://archive.org/details/basic-rendering-effective-drawing-for-designers-artists-and-illustrators-by-robert-w.-gill-1991/page/202/mode/2up

Grombrich, E.H., *The Story of Art* (Phaidon, 16th Ed 2022)

Guptill, A., *Rendering in Pen and Ink* (Watson Guptill Publications, 1997)

Hockney, D., *Secret Knowledge: Rediscovering the Lost Techniques of the Old Masters* (Viking Studio, 2006)

Kedzierski, A., *Artistic Secrets to Painting Tonal Values* (North Light Books, 2000)

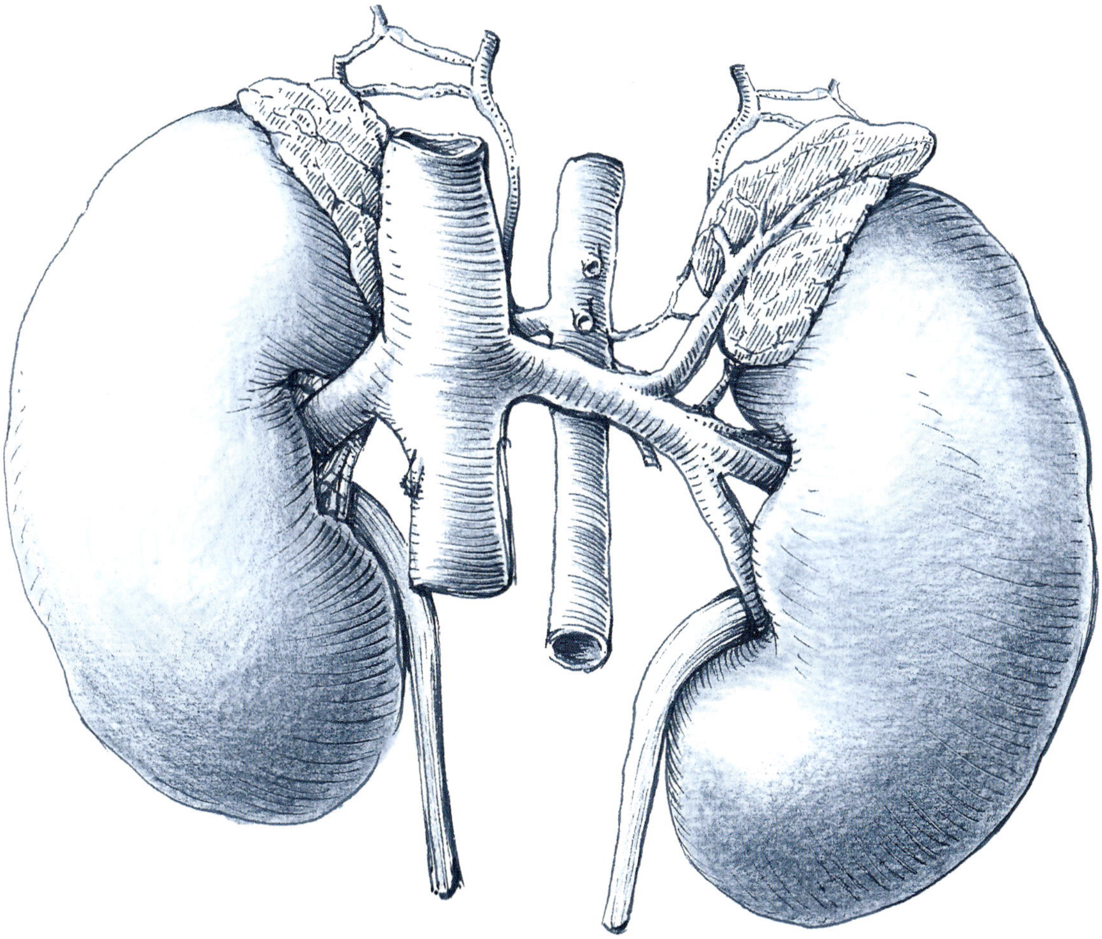

Anterior view of the left and right kidney, including the adrenal glands, ureters and the main blood vessels – the aorta and vena cava. An expressive drawing concentrating on the three-dimensional form. Drawn with a dip pen, with blue-black ink and the addition of coloured pencil, on smooth 200gms cartridge paper.

Lanteri, E., *Modelling and Sculpting the Human Figure* (Dover Publications, 1985)

Logan, J., M*ake Ink – A Forager's Guide to Natural Inkmakin*g (Abrams 2018)

Lumley, J.P.S., *Surface Anatomy – The Anatomical Basics of Clinical Examination* (Churchill Livingstone 1996)

McLarty, M., *Illustrating Medicine and Surgery* (E&S Livingstone Ltd 1960)

Neddo, N., *The Organic Artist* (Quarry, 2015)

Norling, E.R., *Perspective Made Easy* (Dover Publications, 1999)

Petherbridge, D. and Jordanova, L.J., *The Quick and the Dead – Artists and Anatomy* (National Touring Exhibitions, The South Bank Centre 1997)

Roberts, K.B. and Tomlinson, J.D.W., *The Fabric of the Human Body – European Traditions of Anatomical Illustration* (Oxford University Press 1992)

The Royal College of Surgeons of England, *Designing Bodies – Models of Human Anatomy from Wax to Plastics* (RCS, London, 2015)

The author has made every effort to ensure the resources, references and websites are current and correct. If any acknowledgment or reference requires updating, please contact us.

INDEX

Index covers key chapter topics and features.

First published in 2024 by
The Crowood Press Ltd
Ramsbury, Marlborough
Wiltshire SN8 2HR

enquiries@crowood.com
www.crowood.com

British Library Cataloguing-in-Publication Data
A catalogue record for this book is available from the British Library.

ISBN 978 0 7198 4434 8

Front cover illustration
Deep neck and upper back musculature. Watercolour.

Typeset by Envisage IT
Cover design by Sergey Tsvetkov
Printed and bound in India by Thomson Press

Acknowledgements
I am especially grateful and wish to thank all those who have helped shape this book through their invaluable advice, guidance and ultimate generosity and patience in reading all or part of the text, sharing their combined wealth of experience in the field of medical art and anatomy cannot be underestimated. Dr Michael O'Brien MD, FRCP, FRGS, Hon. FMAA, Chairman and Examiner of the MAET. Mr Philip Ball, MA, FMAA, past Chairman of the MAA. Mrs Jenny Halstead, FMAA, PS, Director of the MAET 1993-2001, past Chairman of the MAA. Mr William Edwards, Curator Gordon Museum and Hunterian Society, Kings College London, St. Thomas' Street, London. Mrs Anthea Dendy, Chartered Physiotherapist, Clinical Specialist in Neurology, MSc, BSc, MCSP, HPC reg. Mrs Kate Milne, Principal Physiotherapist, Dip. Phys. Ms Catherine Bone MAA, Director of Education MAET. Dr Wendy Birch, Associate Professor of Anatomy, MBBS Anatomy Academic Lead for Clinical and Professional Practice, University College London.

Also to the many colleague's, tutors and friends, through so many conversation's and demonstrations of their skills have generously shared their expertise and knowledge, for the past, present and future aspiring medical artists.

For permission to include illustrations drawn from the Museum Collections at the Royal College of Surgeons of England, London. Pages 83, 138 and 157.

Professionally scanning a steady stream of artworks, my thanks go to the family run printers Chris Dyer and Sons Ltd, Leatherhead, and to all those who kindly permitted course, museum and further information.

With grateful thanks to all those who supplied or allowed photographs to be taken of external body parts! Those who wished to be acknowledged are:
C Archery, C Bird, J Butler, A Dendy, C Dendy, H Finden-Bowden, S Henson, P Hutchings, B Lane, J Lane, K Milne, M Pearce, T Rankin, D Rutherford, G Taylor, J Turnham and G Wright.

And finally, my indebted thanks to my husband John for the perfect poem written to accompany this book. Alongside his constant support throughout this project and indeed over so many years beside the long and often unpredicable working hours of a freelance artist, engaging in enthusiastic conversations over specimens to my many hours in the studio immersed in drawing.